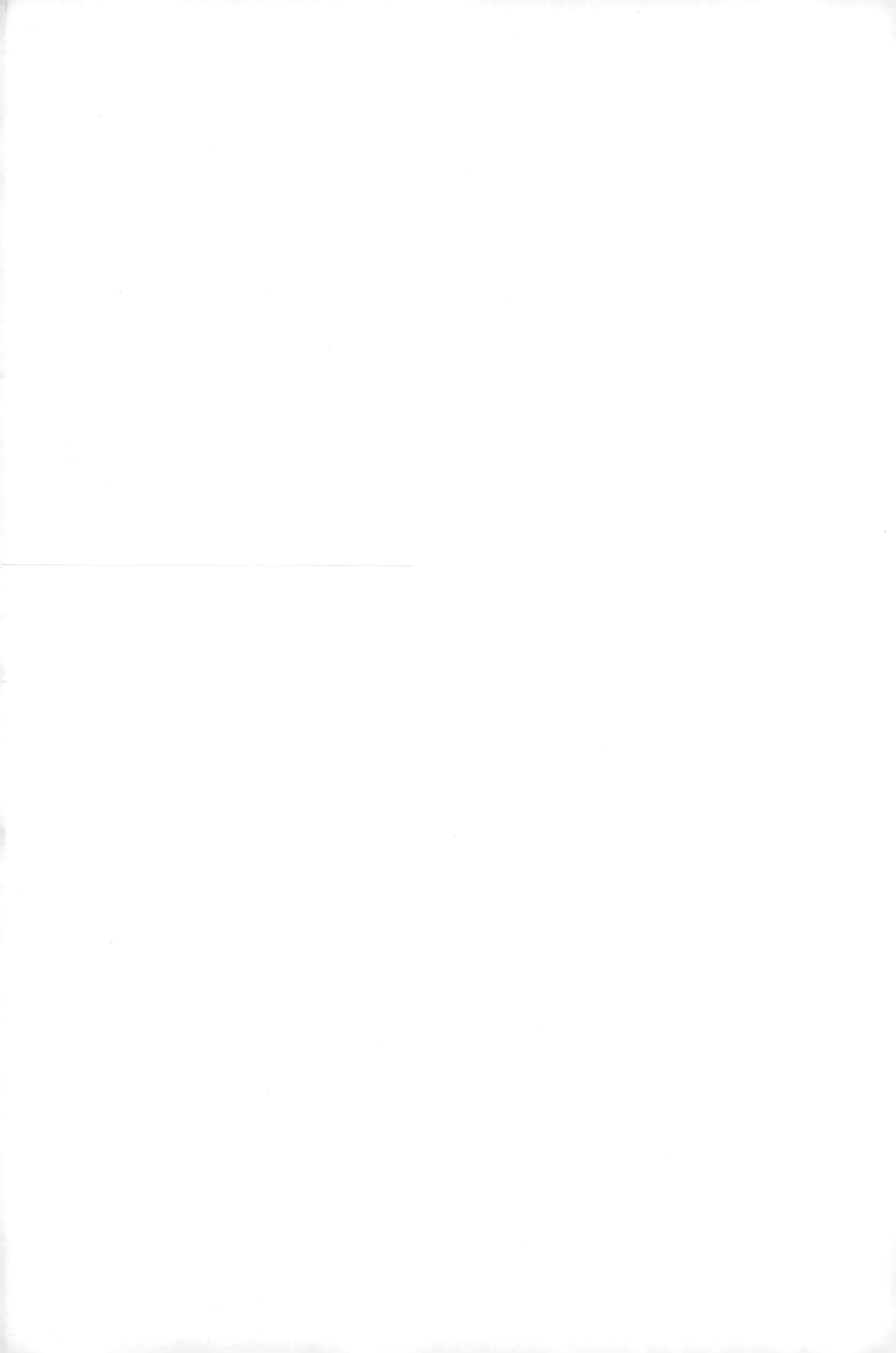

John E. Chaplin
and the RESPECT project partners:
Francis P. Crawley, Liuska Sanna, Adriana Ceci,
David Neubauer, Carlo Giaquinto, Catriona Chaplin and
Monika Bullinger

RESPECT
patient needs

Relating expectations and needs to the participation and empowerment of children in clinical trials

PABST SCIENCE PUBLISHERS
Lengerich

Acknowledgements

The research project **RESPECT: Relating Expectations and Needs to the Participation and Empowerment of Children in Clinical Trials** received funding from the European Union's Seventh Framework Programme (FP7/2007-2013), coordination and support actions, under grant agreement no. 201938.

John Eric Chaplin PhD Leg.psyk.(Project Coordinator)
Göteborg Pediatric Growth Research Center
Sahlgrenska Academy at the University of Gothenburg
Institute of Clinical Sciences, Department of Pediatrics
SE-416 85 Göteborg, SWEDEN
Tel: +46 31 343 51 67
Email: john.chaplin@vgregion.se
Website: www.patientneeds.eu

Bibliographic information published by Die Deutsche Nationalbibliothek
Die Deutsche Nationalbibliothek lists this publication in the Deutsche Nationalbibliografie; detailed bibliographic data is available in the Internet at <http://dnb.ddb.de>.

This work is subject to copyright. All rights are reserved, whether the whole or part of the material is concerned, specifically the rights of translation, reprinting, reuse of illustrations, recitation, broadcasting, reproduction on microfilms or in other ways, and storage in data banks. The use of registered names, trademarks, etc. in this publication does not imply, even in the absence of a specific statement, that such names are exempt from the relevant protective laws and regulations and therefore free for general use.
The authors and the publisher of this volume have taken care that the information and recommendations contained herein are accurate and compatible with the standards generally accepted at the time of publication. Nevertheless, it is difficult to ensure that all the information given is entirely accurate for all circumstances. The publisher disclaims any liability, loss, or damage incurred as a consequence, directly or indirectly, of the use and application of any of the contents of this volume.

© 2012 Pabst Science Publishers, D-49525 Lengerich

Printing: KM Druck, D-64823 Groß-Umstadt
ISBN 978-3-89967-820-8

Contents

 Contributors v
 Abbreviations viii

1 EXECUTIVE SUMMARY 1
 1.1 The Problem 1
 1.2 The RESPECT project: a coordinated action project 1
 1.3 Conclusions 3
 1.4 Empowerment action points 3
 1.5 Main recommendations to stakeholders 4

PART I 5

2 CLINICAL TRIALS 5
 2.1 What is a clinical trial? 5
 2.2 The uncertainty principle – clinical equipoise 9
 2.3 The therapeutic misconception 9
 2.4 Deciding to participate in a clinical trial 11

3 THE NEED FOR PAEDIATRIC CLINICAL TRIALS 13
 3.1 Why adult CTs are not enough 13
 3.2 Off-label prescription 14

4 BARRIERS IN PAEDIATRIC CLINICAL TRIALS 16
 4.1 Structural barriers 17
 4.2 Procedural barriers 19
 4.3 Psychological barriers 20

PART II 23

5 THE RESPECT PROJECT 23
 5.1 The aims of the RESPECT project 23
 5.2 Methods used 24

6 DATA GATHERED BY THE RESPECT PROJECT 28
 6.1 The experience of children and their parents 28
 6.2 The experience of patient organisations 39
 6.3 The experience of CT staff 45
 6.4 The experience of CT networks 52
 6.5 The experience of ethics committees 55
 6.6 The experience of sponsors 59
 6.7 Main conclusions from the reported experiences 62

PART III 63

7 EMPOWERING CHILDREN IN CLINICAL TRIALS 63

7.1 How can children be better mobilised and empowered? 63
7.2 Definitions of empowerment 65
7.3 The gap between the researcher and the family 65
7.4 Reasons for participation 67
7.5 Factors that modify the reasons for participation 71

8 ACTION POINTS FOR INTEGRATING CHILDREN'S NEEDS 75

8.1 Self-determination 75
8.2 Accountability and independent monitoring 80
8.3 Cooperative relationship 87
8.4 Knowledge and understanding 89

9 GETTING CLINICAL OUTCOMES THAT MATTER TO CHILDREN 93

9.1 Children and parents: role and recommendations 93
9.2 Patient organisations: role and recommendations 96
9.3 Principal investigator and CT staff: role and recommendations 99
9.4 Ethics committees: role and recommendations 103
9.5 Sponsors: role and recommendations 105
9.6 Policy makers: role and recommendations 106

10 RESPECT DEMONSTRATION PROJECTS 109

10.1 Self-determination through use of decision aids 109
10.2 Knowledge through an education package for schools 114

11 BEST PRACTICE EXAMPLES OF EMPOWERING CHILDREN 122

11.1 Self-determination 122
11.2 Accountability 123
11.3 Cooperation 125
11.4 Knowledge 129

12 REFERENCES 131

APPENDIX 1 CASE STUDY, SURVEY AND INTERVIEW RESPONSES 141

1a Children and parents 141
1b Patient organisations 166
1c Paediatricians 173
1d CT networks 191
1e Ethics committees 221

APPENDIX 2 RESPECT FAMILY DECISION GUIDE AND WORKSHEET 231

APPENDIX 3 PILOT EDUCATION PACKAGE 257

3a Pilot education package for parents 257
3b Pilot education package for children 271

Contributors

This book was written and edited by **John Chaplin**, **Catriona Chaplin** and **Monika Bullinger** with valued assistance from the RESPECT members below.

Sahlgrenska Academy at University of Gothenburg (coordinating partner)

John Chaplin, PhD. Dr Chaplin is a senior researcher at the Pediatric Growth Research Center, Institute of Clinical Sciences, Sahlgrenska Academy at University of Gothenburg, Sweden. He is a chartered psychologist in the UK and Sweden, and an Associate Fellow of the British Psychology Society. His main research areas are the measurement of the impact of illness and psychological factors in the clinical trials process especially through measurement of cognitive effects and health-related quality of life.

Carola Pfeiffer-Mosesson, RN, CRM. Ms Pfeiffer-Mosesson is a research nurse and clinical research manager responsible for organising and administrating clinical trials at the Pediatric Growth Research Center. She conducted case study interviews for the RESPECT project.

Catriona Chaplin, PhD. Dr Chaplin is a research psychologist at the Pediatric Growth Research Center. Her previous research areas have included public attitudes to risk and cognitive processes in profoundly deaf children. She managed the RESPECT online surveys and project website, as well as coordinating contact among project partners.

Andrea Sandberg, MSc. Ms Sandberg recently graduated from the Dept of Biomedicine, University of Uppsala, Sweden, with a master's degree in Clinical Drug Development. She completed her master's thesis on education needs of families in clinical trials in Gothenburg, as part of the RESPECT project.

University Medical Centre Hamburg-Eppendorf

Monika Bullinger, PhD. Prof Dr Bullinger is the deputy director at the Institute of Medical Psychology, University Hospital of Hamburg-Eppendorf, Germany. She is the coordinator of the DISABKIDS and QoLISSY projects on quality of life and patient-reported outcomes.

Falk Wulf, MD, Dipl.Psych. Dr Wulf is based at the Institute of Medical Psychology and has researched the construction of decision aids for parents of children in clinical trials, as well as carrying out the literature review for the RESPECT project.

Marta Krasuska, MSc. Ms Krasuska is a former Marie Curie fellow whose studies focused on health psychology, organisational psychology and cognitive sciences. She collaborated with Dr Wulf on the literature review for the RESPECT project.

Sylvia von Mackensen, PhD. Dr von Mackensen is a medical psychologist at the Institute of Medical Psychology whose current research focuses on international quality of life issues in children. She interviewed senior paediatricians for the RESPECT project.

Aliaksandra Mokhar, BSc. Ms Mokhar recently completed her bachelor's thesis on willingness to participate in clinical trials at the Center for Psychosocial Medicine in Hamburg, as part of the RESPECT project

European Patients' Forum, Brussels

Liuska Sanna, MA. Ms Sanna is Programme Manager at the European Patients' Forum, Brussels, Belgium. Representation to EU for pan-European and national patients' platforms. She has many years of experience in project and programme coordination and has expertise in managing European projects. She has been acting as a leading driving force behind developing the early involvement of patients as "experts", by promoting their needs and proposing a patient empowerment model ad hoc for paediatric clinical trials.

Gaya Ducceschi, MscEcon. Ms Ducceschi is a Programme Officer at the European Patients' Forum, Brussels, Belgium. She holds a BA in Political Sciences and an MScEcon in International Politics. Before joining EPF, she worked for two years in the NGO sector in Brussels and she has overseas experience in the health sector.

University Children's Hospital Ljubljana

David Neubauer, PhD MD. Prof Neubauer is the head of the Dept of Child, Adolescent and Developmental Neurology at the University Children's Hospital Ljubljana and Board Director of the Foundation of Child Neurology in Slovenia. He has conducted clinical trials with children with epilepsy and mitochondrial disease.

Jana Kodric, PhD, Dipl.Psych. Dr Kodric is a clinical psychologist at the University Children's Hospital Ljubljana and the Foundation of Child Neurology, Slovenia.

Ana Fakin, MD. Dr Fakin is a recently qualified medical doctor. She conducted case study interviews for the RESPECT project.

Viktorija Kerin MD. Dr Kerin is a recently qualified medical doctor. She conducted case study interviews for the RESPECT project.

Good Clinical Practice Alliance Europe, Brussels

Francis P. Crawley, PhL. Mr Crawley is a philosopher specialising in ethical, legal, and regulatory issues concerning health research, He is the Executive Director of the Good Clinical Practice Alliance – Europe (GCPA) and a World Health Organization (WHO) Expert in ethics.

Consorzio per le Valutazioni Biologiche e Farmacologiche, Pavia

Adriana Ceci, PhD. Professor Ceci was the coordinator of the project TEDDY (Task force in Europe for Drug Development for the Young) Network of Excellence. She is a professor of paediatrics and has been a member of the EMA Paediatric Committee since 2008.

Annagrazia Altavilla, PhD. Dr Altavilla is a lawyer and associate senior lecturer at the Université de la Méditerranée, Faculté de Médecine, Espace Éthnique Mediterranéen, Marseille, France. She was the coordinator of the activities in the field of ethics in the project TEDDY (Task force in Europe for Drug Development for the Young) Network of Excellence and has been a member of the EMA Paediatric Committee since 2008. She conducted the joint TEDDY-RESPECT inventory of ethics committees.

Cristina Manfredi. Ms Manfredi has collaborated within the TEDDY project on reporting key questions concerning paediatric drug use. She conducted surveys of CT networks for the RESPECT project.

University of Padua

Carlo Giaquinto, PhD MD. Dr Giaquinto is Head of the Referral Centre for Paediatric HIV Infection in the Department of Paediatrics at the University of Padua, Italy. He chairs the steering committee of the Paediatric European Network for Treatment of AIDS (PENTA) and is the Principal Investigator of the EU GRIP project, Global Research in Pediatrics.

Pia-Sophie Wool, MD. Dr Wool is a paediatrician with an interest in infectious diseases. She has worked in Africa with HIV-infected children, as well as for the World Health Organization (WHO) on the Polio eradication project (STOP). She has collaborated with Dr Giaquinto in various research projects and clinical trials involving children with HIV.

External advisors

Ken J Rotenberg, PhD. Professor Rotenberg is a social psychologist based at the School of Psychology, Keele University, UK. He is widely published and conducts research on, among other areas, the implications of children's trust in health professionals for medical treatment.

John Bowis, OBE. Mr Bowis is a former Member of the European Parliament for London and spokesperson on the Environment, Health and Food Safety in the European Parliament. He has also served on the Council of Health Ministers.

Abbreviations

ADR	Adverse Drug Reaction
CRO	Contract Research Organisation
CT	Clinical Trial
EMA	European Medical Agency
Enpr-EMA	European network of paediatric research at the EMA
GCP	Good Clinical Practice
ICH	International Conference on Harmonisation of Technical Requirements for Registration of Pharmaceuticals for Human Use
NGO	Non-Governmental Organisation
PIN	Patient-Identified Need
PIP	Paediatric Investigation Plan
PO	Patient Organisation
PRO	Patient-Reported Outcome
RCT	Randomised Controlled Trial
RESPECT	Relating Expectations and Needs to the Participation and Empowerment of Children in Clinical Trials.
SACK	Self-determination, Accountability, Cooperation and Knowledge
SPC	Summary of Product Characteristics
WHO	World Health Organization

1 Executive Summary

1.1 The Problem

"More than 50% of the medicines used to treat children have not been tested and authorised for use in children." Statement from the European Confederation of Specialists in Paediatrics to the European Parliament (CESP, 2005). This issue is the basis for a recent European Commission directive, Regulation (EC) No. 1901/2006 on Medicinal Products for Paediatric Use, requiring paediatric medicines to be tested in children.

1.2 The RESPECT project: a coordinated action project

The European RESPECT project set out to explore the expectations and needs related to the participation and empowerment of children in clinical trials. It responded to a call from the EU Seventh Framework programme for a coordination study concerning **Identifying patients' needs in the clinical trials context (HEALTH-2007-4.1-4).** This call requested that three questions be answered:
- How can patients be better mobilised and empowered?
- How can patients get the clinical outcomes that really matter to them?
- How can their needs be integrated into clinical trials?

The RESPECT project specifically investigated children's participation in clinical trials. The objective was to determine whether there are opportunities to improve recruitment through empowering the children and their parents. The reasons families give for participation were investigated and are summarised below.

- Most respondents believed that they would receive the newest and best medication by participating in a clinical trial.
- Families believed they would get the opportunity for additional monitoring and specialist care.
- There is a wish to pay back the health care system for previous health care received. Connected to this was the belief among the parents that their child's contribution was meaningful and would be helpful to other children; it was important to them that the research should have a value for the patient group to which they belong, including future generations of that group and, indeed, future family members (their children's children).
- To a lesser extent, parents put their children into clinical trials in order to learn more about the child's health condition. This reflected a need to be actively involved in the care of their child.

These reasons were modified by several other factors related to the trust that they had in the doctor or medical profession and the fear of missing out on what was best for the child. The ease of participation played a major role, as did the feeling that there was minimum risk involved.

Previous participation was not likely to increase the chances of subsequent participation, except where parents had received the results of the previous study and acquired additional knowledge about the health status of their child.

The paediatric clinical trial is an opportunity for the clinical staff but it should also be an opportunity for the participant; the clinical trial should be a team effort between clinician, sponsor, family and child. In order to foster this collaboration, the trial needs to be designed in a more holistic way, taking into account how it will affect the child.

Additional outcome measures are needed to establish what the family and patient group want to gain from participation. This could be achieved, for example, via peer meetings prior to the study start, enabling the investigator to ensure that the patient group's needs are respected.

Information has to be tailored to the needs of the child and the parents. Understanding of risk and how risk levels are conveyed are also important factors influencing the family's ability to make a decision about participating in a clinical trial. Once the decision to participate has been made, there should be opportunities to actively contribute to the research beyond being the subject of the research.

By incorporating these needs into the planning process of a clinical trial, a partnership model of empowerment emerges, based on four elements:

- **S**elf-determination through active involvement;
- **A**ccountability and transparency;
- **C**ooperation and mutual respect;
- **K**nowledge and access to information.

Figure A: The RESPECT project's SACK model of empowerment.

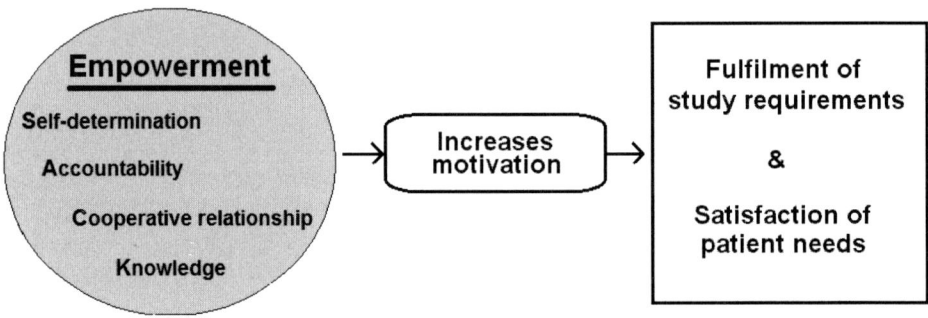

1.3 Conclusions

In conclusion, the challenge is to empower children and parents to be active in the process of seeking information about the trial before making their decision, as well as making practices transparent; to this end, the child's views should be taken into account as far as possible. Increased involvement can be achieved by reaching beyond informed consent to improved education and a shared decision-making process that is needed to prepare families for participation. Older children should be fully included in the process and younger children should be involved according to their competence. By moving towards the realisation of the SACK empowerment model in clinical trial research, the child's needs are met and improved participation and compliance are possible.

Given the need to incorporate the principles of empowerment into the clinical trial process, action points based on the SACK model are listed below. This is followed by the main specific recommendations to children and their parents, patient organisations, investigators and CT staff, ethics committees, sponsors and policy makers. These recommendations are the key results of the research and discussions carried out within the RESPECT project. Detailed discussion of these issues and practical proposals for improvements are found in chapters 7, 8 and 9.

1.4 Empowerment action points

- Self-determination
    - ✓ Families should identify the trials that matter to them.
    - ✓ Families should be in control of decision-making.
    - ✓ Children and parents should use the trial to gain skills and knowledge.
- Accountability
    - ✓ Increased transparency should be included in the development of protocols, and in ethics committee procedures.
    - ✓ Patient-reported outcomes should be incorporated as a method of providing feedback from the child participant to the trial investigators.
    - ✓ The support given in the case of adverse consequences of participation should be clearly communicated to clinical trial participants within the informed consent process.
    - ✓ The investigators should develop procedures to monitor the child's experiences.
- Cooperation
    - ✓ Patient representatives, sponsors and investigators should work together to ensure that clinical trial protocols represent the needs of the participants alongside the purely scientific goals.
    - ✓ Training in person-centred care should be provided to all CT staff in order to ensure that participants are treated in uniformly inclusive manner in all CTs. This is of particular importance with child participants.
    - ✓ A strategy should be developed for cooperation between CT investigators and patient organisations.

- ✓ There should be possibilities for families to be involved in all stages of the CT design.
- Knowledge
    - ✓ Access to information about the trial and the drug should be available to the participants and potential participants. This should include summaries in non-scientific language and scientific journal articles presenting the results of the CT.
    - ✓ The informed consent procedure should be viewed by the CT team as a continuous process of informing and teaching about clinical trials methods. The participants should view informed consent as an opportunity to ask questions and gain information.

1.5 Main recommendations to stakeholders

The main recommendations are described in the figure below. A full description and discussion of these recommendations is found in chapter 9.

Figure B: Main recommendations based on the RESPECT findings

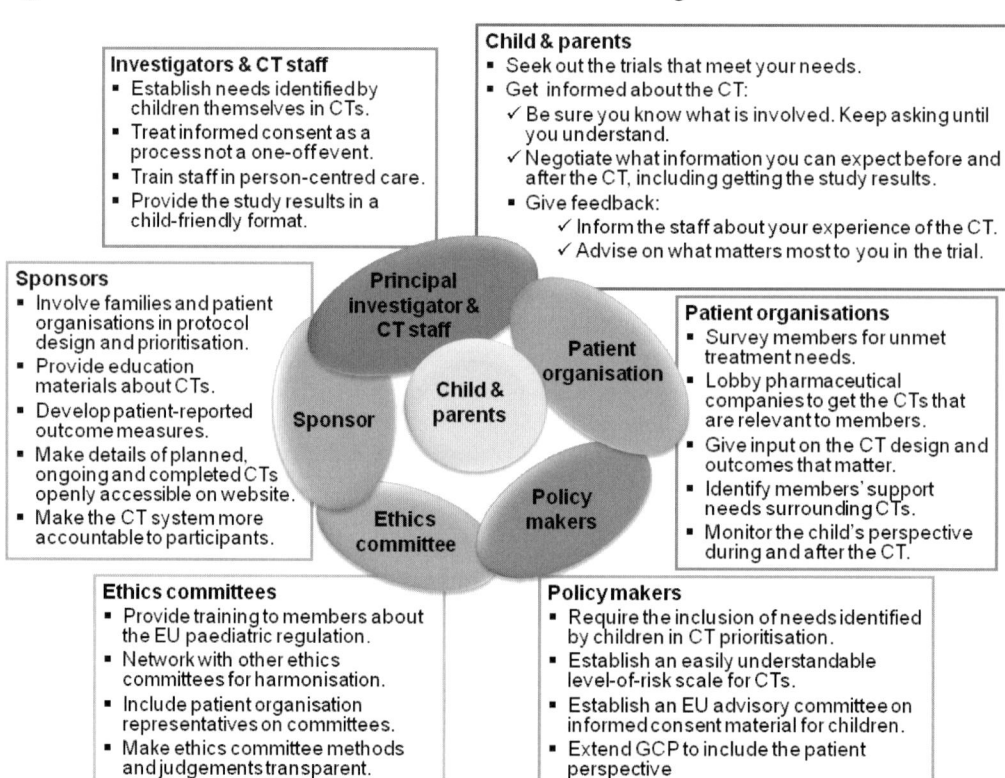

PART I

2 Clinical trials

2.1 What is a clinical trial?

Clinical trials (CTs) are, in the broadest sense, structured investigations into the effects of medicines on relevant outcomes. The drug-development process will normally proceed through several phases over many years. Each phase is treated as a separate CT. If the test drug successfully passes through Phases I, II and III, it will usually be approved by the national regulatory authority for use in the patient population for which it was developed. Phase IV trials are surveillance studies conducted after the drug has been approved and a licence is granted for it to be sold.

2.1.1 Phases of drug development

Pharmaceutical companies conduct extensive pre-clinical studies before starting CTs of a drug under development. These involve *in vitro* (test tube or cell culture) and *in vivo* (animal) experiments using wide-ranging doses of the test drug to obtain preliminary information on efficacy, toxicity and pharmacokinetics.

Phase 0 is a recent term used for exploratory, first-in-human trials, which include the administration of a single sub-therapeutic dose of the test drug to a limited number of healthy volunteers, usually involving 10 to 15 people, to gather preliminary data on both pharmacodynamics (what the drug does to the body, both desirable and adverse effects) and pharmacokinetics (what the body does with the drug, including absorption, distribution, metabolism and excretion).

Phase I trials involve a small group of healthy subjects, usually 20 to 100 people. This phase includes trials designed to assess the safety, and tolerability, as well as pharmacodynamics and pharmacokinetics of a drug. These trials are ideally conducted in an inpatient clinic, where the participants can be observed by full-time staff.

Phase II trials are performed on larger groups, usually ranging between 20 and 300 participants with the medical condition that is the target for the test drug. Phase II trials are only carried out once the initial safety of the test drug has been confirmed in Phase I trials. They are designed to assess how well the drug works, as well as to continue Phase I safety assessments in a larger group. If the development of a test drug is aborted, this most frequently occurs during Phase II trials.

Phase III trials are multicentre randomised controlled trials (RCTs) on large patient groups (300–3000 or more, depending upon the medical condition studied) over a longer period than phase I or II trials. In a RCT, the benefit, safety and efficacy of the test drug is measured against the standard treatment and/or alternative treatments (see **2.1.3 *Randomisation***). These trials are considered the definitive assessment of how a novel medication compares with current standard treatment. Because of the number of participants and the long duration, Phase III trials are the most expensive, time-consuming and difficult trials to design and run, particularly in therapies for chronic medical conditions.

At the end of phase III all the necessary evidence for a licence application should be available for submission to the medical licensing authority. It is at this stage that the label identifying the criteria for the target patient group is written. There must be sufficient evidence from phase III to justify the use of the new medication in this group. The success of the phase III trial will determine the licence criteria.

Phase IV trials are post-marketing surveillance trials. Once the drug is in use, the safety aspects (pharmacovigilance) continue to be monitored. This is because the drug needs to be assessed with a more representative population including previously controlled factors, such as co-existing medical conditions and combinations of medicines that could affect the safety of the new drug.

2.1.2   Who conducts CTs?

The **sponsor** of a CT may be an individual, company, institution, or organisation that takes responsibility for the initiation, management and/or financing of a CT. The sponsor designs the study *protocol*, which describes the scientific rationale, objective(s), methodology, statistical considerations, and organisation of the planned trial. The sponsor is also responsible for accurately informing the local site investigators of the safety record of the test drug, and of any potential interactions with already approved medical treatments. Throughout the trial, the sponsor is responsible for monitoring the results of the study and collecting adverse event reports.

A **contract research organisation** (CRO) is an organisation (commercial, academic, or other) contracted by the sponsor to perform one or more of the sponsor's trial-related duties and functions. This may include planning, organising and conducting the CT.

A **principal investigator** (PI) is usually the physician responsible for conducting the study at the study site and for supervising the CT staff according to the protocol throughout the duration of the study. The PI helps the sponsor to produce site-specific informed consent material that informs the potential participants of what the study will involve if they consent to participate. The PI has the ultimate responsibility to ensure that potential subjects in the study understand the risks and potential benefits of participation.

2.1.3   Randomisation

The randomisation process in Phase III trials involves randomly allocating subjects to different treatment groups (known as the *arms* of the study) – which can include standard treatment, no treatment or placebo – and measuring the clinical differences between the groups. Randomisation is importance because it guarantees that the CT participants all have the same chance of being allocated to the respective treatment arms, thus avoiding systematic selection bias. In *single-blind* study designs, the physician knows which drug is given to each patient whereas, in *double-blind* designs, neither the patient nor the physician is informed which drug is given to which patient.

Randomisation is only justified if there is true uncertainty about the superiority of the test drug compared to the alternatives. If interim analysis of the CT results indicates a better outcome in one of the treatment arms, the trial has to be stopped.

2.1.4 Sample size and statistical power

Statistical power refers to how much the results of a study can be relied upon to give an accurate estimation of the intervention in the whole population. Power is determined by the relationship between the number of patients enrolled in a study and the number of treatment arms and variables studied, and by the magnitude of expected differences between the test drug and the alternative treatments. In general, the larger the sample size or number of participants in the trial, the greater the statistical power of the trial, in terms of whether it is possible to accept or reject hypotheses about the effects of the test drug.

2.1.5 Ethical review

Ethical principles and strict regulations in terms of good clinical practice (GCP) guide the conduct of all CTs, according to the three fundamental ethical principles for the protection of human subjects in research: respect for persons, beneficence, and justice.

A CT proposal has to be submitted to an ethical committee for review and successfully pass this scrutiny. The ethics committee considers the potential ethical issues that the CT protocol raises; in the case of paediatric CTs, there is a particular focus on the need to minimise children's pain, discomfort and fear and on the responsibility to protect this vulnerable population from harm beyond a defined acceptable minimal risk (Gill et al., 2003).

2.1.6 Informed consent

A paediatric CT can only be conducted if someone with parental responsibility has given prior informed consent and the child has assented to participation. Informed consent refers to a declaration (which must be written, dated, and signed) indicating that the person with parental responsibility has understood what will take place and what will be expected of the child in the CT. The child and parent should be informed that:

- this is a request to participate in a clinical study, what will happen in the trial and how this is different from normal medical treatment;
- participation is voluntary;
- they have the right to withdraw from the study without needing to give an explanation and that withdrawal will not affect their normal treatment;
- the parent or legal guardian has to give written consent to the child's participation in the trial;

- the study protocol has been approved by an ethics committee;
- appropriate paediatric expertise is available at the trial site;
- efforts will be made to minimise the child's pain, discomfort and fear;
- arrangements for fair compensation in the case of damages are provided;
- they have the right to access the global results of the study after it is completed;
- participants have the right to the respect of confidentiality of personal data;
- participants have the right to a reference person for psychological support, to clarify doubts or to be helped in other ways.

After being duly informed of the trial's nature, significance, implications and risks, informed consent has to be freely given by the child if capable of giving consent. Where a child is below the age of consent, the parent or legal guardian is responsible for giving consent; however, the child's assent is expected. In the case of a difference of opinion between the child and the parents, the child's opinion is respected.

Faced with any treatment decision, the doctor must establish whether the child has the capacity to give consent. This is usually based on the legal age of *automatic competency*, which varies across countries between 16 and 18 years.

In some countries, even children under the age of 16 are considered legally competent if they have 'sufficient understanding and maturity to enable them to understand fully what is proposed' (British Medical Association, 2001); however, parental authority is still required (ICH E11, 2000). A young person who has the capacity to consent to straightforward, relatively risk-free treatment may not necessarily have the capacity to consent to a complex CT which involves elevated risk levels above their normal treatment. In the context of medical research, a higher level of risk should be assumed compared to standard, well-established treatments, in the light of the fact that the effectiveness of an untested drug is by definition unknown.

Paediatric researchers have to be creative in designing strategies to ensure participants' adequate comprehension of study goals, procedures, risks and benefits. This may require implementing educational interventions before consent or developing methods for determining a child's comprehension of the study objectives.

2.1.7 Assent

Even where the research may have a therapeutic value, GCP guidelines state that the child should give assent in the absence of competence to give consent. Assent is the expression of a minor's will to participate in a CT; this is to be obtained in addition to the parent or legal guardian's signed informed consent.

An assent discussion with a child should contain at least an overview of the basic study procedures, a disclosure that participation is voluntary, and an explanation that the child is being asked to agree to research rather than medical care per se (Kon, 2006). Some advice on GCP simply states that the child should not 'object' to the research activity (RCN guidance for nurses 2011) and it may be left in the hands of the parents to make sure that their child fully understands his or her part in the CT process.

The assent process has been described as *quasi-consent* if investigators mirror the informed-consent process and disclose all information that they would discuss with potential adult research participants (Kon, 2006). How this information is conveyed to the child will depend on the age and maturity of the child.

There exists a legal distinction between *therapeutic research* (such as an untested treatment that might be better than the existing treatment) and *non-therapeutic research* (for example, taking additional blood samples with no therapeutic benefit to the child). In the case of therapeutic research, European legislation states that a person with parental responsibility – or the child, if competent – gives consent to the child's participation. In contrast, a non-therapeutic procedure cannot go ahead if the child withholds assent, irrespective of age and of the consent of those with parental responsibility (Lynch, 2010).

2.2 The uncertainty principle – clinical equipoise

The ethical basis for entering patients in RCTs of *therapeutic research* is the uncertainty of the benefits of the new treatment over those of the patient's standard treatment; this is known as *clinical equipoise* (Weijer & Shapiro 2000). If the doctor were certain of the best course of treatment for the patient then it would be unethical to randomly assign the patient to a different treatment. However, there is debate as to whether clinical equipoise should be defined as the individual doctor's uncertainty or as a collective uncertainty of the medical profession. At the individual level, the burden of proof of uncertainty is placed on the individual physician's opinion of a substantial or reasonable uncertainty. The collective approach is based on the idea that it is the clinical community that establishes standards of practice and therefore there should be evidence of uncertainty within the clinical community before random allocation of treatment takes place.

These two definitions of clinical equipoise highlight the fact that there can be disagreement concerning equipoise. There can be evidence in the clinical community of uncertainty whereas individual physicians may be certain of their choice of treatment. The opposite is also possible: that the community can be certain but individual physicians remain unconvinced. This difference in opinion also occurs when a new drug has been tested in adults and proven useful but not proven in children. There may be no evidence for the usefulness of the drug in paediatric cases and therefore genuine uncertainty as to its effectiveness compared to current therapies. However, the evidence from adult studies may be sufficient to convince individual physicians of the paediatric benefits, in which case, the study team and the individual physician have to decide whether clinical equipoise exists and whether children should be entered into a RCT.

2.3 The therapeutic misconception

The therapeutic misconception arises wherever participants in medical research misunderstand the primary purpose of a CT and believe that participation will lead to an individual therapeutic advantage. It could be argued that that therapeutic *research* can be equated with therapeutic *treatment*; in other words, both are in the child's best interest, with the benefit outweighing the risk. However, this does not take into account the fundamental principle of clinical equipoise: that the benefits and risks of the test drug in comparison to the standard treatment are unknown. If there were a clear and documented benefit over that of the standard treatment, it would be unethical to assign a child to the standard treatment in the control arm of a RCT. Indeed, if the test drug were already known to be safe and therapeutically effective then a CT would be unnecessary.

It is thus a misconception that the test drug is guaranteed to be better than the standard treatment. The misconception was first described in an article by Appelbaum, Roth & Lidz (1982), who described the problems of creating research ethics guidelines in which the boundaries between research and standard clinical care were misunderstood. Appelbaum labelled the phenomenon the *therapeutic misconception* (Henderson et al., 2007).

It is not surprising that a misconception exists, since patients are aware that the primary duty of a physician is to the patient's welfare. Although the physician is also an investigator with additional priorities, such as recruitment and retention in a CT, the patient may reasonably believe that their doctor would only recommend any treatment that is in the patient's best interests, regardless of random assignment.

A major issue regarding CT research is the parallel nature of the health care provider, who is also a member of a clinical research team. We as a society believe in the 'good doctor' who always advises us to do what is in our best interests. This of course becomes less certain when the doctor represents a CT in which the efficacy of the test drug is, by definition, not certain.

Despite all efforts by the CT staff to follow informed consent procedures and make the nature of the trial clear to the child and to the parent signing the informed consent form, some confusion over how the CT fits into the child's personal treatment plan can still exist. Indeed, if the trial takes place over several years, as may be the case in the longitudinal study of a test drug in a paediatric population, health care and CT participation can become indistinguishable to the participant. In many respects, the trial appears to be the same as their treatment: the participants attend the same clinic, meet the same staff; they are called to appointments in the same way and are treated alongside other people who are not in a trial. The difference is usually that they attend the clinic more often and that the investigations are more extensive and time-consuming. Over time, CT participation is incorporated into their normal health care routine.

The therapeutic misconception is key to understanding some of the ethical dilemmas facing the development of empowerment policies in this area and will be referred to in the chapters below.

2.4 Deciding to participate in a clinical trial

2.4.1 Stages of change model

A *stages of change* model (Prochaska & Velicer. 1992) can be applied in order to understand the process of agreeing to participate in a CT. The model identifies six stages, as outlined below. See also Figure 1.

1) **Pre-contemplation** (not aware of the possibilities). Most children attending a clinic are likely to be at this stage. Not all clinics are involved in CTs; there are only trials on certain conditions and very few on mild conditions. Recruitment is not continuous and therefore, patients may not be aware of the existence of CTs. Even where families are attending an active CT clinic they may be unaware that they could join a trial.

2) **Contemplation** (considering participation once informed of a possible CT). Once informed about the CT, the family starts to consider what this might mean in terms of medical risks and practical burdens. Parents or the child may seek advice from previous participants in CTs or from medically knowledgeable people, as well as making use of internet or library. Families will seek reassurance that they are making the right decision by balancing the burdens against the risks and by building up expectations for the experience. It is at this stage that the therapeutic misconception is likely to be more apparent.

3) **Preparation** (intention to participate within a short period of time). Certain things may need to be arranged, such as regular time off work for an accompanying parent, time off school and childcare for siblings. The family will also need to prepare psychologically for the first meeting with the medical team. Practical issues start to be apparent.

4) **Action** (initial participating in a CT). Attending the first clinic visit is a significant stage. The reception received by the child at this first visit may determine the family's attitude for the rest of the CT. The emotional aspect of participation becomes important.

5) **Maintenance** (following the protocol and attending the clinic). The family and the child may experience no direct benefit from participation, in which case motivation is maintained via belief in the importance of the research or acceptance of the 'agreement' to participate. If the experience does not match what was anticipated, motivation is reduced.

6) **Completion** (ending the CT participation). Completion may be greeted with relief that at last the trial has finished, disappointment that their expectations were not fulfilled or sadness that the personal contact with the research team is ended.

Figure 1: Stages of Change model showing the first five stages and the core factors influencing these stages

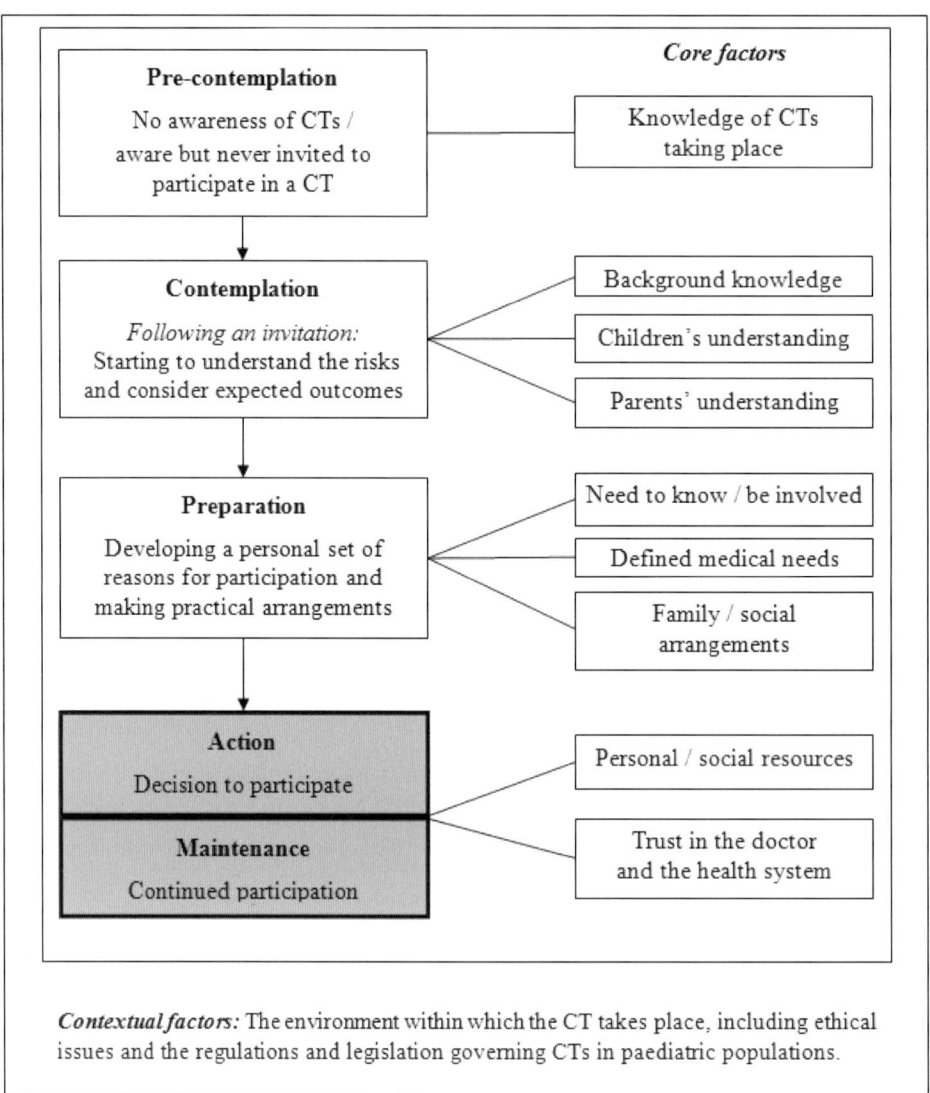

Contextual factors: The environment within which the CT takes place, including ethical issues and the regulations and legislation governing CTs in paediatric populations.

Conducting state-of-the-art paediatric CTs depends not only on appropriate legislations and guidelines, but also on children's and families' decision to participate or not. In order to improve CTs with children, we have to understand not only why some children do not participate but also why others do participate. If we can understand the reasons behind these decisions for and against participation, then we can adapt the CT process to children's needs and thereby improve paediatric CTs and ultimately the medicines produced.

3 The need for paediatric clinical trials

3.1 Why adult CTs are not enough

Studies have shown that over 50% of the medicinal products used in children may not have been tested or authorised for use in this age group (Pandolfini & Bonati, 2005).

The EU regulation (EC No. 1901/2006 on Medicinal Products for Paediatric Use) came into effect in January 2007 to ensure that medicinal products that are researched, developed and authorised in Europe can only be authorised for paediatric use if they are also tested in CTs on children, to ensure that children's therapeutic needs are met. This is expected to lead to an increased demand for children to participate in CTs of new medicines.

The lack of CTs on children has serious consequences, notably that:

- children may be given ineffective treatment or inaccurate dosing;
- children may receive medicines with unknown and possibly harmful effects;
- children are denied access to new breakthroughs that are made available to adults only, leaving children to be treated with older and less efficacious products

Paediatric CTs are necessary even where successful adults CTs have been carried out. The pharmacodynamic and pharmacokinetic properties of drugs are different in adults and children and, for a majority of drugs, a relationship between these factors exists. Because of their immature organ development, children rarely respond to a drug in the same way as adults do. The pharmacokinetic properties fluctuate during organ development and it is important to understand, and be aware of, these changes when developing new drugs (Yaffe et al., 2000). The following issues regarding the use of medicines for adults in children have to be taken into account:

- Absorption characteristics are unknown
- Efficacy in children cannot be assumed to be the same as compared to adults
- Difference in adverse reactions may exist
- Effects on growth, development and maturation may exist which are unseen in the adult population.

Furthermore, while drugs tested on adults are applicable in almost any adult, this is not the case for children. The paediatric population cannot be considered as a homogeneous group because children go through various stages of development and each stage has its own physiological prerequisites. This may result in efficacy differences in different age groups, due to changes in organs and body tissue.

In the light of these factors, it is increasingly considered dangerous to treat children with drugs based on data derived from CTs performed in adults.

3.2 Off-label prescription

When a test drug proceeds successfully through all the CT phases, it is a requirement for EC authorisation that an approved summary of product characteristics (SPC) is included in the registration dossier for the medicinal product. The SPC is the definitive description of the product, both in terms of its chemical, pharmacological and pharmaceutical properties and the indications for clinical use. It is the basis of the labelling on the product container and packaging, as well as for the patient information leaflet inserted in the packaging, including the product name, its indication, form of administration, dose, known side effects and whether it is intended for babies, children or adults (where applicable).

The manufacturer cannot by law recommend or market the medicinal product for use beyond its indication or for use in a population for which there is no authorisation. Indeed, many drugs licensed for adult use carry disclaimers in the SPC such as: 'Clinical studies have been insufficient to establish any recommendations for use in infants and children', and warnings on the product label such as: 'Should not be given to children'.

Off-label prescribing refers to physicians prescribing a medication for an indication, age group, dose, or form of administration that is not included in the approved SPC for that product (Stafford, 2008). Whereas off-label marketing is illegal, off-label prescribing is not; indeed, it is common practice among physicians and it is undertaken in order that patients should have access to drugs that, through experience, have shown a wider application than is indicated in the labelling. Physicians have a responsibility to use the medications that they believe are for the benefit of their patients; given the lack of scientific data on the use of medicines in children, as well as limited research into new medicines for paediatric conditions, their only alternative would be to deprive children of treatment that has proven efficacy in clinical practice. Shirkey (1968) described children as *therapeutic orphans* when a paediatric CT is not carried out because an adult trial is used as a proxy.

In the absence of paediatric labelling, physicians have to decide themselves whether the drug is appropriate for their paediatric patients and, if so, extrapolate suitable dosages without having evidence derived from a CT (John, Hope et al. 2008, Neubert, Wong et al. 2008). Shirkey argued that to test these drugs in the therapeutic setting, rather than in the controlled conditions of a CT, is testing "by ordeal" and unnecessarily exposes children to the risk of inefficacy and adverse reactions (Shirkey, 1999).

It has been estimated that two thirds of children in hospitals and 90% of sick newborn infants receive medicines off label. A recent survey covering all paediatric hospitals in Sweden reported that half of all administered prescriptions were not documented for use in children (Kimland et al., 2012). It is also known that the off-label prescription of drugs in paediatric settings tends to be associated with a more frequent incidence of adverse drug reactions (ADRs) than using drugs indicated for this age group (Sammons, Gray et al. 2008; Ufer, Kimland et al. 2004). A major concern regarding ADRs in children is their effects on growth and other developmental processes. Health conditions associated with ADRs in children include: tooth discoloration, skin reactions, growth reactions, hepatotoxicity, Reye's syndrome and "grey baby syndrome" (McIntyre, Conroy et al. 2000). Such ADRs are a major cause of hospitalisation and have resulted in drug-related deaths in the paediatric hospital setting. Still, it is reported that every second ADR might be preventable (Easton 1998; Samoy, Zed et al. 2006). This high frequency necessitates a more careful risk-benefit analysis when prescribing a drug to a young person.

The equivalent percentage of off-label use in adults has been estimated to be 20% (EURORDIS (2010). See Figure 2.

Figure 2: On- and off-label prescription drug usage.

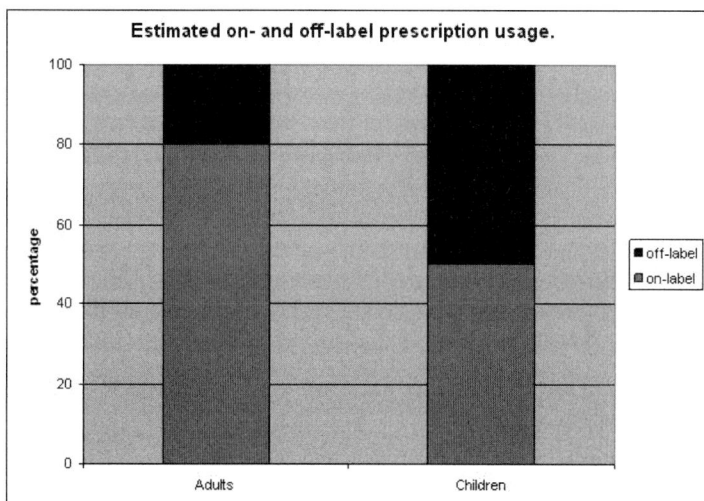

By conducting adequate CTs adapted to children, documentation of ADRs and improved safety of medicines in paediatric health care can be attained.

4 Barriers in paediatric clinical trials

CT data are used in the submission of a request to license a medicine (or other medical product). These data are also used to assist in the determination of how the medicine will be labelled for use in specific populations, including the recommended dose. If no paediatric CT is conducted for a new medicine, then there will be no evidence on which to base labelling and dosage for use in children.

The Paediatric Regulation (EC) No 1901/2006 (European Parliament 2006a) aims to ensure that all new medicines that could be used in paediatric populations will be registered for use in children and therefore tested in a CT with children before a licence is issued. However, the practical difficulties of conducting CTs with children remain.

There are barriers to paediatric CTs that include **structural** barriers that are particular to testing children, **procedural** barriers and **psychological** barriers that apply to the children but also to the parents of children who might enter a CT, as illustrated in Figure 3.

Figure 3: Barriers to participation

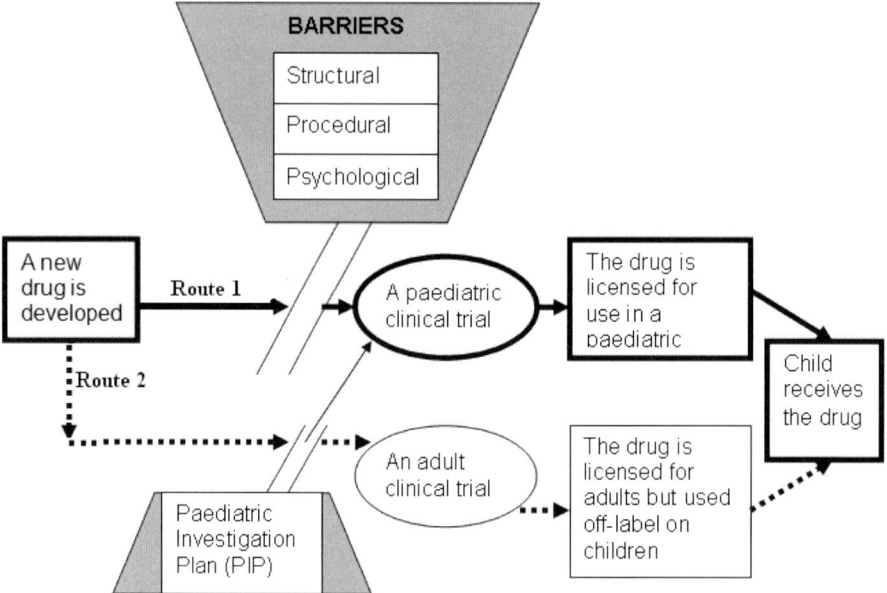

Following its initial development, a new drug will be tested in a series of CTs in order ensure that the drug is safe to use and effective for the targeted condition in the intended population. For a drug aimed at treating children, a paediatric CT is initiated and the results submitted to the licensing authorities (route 1).

Where a medication may be efficacious both in children and adults, the adult route is usually followed first (route 2), as this presents fewer barriers and takes less time to complete, thereby being more cost effective. Following a successful adult CT and the drug being marketed for adults, it can still be used in children, but it will be used off label and the manufacturer cannot recommend it for use in children or market it as a paediatric medicine. Due to the commercial nature of drug development, the financial argument for then conducting a paediatric CT may not be strong enough for the initiation of a paediatric CT. Information about the efficacy of a drug in children is then reliant upon published case reports, anecdotal reports, uncontrolled studies, studies that are not published or peer reviewed and physician experience. Such poorly controlled evidence based on non-representative sampling and non-blinded studies increase the chances of bias, as negative studies are less likely to come to light.

Following route 2 and using the drug off label in children means children are not warranted the same safety as adults. A recent attempt to secure paediatric CTs has been the introduction of the *paediatric investigation plan* (PIP), which forces the manufacturer to provide evidence either that the drug has no paediatric relevance (in which case a waiver is granted) or, if it could have potential for use in children, how and when the paediatric CT will take place.

4.1 Structural barriers

Where the inclusion criteria are strict, recruitment can be problematic; of the over 5000 CTs in the new EU Clinical Trials Register (https://www.clinicaltrialsregister.eu/) as of March 2011, a disproportionately small percentage were trials on children, indicative of structural barriers.

Many trials are abandoned because of difficulties recruiting the required number of children to the trial (Easterbrook & Matthews, 1992). As reported in pharmaceutical conferences, the problem of recruitment to some trials is not difficulties persuading parents to allow their children to participate in a trial, but rather that the inclusion criteria are so narrow that there are too few children to ask.

There are several structural aspects of a paediatric trial that present barriers, as outlined below.

Size of the population
There are fewer children than adults, paediatric populations are more heterogeneous because they are undergoing different stages of physiological development (Kern, 2009) and they have different behavioural characteristics; this makes it a challenge to reach adequate statistical power to detect small or moderate differences in treatment outcomes (Smyth 2001). Specific protocols must be devised for different age groups (compared to one broad age group in adult research). At least six different developmental groups can be identified:

- Premature newborn infants (less than 36 gestation weeks)
- Term newborn infants (0-27 days)
- Infants and toddlers (28 days – 23 months)
- Small children (2-5 years)

- Schoolchildren (6-11 years)
- Adolescents (12-18 years)

All of these require a different approach when considering CT participation.

Age-specific needs
In addition, paediatric drug trials require specific age-appropriate formulations, for example liquid preparations especially for younger children. Frequently, these formulations are not readily available (Mulla et al 2007), thus requiring additional costs and time to develop them. In order to be able to develop appropriate paediatric formulations, these must be based on pharmacokinetic studies done prior to the CT, thereby adding additional expense to the development of the drug.

Blood sampling procedures
Some procedures that might be acceptable in adults require specific justification in children, as they are not able to give consent. Less invasive sampling procedures are always sought; however, these require further effort to develop and adapt to a paediatric population (Conroy et al., 2000) and require strategies and expertise that may not be available at the CT site.

The volume of blood in neonates and infants necessitates small blood sample volumes compared with studies in adults. This produces limitations on the data analysis possibilities that are not found in adults (Kern, 2009).

Different types of medical conditions
Many diseases, such as arthritis or diabetes, are less common in children and other conditions such as cerebral palsy and Down syndrome occur only in children. Genetic disorders that may lead to serious disability or death in childhood are also rare. This implies that specific product lines directed at child conditions need to be developed.

Lack of objective diagnosis
Some diseases are common in children but rely upon subjective diagnoses, such as with asthma. Asthma in young children (aged 0 to 5 years) can be hard to diagnose. Symptoms of asthma also occur with other conditions and many young children who wheeze when they get colds do not go on to have asthma after they are 6 years old. This then poses problems when establishing selection criteria for CTs.

Relevant outcomes
Quality of life is an important outcome in many conditions; however, it has not been until recent years that reliable methods of measuring quality of life in children have been available and these are still not routinely used in paediatric CTs (Bullinger et al 2009; Ravens-Sieberer 2007).
See **8.2.2 *Empowerment through patient-reported outcomes***.

The cost of drug development
The huge investment required for new medicines to be developed and brought to patients inevitably calls for the involvement of the pharmaceutical industry. The nature of industrial involvement is, however, that pharmaceutical development and production is a commercial process with financial pressures upon companies to make a profit.

There is a smaller return on investment if the market for the new product is small, even if the need for a new medicine is great among a narrowly defined population. Paediatric CTs are less profitable because the paediatric population is smaller than the adult population and therefore the proportion of patients available to participate in a CT is smaller. Recruitment can take much longer and thereby increase budget costs. Pharmaceutical companies are thus reluctant to bear the costs of CTs for the smaller and less profitable paediatric market (CESP, 2005; Shirkey, 1999; Wilson, 1999). Developing medicines for the adult market generally provides a much better return on investment.

Awareness of ongoing CTs
People are generally only aware of a CT if they attend the clinic where the trial is being held. From the patient perspective, there is a general lack of awareness of what trials are taking place. A number of attempts have been made to overcome this barrier through CT databases and websites where people can sign up for future CTs. None of these databases have external monitoring, so it is not possible to say how many people sign up or how many are actually recruited to a CT by this route. We have no published evidence that these databases have been used in the recruitment of children to phase III trials.

4.2 Procedural barriers

The application of the principle of minimal risk
The application by ethics committees of a minimal risk threshold for paediatric research acts as a procedural barrier. Non-therapeutic research is necessary for improving paediatric care but carries with it a potential risk of harm to the participants. The application of the principle of minimal risk to paediatric research can lead to the rejection of important research proposals. The difficulty of getting approval, it has been said (Conroy et al., 2000), has resulted in the pharmaceutical industry being reluctant to propose paediatric CTs due to uncertainly of ethics committee approval. The European Paediatric Regulation seeks to address this by requiring that the need for paediatric research is assessed for all new medications in Europe. The principle underlying the Paediatric Regulation is that it is unethical to give to children drugs that have never been tested on that age group in a controlled CT, which is the method by which we are most certain to generate reliable evidence of the efficacy and safety of the drug. In a recent survey (Altavilla et al., 2012), ethics committees in Europe were found reluctant to engage in discussions about how they have adapted to the new paediatric regulation and those that responded to the survey indicated that they wanted more training in dealing with assessing paediatric trials. This gives the impression, at least, that ethics committees have limited knowledge and understanding of the current paediatric regulatory framework and that things have not changed from the perspective of ethics committees (Altavilla, et al 2012). There is still a reluctance to include children in CTs.

In order for a paediatric CT to be approved by an ethics committee, it is expected that the CT will involve 'minimal risk' to the child; however, the definition of minimal risk is complex. In the United States, the definition of minimal risk is that *'the probability and magnitude of harm or discomfort anticipated in the research are not greater in and of themselves than those ordinarily encountered in daily life or during the performance of routine physical or psychological examinations or tests'* (US Dept of Health and Human Services, 2009).

This definition has also been adopted by the EU working group proving guidance to the European Clinical Trials Directive with the guideline document *Ethical considerations for clinical trials on medicinal products conducted with the paediatric population* (EC Directorate-General for Health and Consumers, 2008). Applying this definition means that if a study is approved on the basis of minimal risk, the child participant is being asked to agree to undergo procedures that carry no more likelihood of harm than their daily activities.

The difficulty of obtaining true informed consent
In most cases of medical research involving human subjects, the basic principle of respect for the individual requires that participants enter into the research voluntarily and with adequate information. In some situations, however, application of this principle is not obvious. The involvement of children in research is such a case, where the child is deemed to be unable to consent to participate themselves and this responsibility is given to someone else on their behalf. The fact that children may participate based on assent rather than consent makes some researchers believe that research on children cannot ethically be carried out. Informed consent is seen as the cornerstone of ethical practice in medical research and, if informed consent cannot be obtained, then they argue that the research should not be carried out. See **2.1.6 *Informed consent*** and **2.1.7 *Assent***.

The principle of voluntary participation based on adequate information and understanding may take some time to apply. Informed volunteers are sometimes difficult to find; therefore, the application of true informed consent and how this is carried out in the CT can act as a procedural barrier to research where in every situation, paediatric researchers have to pay attention to ethical issues arising from the fact that informed consent is not obtained from the child.

4.3 Psychological barriers

There are risks in testing new medicines, regardless of the age of the CT participant. However, these risks are considered more acceptable if the individuals being asked to participate are informed of the risks and understand the implications.

As the literature on decision-making in medicine shows, many factors are expected to play a role in this process (Frosch & Kaplan 1999). It is essential to acknowledge that participation or non-participation in a CT is a psychological process that applies to both the child and the parents.

Their attitudes to medical research in general, solidarity with other children having the same condition, trust in the individual clinician inviting them to participate and the child's personal medical needs are all crucial elements in the family's decision-making, as illustrated in Figure 4.

Figure 4: Attitudes, needs and medical research

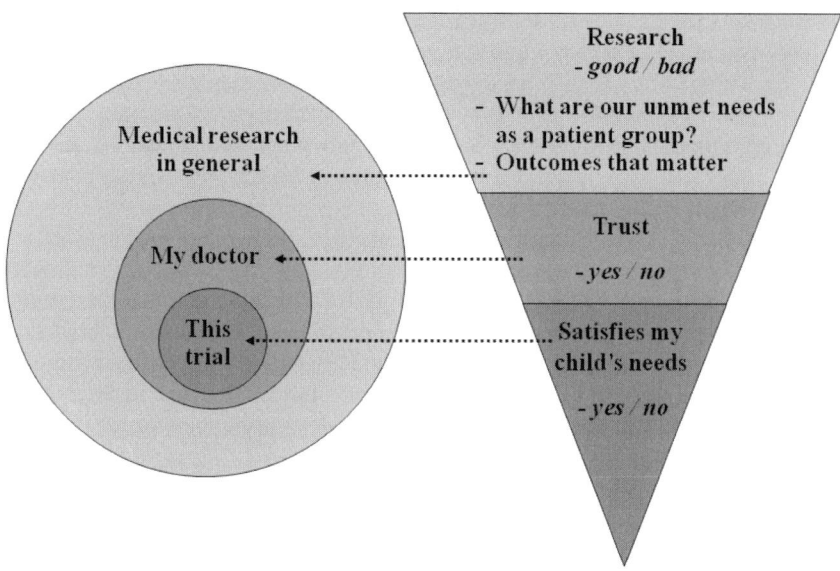

Happy with current medication – no need to change
In general, parents do not enter their child in a CT if they are satisfied with the current medication. These parents are not looking for a trial. Perceived health status is also a reason for premature withdrawal from participation. The withdrawal rates will rise if participants perceive an improvement of their health status (Sederberg-Olsen et al., 1998). In diseases that remain asymptomatic for a long time, the probability of a higher attrition rate among participants increases (Gómez-Marín et al., 1991; Crom et al., 2006).

Change of routine
Some families may see any change in routine as unwelcome. There is uncertainty in the unknown and to change an established treatment routine may involve some unforeseen consequences.

Time and inconvenience
Studies of adolescents' reasons for declining participation have highlighted these factors: increased clinic visits, increased number of treatment interventions (Tercyak et al 1998), increased frequency of diagnostic procedures and transportation issues (Dolan et al 2008, Tercyak et al 1998). Frequent reasons for premature withdrawal from a study are long delays to follow-up or family constraints (Crom et al 2006, Reitamo et al 2008).

Fears regarding the randomisation process: the risk-benefit ratio
It has been reported that parents tend to decline participation if they wanted a specific treatment for their child and are opposed to randomisation. It is common for the experimental treatment to be perceived as superior to the control or standard treatment (Sammons et al 2007) and thus parents do not want to take the risk of randomisation.

Use of needles as a part of blood sampling
Children who dislike participating in CTs often report that it is because they do not like the needles (Sammons et al 2007). In many cases, the main procedures in the CT are not as painful as the blood tests that are carried out for monitoring purposes.

Many children already object to blood tests that they have to undergo as part of their treatment plan and health care staff have to find ways to overcome their young patients' fear of this unavoidable pain. In contrast, where the child is in a CT – in which withdrawal is always an option – the obligation to accept this pain is less clear (Sammons et al 2007, Stuijvenberg et al. 1998; Pletsch & Stevens 2001) and putting children through pain not related to their health treatment becomes more ethically questionable.

Being overwhelmed
The literature suggests that some parents report a feeling of being overwhelmed by the information or have expressed that they did not understand the options being offered to them. The feeling of being overwhelmed depends upon the amount of information and the use of technical language. The easiest response is to say no, thus reducing the number of decisions that have to be made.

PART II

5 The RESPECT project

The European RESPECT project set out to explore the expectations and needs related to the participation and empowerment of children in CTs. The RESPECT consortium consisted of experts from the fields of clinical research, patient representation, and European paediatric research ethics and regulation. The following organisations were partners in the project:

- **Sahlgrenska Academy at University of Gothenburg, Göteborg Pediatric Growth Research Center.** The coordinator of the project. An academic and clinical partner conducting CTs with children.

- **Good Clinical Practice Alliance - Europe.** A consultancy group active in the area of ethics as related to CTs and medical research.

- **University Medical Centre Hamburg-Eppendorf.** An academic partner with access to trainee medical staff who will in the future conduct CTs with children.

- **European Patients' Forum.** A European umbrella NGO representing 44 chronic disease-specific patient organisations operating at EU level and with national coalitions of patients organisations.

- **University Children's Hospital Ljubljana - Dept of Paediatric Neurology.** A clinical partner conducting CTs with children, particularly children with epilepsy and mitochondrial disease.

- **Consorzio per le Valutazioni Biologiche e Farmacologiche.** A clinical research organisation (CRO) conducting and monitoring CTs, particularly with Thalassaemia patients, and coordinator of the TEDDY European Network of Excellence.

- **Azienda Ospedaliera di Padova - Dept of Pediatrics, University of Padua.** A clinical partner conducting CTs with children with a focus on HIV. Leads the steering committee of the PENTA paediatric CTs network.

5.1 The aims of the RESPECT project

The RESPECT project aimed to identify, firstly, the needs and motivations of children and their families making the decision to participate or not participate in CTs of drugs under development in Europe. The second aim was to identify methods by which children's needs can be translated into empowering and motivating them in future CTs.

The aims of the project were realised though three objectives, of which the first was to construct a common basis for understanding. The second objective was to collect and analyse the experiences of those families invited to participate in paediatric CTs, as well as the various approaches to recruitment and current practices in running CTs involving children in different medical areas and conditions. The third objective was to disseminate our findings and conclusions in order to widen the debate and encourage the adoption of better empowerment and recruitment methodologies for children in CTs.

The project consortium contacted children in Europe who had participated or might participate in CTs, their parents, patient organisations, clinical staff, pharmaceutical companies and ethics committees, to gather their insights and suggestions. In addition, a wide consultation was conducted among other European research projects in this area as well as European academic, industry, and regulatory experts. Further consultation and research was also included from the global CT community.

By drawing together different actors, the project opened the debate on how to contribute to the empowerment of European children and their organisations in CTs. Together with the partners in the project, who represented both the research side and the patients' perspective on involvement in paediatric CTs, a strong, integrated, and fruitful coordination was fostered.

The dissemination activities of the project were intended to assist all stakeholders in defining more appropriate strategies to improve the participation of children in paediatric CTs within Europe and to contribute to the further development of European paediatric research policy.

5.2 Methods used

The project employed a variety of methodologies to explore the issues raised by children's participation in medical research. These methods were chosen and adapted according to the specific groups studied and the needs of the project.

Case study interviews and surveys were employed for child participants and potential participants in CTs, including at times the parents of such children; focus groups were used to evaluate clinical staff views on children in CTs; interviews were employed to understand industry views on children in CTs; group exercises in schools were conducted among children in schools and surveys were undertaken among members of ethics committees and of patient organisations. The disease areas focused on were epilepsy, growth problems, diabetes, mitochondrial disease, HIV, Thalassaemia, and cancer.

The main emphasis was on obtaining qualitatively rich data that includes the families' own stories of why they agreed to participate and why they continued to participate. All centres were also strongly encouraged to consult with local and national research groups and companies involved in CTs.

Interviews
* Case study interviews: CT participants (63 responses)
* Focus groups: CT participants (5 responses)
* Paediatrician interviews (4 responses)
* Focus groups: CT staff (16 responses)
* Pharmaceutical industry interviews (4 responses)

Surveys
* Child-Parent survey (110 responses)
* Healthy Child survey (38 responses)
* Patient organisation surveys (30 responses)
* Paediatrician survey (10 responses)
* CT networks survey (7 responses)
* Ethics committee survey (77 responses)

Workshops
Workshops were held in each of the participating partners' countries. These helped us to establish a 'common knowledge' with a wider audience and to identify the operating procedures needed to encourage empowerment and increase motivation for participation in CTs. The project workshops were open to other participants invited to contribute to the topics discussed, thus providing another means by which networking can be progressed.
* Methodology workshop (October 2008)
* Trust seminar (November 2009)
* Paediatricians seminar (January 2010)
* Patient organisation workshop (April 2010)
* Pharmaceutical industry seminar (May 2010)
* Ethics workshop (June 2010)
* Harmonisation workshop (June 2010)
* Decision aids workshop (December 2010)
* Dissemination meeting (May 2011)

The project management (Work Package 1) was provided by the project coordinator (University of Gothenburg), responsible for the overall planning and monitoring of the work of the project. Regular meetings were held and a web-based coordination tool was developed as a platform for cooperation between the partners.

The initial project meeting took place in Gothenburg and this was followed by two workshops, which took place in Hamburg and focused on developing the methodology for the project and training in case study description (Work Package 2). The study plans, interview questions, case study manual and questionnaires were developed and finalised. The second workshop was a knowledge-base workshop to present the information collected and identify the issues for further consideration in the harmonisation stage. This workshop gave the partners an opportunity to discuss the emerging issues and raise further areas for consideration by the project. As part of this work package, a literature review was undertaken.

The first qualitative data collection was undertaken in Work Package 3, in which the objective was to explore the existing procedures for identifying and satisfying patient needs in CTs. The aim of WP3 was to deepen and extend the knowledge of patient needs, attitudes, expectations, motivations and perceived barriers to participation in CTs. The first source of information was case studies of normal and benchmark best practice in the participating CT centres. Following approval by the local ethics committee, interviews with families and children currently participating in CTs were undertaken. Information was collected on how families get involved in CTs and what their expectations and wishes were for their participation.

A complementary part of WP3 was to solicit and collate opinions from CT researchers via focus groups, interviews and surveys, as listed above. In addition, telephone interviews were undertaken with representatives from the pharmaceutical industry and ethics committees.

Web-based surveys of patient organisations (POs) throughout Europe were conducted in Work Package 4. In addition, an empowerment workshop was held in Brussels in order to identify the concerns and needs of POs and their recommendations as to how empowerment of their members in the CT landscape could be achieved.

From this integrated sequence of approaches, the RESPECT project was able to obtain improved understanding of children and their families' needs concerning CTs. In Work Package 5, the survey data and opinions generated from the earlier work packages were brought together in order to draw conclusions that can contribute to recommendations for the future development of child-focused CTs. These conclusions were finalised at the WP5 harmonisation workshop.

WP5 included two demonstration projects based on the findings of the RESPECT project. The first was a decision aid to provide a structure for children and their families who are thinking about participation in a CT. A pilot decision aid was developed and tested.
See **10.1** *Self-determination through decision aids*.

The second demonstration project was a CT education package for parents and young people, based on the information needs that emerged from the RESPECT data sources. A pilot education package describing the need for CTs and the ethical issues concerning research with children was developed and tested in a school environment. See **10.2** *Knowledge through an education package for schools*.

The final work package (WP6) involved dissemination of the RESPECT findings in order to facilitate collaboration and information exchange between different actors in the CT landscape and to ensure that the results of the project influence the research community and persist in the public domain. One avenue of dissemination, our public website, will continue to be maintained in the years that follow the project. In addition to a dissemination conference held in Brussels, this book has been produced as one of the main channels for wider public information and dissemination of the project's findings and conclusions. Our ambition is to raise awareness of how to empower children and their parents and respect their interests, to motivate their participation in future CTs.

The stages of the RESPECT project are summarised in Figure 5.

Figure 5: Work package overview

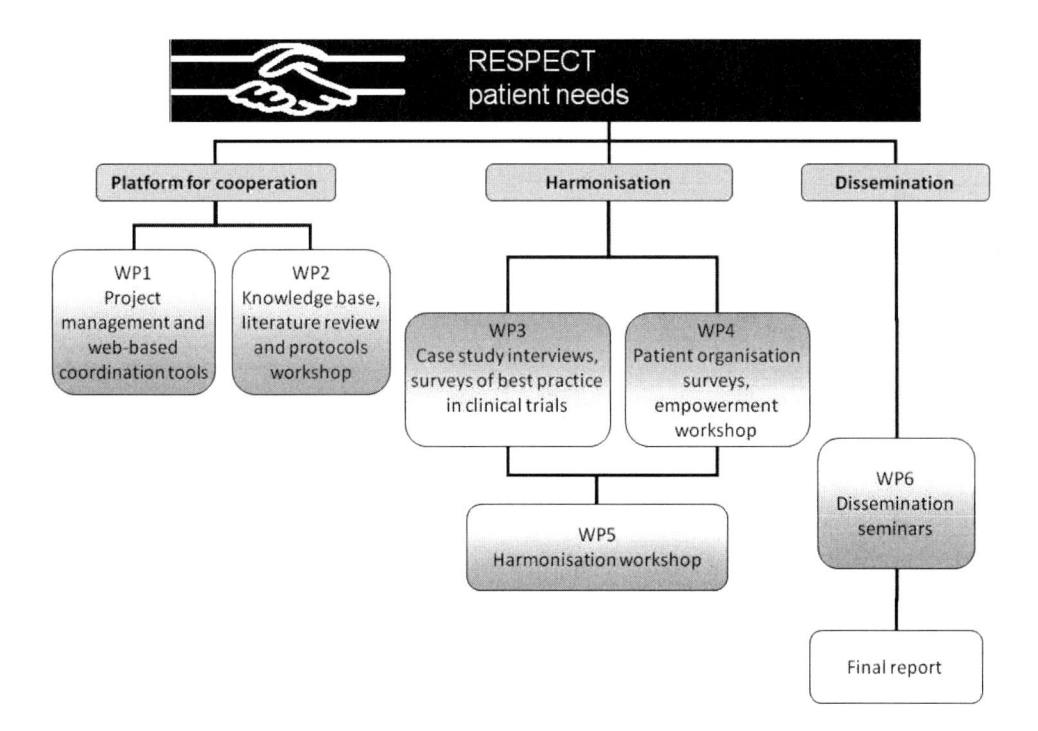

```
                          RESPECT
                          patient needs
        ┌───────────────────┼───────────────────────┐
  Platform for cooperation     Harmonisation        Dissemination
     ┌────┴────┐            ┌──────┴──────┐              │
    WP1       WP2          WP3           WP4             │
  Project  Knowledge   Case study    Patient             │
 management base,      interviews,  organisation         │
 and web-   literature surveys of   surveys,             │
 based      review and best practice empowerment         │
 coordination protocols in clinical  workshop            │
 tools      workshop   trials                            │
                          └──────┬──────┘               WP6
                                WP5                  Dissemination
                           Harmonisation              seminars
                             workshop                    │
                                                    Final report
```

6 Data gathered by the RESPECT project

6.1 The experience of children and their parents

The RESPECT project is not a quantitative study but rather a 'coordinating action' exploring and sharing the opinions of the stakeholders surrounding CTs on children. As part of this process, we conducted structured interviews and some small-scale surveys of parents and children in hospital outpatient settings in Slovenia, Sweden, Italy and Germany. For more details on these results, see **Appendix 1a**.

Various groups of CT participants were interviewed: diabetes, HIV, epilepsy, mitochondrial disease. The majority of participants who participated in CTs were families who were being treated for their health care needs at the trial site. In the majority of cases, the participant was invited to participate by their health care physician. Most of our respondents were in an ongoing CT and thus represented the *maintenance* stage of participation (see **2.4.1 Stages of Change model**).

6.1.1 Slovenian parents of children in CTs

Case study interviews were conducted with 30 parents of patients in one CT and 14 parents of patients with a more severe condition participating in another CT in Slovenia. A general pattern was that parents of children with the more severe condition gave more positive responses than those with the less severe condition. They saw the study in a more positive light: more worthwhile and more likely to help their child or others in the same position, which compensates for the extra discomfort the child incurred in this CT. It is possible that this reflects the severity of this condition and the limited treatment options currently available to these families.

Themes that emerged

- **Benefit to the child personally:** Many of the parents talked about the trial as an opportunity to get more information on their child's condition. They referred both to the chance of a more precise diagnosis from the additional medical procedure involved in one of the two CTs but also to the fact that they learned more about their child's condition and wanted to do anything that could improve the child's chances of improvement, even if the benefit was only in small increments or not until a more distant future. This was also their motivation to participate in other trials, if asked in the future.
- **Altruism:** Apart from wanting the best for their child, the parents spoke of a duty towards all children with a similar condition. Some considered their own child unlikely to benefit but believed that other children may do.
- **Increased knowledge:** The vast majority of the parents were (or became) interested in the research and wanted to learn more. Some parents searched the internet for information on the disorder; the majority wanted to know the outcomes of the study.
- **Pain & discomfort:** Many parents observed that the procedures were unpleasant for the child, particularly if general anaesthesia was involved. Some drew the line at accepting

general anaesthetic or an additional medical procedure that was being conducted for research purposes rather than for the child's therapy, seeing what discomfort it caused the child. They also found it hard to watch their child's distress when giving blood samples.

- **Inconvenience:** Some reported long journeys to the hospital and long waiting times once there. It could be hard to get the time off work for this. Nonetheless, the vast majority expressed the feeling that the study warranted the amount of their time it demanded. Some felt that it was no more inconvenient than a normal visit to the hospital paediatrician.
- **Informed consent:** The parents did not always understand what the study was about. The specialist language (including Latin terminology) in the informed consent material made it harder for them and they wanted the information to be presented in non-technical language. It was notable that they did not consider the use of their personal information by the researchers to be an issue; this relates to the hope to get personal benefit for their child if possible.
- **Trust in the child's doctor:** Despite not being sure of what the study was about, these parents usually consented to the full procedure and did not feel under pressure to consent. The vast majority liked the clinical staff and felt that they were serious and responsible people. This suggests that they could put their trust in these individuals without having to understand all of the facts.

6.1.2 Swedish CT - children and parents

Case study interviews with 15 paediatric patients and their parents participating in a Swedish CT were conducted.

Themes that emerged

- **Trust:** Parents often assume there are no risks involved in a trial. They trust the doctors and rarely refuse to participate. ("It's good that it's the same doctor at the same hospital. It feels safer here.")
- **Altruism vs. personal benefit:** Parents say it is worth the time and trouble as long as somebody's child stands to benefit. In practice, they hope for direct benefit to their own child. They do not want their child to get the placebo or miss out on the latest treatment.
 Understanding: For both the parents and the child, it is not clear what the trial will involve. It often comes as a surprise that it is time-consuming or painful or that there may be side effects.
- **Pain & distress:** No-one wants their child to suffer. Needles are particularly distressing. ("I wouldn't let my son be used as a 'guinea pig' in an experiment that could harm him.")
- **Assent:** Parents vary in the degree of autonomy they give the child to make the decision. Most often, the child does not have much say in the decision and trusts that the parents have understood what the research involves. ("It's easy to agree to something if you don't know what it actually involves.") The child often wants to stop at first but is persuaded to continue. Some of the children say they have now adjusted to the discomfort while others say they would refuse if asked again.
- **Information seeking:** Some parents sought information independently (often reading journal articles) before deciding to participate. Parents repeatedly express an interest in

receiving feedback on the study findings but rarely get any. ("We definitely want some report of the results: we want to know which group he was in, but also what this study found.")

6.1.3 Italian paediatric patients and their parents

The case study questions were presented to children and their parents: Only one of the families had been involved in a CT. Those who had not participated in CTs were asked questions about their needs and what would be important to them when thinking about participation in a CT. In general, because the families were aware of having seen enormous progress in medical treatment of this condition, all the families expressed their willing to participate in CTs and all had a good knowledge of what is required of participation in a CT. This gave us their perspective at the *pre-contemplation* stage.

Themes that emerged

- **The distribution of results** and progress made through trials were particularly relevant to willingness to participate.
- **Access to information:** The importance of having access to all the available information was stressed.
- **Openness:** Respondents wanted the possibility to feel free to ask questions.
- **Not feeling forced** to participate was essential.
- **Time commitment:** Time lost (off school or work) was not an issue for this group.
- **The importance of the collective good** of the CT took precedence over that of the good of the individual child.
- **The rapport between the doctor and patient** were important for participation although it was stated that if a study were proposed by an unknown doctor, a rapport would have to be created before the family would feel comfortable about participation.
- **An interest in medicine** had arisen out of the experience of having the illness and frequenting the hospital environment.

6.1.4 Swedish interviews exploring understanding of CTs

In order to survey the needs that may exist for a child to participate in a CT, what level of knowledge parents and patients have about their child's trial and the principles it is built on, we interviewed children and their parents participating in a CT in Sweden, with a particular focus on their understanding of CTs

The parents were all aware that their child was a participant in a trial but the parents of younger children admitted that their child was probably not aware of the research part, being a minor at the time of enrolment.

Themes that emerged

- **General knowledge of CTs:** When they were asked to define the aims of the CT, all of them were able to identify the objectives but hesitated when asked to explain, in their own words, *what is a clinical trial*? All of the interviewed people expressed their lack of knowledge about the fundamental aspects of a CT, particularly the way it is conducted.
- **Information overload:** All parents seemed to remember signing a consent form, but did not remember the details. They described the information as "too much" and hard to understand. They said that it would probably have been better if all parts were described more clearly and simply. None of them said they were reminded that they were in a trial.
- **Randomisation:** Most of the parents seemed to be aware of the term *randomisation* and what arm their child belonged to and they accepted the procedure. However, it was not clear for everyone that this is used to compare groups against each other. They consented to participation because both arms in the trial received the same medicine, but in fixed or individual doses. They were all satisfied with the trial and would recommend others to participate; they felt inclined to include their children in future trials if it were to their personal benefit.
- **Unpleasant procedures:** The extra blood tests were unpleasant but the children were able to cope because they thought they would benefit from the study.
- **Positive experiences of participation:** They stated the following positive outcomes of being in a CT:
  ✓ the clinicians and the nurses give more time to examining each patient and answering questions that might arise;
  ✓ the positive benefit of helping others and hopefully themselves (or their child);
  ✓ the trust that they placed in the clinicians and the test drug, due to the safety requirements, the careful observations that would be conducted and the adverse event reporting.
- **Sample size requirements:** They knew that their child would receive their standard treatment if they decided to withdraw, but they were not aware of the negative outcome for the study that would arise if a major part of the participants did withdraw.
- **Being informed of results:** They were eager to see the outcome of the study in total, but were not aware if there was such an opportunity or how they would receive the information.

RESPECT

6.1.5   Child-Parent survey (Italian patients)

RESPECT received responses from Italy to the online survey. Most of the children (8 of 12) had participated in a CT.

These results were interesting because there was a mix of responses from children and parents.

Themes that emerged

- **No burden of participation:** These patients were attending hospital regularly for blood transfusions and thus did not experience the CT as an extra burden because they had to come for appointments anyway.
- **Benefit to the child:** It was thus like a continuation of their treatment and they saw a definite benefit for the child. They also noted the potential benefit to other children but this may have been of secondary importance to them.
- **Positive evaluation:** They understood that this was a CT and felt it had been clearly explained to them and that it was a worthwhile study.
- **Receiving the results:** They wanted to receive a report on the results after the CT.
- **Trust:** They expressed trust in the clinical staff and most felt appreciated for their contribution and would participate again if asked.

6.1.6   Child-Parent survey (German parents)

The German responses to the online survey gave a different perspective because eight of the nine parents who responded had never been asked to participate in research at a hospital, so they gave the *pre-contemplation* point of view (see **2.4.1 Stages of Change model**). These patients were more hesitant at the prospect of participating in a CT.

Themes that emerged

- **Burden:** It would be a burden to them because they would not otherwise come to the hospital regularly; most indicated that this inconvenience would not be great but they would expect some kind of payment and practical help. (This may refer to travel expenses.)
- **Not obliged to participate:** They did not feel any obligation to the clinical staff and indicated that there would have to be a positive relationship for them to agree to participate.
- **Risk:** They were not totally against the risks involved in a CT and were not particularly interested in having this explained to them.
- **Being used as a 'guinea pig':** They were against the child being used as a 'guinea pig' for research. They wanted to know how the results would be used.
- **Testing new medicine preferred to building scientific knowledge:** They were unwilling to have their child assigned to a control group and did not want to be tied to one treatment and miss other options because of the CT. This indicates that they did not

appreciate the basic principles of clinical research and the importance of randomisation; they expected more personal benefit.

6.1.7 Child-Parent survey (Slovenian parents, study A)

Half of these parents completing the online survey gave responses concerning participation in this study, while the other half were at the *pre-contemplation* stage and gave their thoughts on potential participation in a CT. This was a long-term study and the parents were aware that they were participating in research and volunteered their child freely without feeling any pressure. There was no immediate advantage to the child (such as better treatment) and the families only attended the hospital to participate in the CT;

Themes that emerged *(participating in this study)*

- **Burden (special arrangements):** they had to make special trips for the study but did not find this a problem.
- **Altruistic motivation:** They were motivated by interest in worthwhile research that could help all children, including their own, as well as showing a desire to 'pay back' to the medical profession for help already received.
- **Respect:** They indicated respect and trust in the staff but did not feel especially valued for their contribution.
- **Receiving the results:** They wanted to receive the results at the end of the study.
- **Future participation:** They would participate in other studies if asked.

Themes that emerged *(potential participation in CTs)*

- **Anticipated motivation:** Altruism, gratitude and an interest in research featured in these responses too.
- **Worthwhile research:** The parents would want a lot of information when considering participation. They wanted to see whether it was a worthwhile study and to know exactly what would be expected of the child, as well as the risks and benefits.
- **Being used as a 'guinea pig':** The parents would not expect a direct benefit to their child but, on the other hand, they did not want their child to end up in the control group and thus effectively be a 'guinea pig' in the research.
- **Receiving the results:** They would want a report of the results at the end of the study.

6.1.8 Child-Parent survey (Slovenian parents, study B)

A shorter version of the child-parent questionnaire was filled in manually by 52 Slovenian parents (mostly mothers) of control group adolescents who have been included many times in longitudinal follow-ups in a neonatal outcome study. These children were born in 1987-1989 and were included at birth in the research study. Later on they were included in two different follow-up studies, around age 4 and age 7, then some of them were included at the age of around 15 years, and finally at the ages of 16 years and 20 years respectively in two further studies. The questionnaire was distributed to parents by the adolescents included in the study.

Themes that emerged

- **Altruism:** The parents indicated that participating was of no personal benefit to the child but that they felt a duty to participate for a worthwhile cause.
- **Pressure to participate:** One quarter of the respondents felt that they could not refuse to participate.
- **Benefits outweighing disadvantages:** They did not find it painful or difficult and, although it was time-consuming, they were willing to volunteer the time necessary for the research.
- **Positive attitude:** One third indicated that it was fun to take part in the research and most respondents were interested to see what the research was about.

6.1.9   *Healthy adolescent survey (Swedish)*

The Swedish version of the healthy child survey was sent by email to healthy adolescents.

The majority (30 of 38) had not even heard of the concept of a CT, so their views were interesting to us to get a snapshot of adolescents at the *pre-contemplation* stage (see **2.4.1 *Stages of change model***) and their potential reactions to being invited to participate in a trial.

Themes that emerged

- **Trust:** The response that surprised us most was that they were generally comfortable with the idea of being a 'guinea pig' for medical research, as long as the risks were minimised. This suggests a trust in the medical profession.
- **Importance of medical research:** They could see the benefits for the progress of medical knowledge, showing an altruistic attitude to societal benefits. (As healthy adolescents, they had no personal need of new medicines, which is often the motivating factor in our other groups studied.)
- **Tokens of appreciation:** They were not motivated by payment or other rewards, apart from some token gesture of appreciation.
- **Altruism** was a stronger motivation than personal benefit.
- **Sufficient information:** There was striking agreement that they would only participate if they were given a lot of information about the trial.

6.1.10 German follow-up study: the 'willingness to participate' construct

In the RESPECT project, one aspect of the different approaches to understanding participation in CT was a closer investigation into the 'willingness to participate' construct. In a pilot study, questions specifically regarding willingness to participate were extracted from the RESPECT online survey for parents and children; these were then presented to a convenience sample of medical students, health sciences students and hospital outpatients (thus, also at the *pre-contemplation* stage). In total, 215 questionnaires were returned and psychometric analysis of these responses was carried out to identify the largest explanatory factors for willingness to participate in CTs.

The analysis suggests that the general willingness to participate in clinical research is influenced by the patient's interest and the effort involved. The decision to participate in a study depends upon having a basic general knowledge of clinical research and an interest in such projects.

The prospect of benefit to others emerged as of great importance but the degree of willingness to participate depends on the extent of personal gain the respondent can derive from participation.

These respondents wanted to be given access to all the information on the use of the study data and the results, indicating that they were a lot more confident about understanding this information than the average CT participant. They also indicated that they wanted to have a say in the study as part of their participation. However, this expectation may reflect the fact that 80% of the respondents were medical or health science students, not children or parents.

In planning a CT, the responses indicate that it is important, even before the implementation of the study, to provide information about possible risks and side effects of the test drug, or potential negative consequences from participating in the study.

Themes that emerged

The identified factors were interpreted in terms of factor one (***control***), factor two (***general concerns about participation***), factor three (***general interest in clinical research***) and factor four (***personal benefits of participation***).

The first factor is mainly about a sense of **control** for the trial participants. These respondents are not only interested in basic information about the clinical research, but also in a precise description of the smallest details of the study and its implementation. We also note that the anonymity of the participants is very important to these respondents; they do not want to be identifiable, thus removing fear of uncontrolled dissemination of the results.

Factor two describes more **general concerns** that lead to participation or non-participation in a CT. The corresponding items concern fears and anxieties of the respondents. This factor also describes the aspect of the time required for participation in a trial, including easy accessibility of the research site.

The third factor is a **general interest in clinical research**, with an altruistic attitude being linked to participation. This depends on the person's own experience with clinical research projects, or at least general knowledge about clinical research. The more points of contact there are in this respect, the more likely is a commitment to participate.

The fourth factor identifies the **personal benefits** to be crucial for a commitment to participate in a CT.

6.1.11 Trust in doctors: discussion with an expert on the trust concept

During the RESPECT project, doctor-patient trust emerged as an important factor in why people participate or refuse to participate in CTs. Therefore, RESPECT carried out a workshop on trust with an invited expert in this area.

Doctor-patient trust is a crucial element for participation in CTs. In the absence of an established relationship between the doctor and patient, willingness to participate is markedly lower according to our observations. So how can we increase the level of trust so that, if there is only a weak relationship between the doctor and patient (or the parent making the decision), the patient might still feel safe in agreeing to participate? Should we generate more trust or ensure that the family can make a truly informed decision that is not so dependent on the doctor's influence?

Most research on trust focuses on interpersonal relationships, but in the case of CT research it is also interesting to consider the power imbalance of doctor-patient and adult-child relationships. A paediatric patient is weaker on both scores. The CT should be entered into voluntarily and therefore it would be dishonest to use or allow the imbalance of power to promote participation. The informed consent process is very clear in pointing out that the potential participant is informed of the voluntary nature of the research. Where this is not stressed, trust will break down.

Themes that emerged from the workshop

Trust is a multidimensional concept. Important aspects established in the literature are summarised below.
- Trust judgements take into account **honesty** (telling the truth), **reliability** (promise fulfilment) and **emotional respect** (avoiding criticism, not causing embarrassment). These elements are independent: you may for example trust someone to be honest but not that the same person will keep their promises.
- Trust is dependent on **beliefs** (gut feeling), **trusting behaviour** (tendency to trust others) and **trustworthiness** (demonstrating honesty, reliability and emotional respect).
- Trust is **reciprocal** (mutual) - the patient needs to trust their doctor but the doctor also has to trust the patient (to be honest, to adhere to the treatment regime or protocol, come for check-ups, etc.). Even children of 5 or 6 yrs appreciate reciprocal trust.
- Trust is **dynamic** - it may build up gradually or initial trust may be weakened over time, as it is reassessed based on experience.

- Trust is shown in all levels of society, from trust in family members, to trust in doctors, to trust in the government, and our trust may be directed at a specific person, a group or a generalised other. We need to trust others in all walks of life to be able to function.
- Rotter (1980) showed that higher-trusting people are not gullible. They are good at judging trustworthiness and will look for reliable information to help them make a decision. Low trusters will reject information; their mind is already set to be cynical.

Trust in clinical trials

There are three relationships of trust, related to the CT experience, which can be identified:
- trust beliefs **between the parent and child**;
- trust beliefs **in physicians**; and
- trust beliefs **in medical treatment**.

Within these three relationships there are both spoken promises and unspoken promises. For example, spoken promises are made as part of the informed consent process, i.e. what will happen during the trial. Unspoken promises are also made, primarily that of not doing harm. This applies to the personal relationships but also to the third relationship: namely, an unspoken promise that medical treatment is a good thing and will not cause harm. Honesty is crucial to trust; where spoken promises are made, it is vital that the physician or parents are honest to the child about what will happen and what else might happen. Where medical research has broken the unspoken promise of doing no harm, the willingness to participate at the *contemplation* stage (see **2.4.1 *Stages of change model***) is reduced. Note that fear is a separate dimension: a child might be afraid of needles, just as some children are afraid of the dentist, but the child may still trust that this pain is necessary and for a good reason.

Being empowered to decide (or not) at the *contemplation* stage seems strongly related to how much information the family has and their level of trust. Where they do not have sufficient information trust fills the gap. If the parents and children do not have enough information, they make a judgement (sometimes described in the interviews as a gut feeling) about whether they trust the doctor and the medical profession enough to participate. At a later stage, the participants may re-evaluate this decision and, on the basis of this, decide to stay in the CT or leave. Over time the participants have the opportunity to evaluate the veracity of the promises made to them concerning the pain and inconvenience of being in a CT. In the majority of cases, the RESPECT project found, that the families in the *maintenance* or *completion* stage of a CT had high levels of trust in the investigators and the CT process.

6.1.12 Conclusions on the experience of children and parents

We gathered the comments of families who agreed to participate in CTs and individuals who had never been asked, but it should be noted that we did not get any responses from those who refused when invited to participate or those who withdrew from an ongoing trial. Thus, some of our material sheds light on how people at the *pre-contemplation* stage think they would respond to a hypothetical invitation to participate, while those at the *maintenance* or *completion* stages of CT participation could reflect on why they consented and how they experienced it.

Many of the parents we interviewed saw the CT as a way to get the latest and best medicine for their child (thus misunderstanding the principle of equipoise that is fundamental to CTs). They are disappointed that their child might get the placebo and thus miss out on the latest treatment. A child placed in the control group was seen as a 'guinea pig' in the research, whereas being given the test drug was not seen in this light. This indicates that they did not appreciate the importance of randomisation; expecting more personal benefit (which is the normal role of the medical profession). Only the healthy adolescents we surveyed were comfortable with the idea of being a 'guinea pig' for medical research, on the assumption that the risks would be minimised.

Families generally reported that participating in the CT was inconvenient, apart from those who had to come for appointments anyway. Parents said it was worth the time and trouble as long as somebody's child stands to benefit, but we saw repeatedly that the greatest altruism came from those who had not actually been in a CT or whose participation had not been painful or unpleasant. There was clearly a 'tipping point' if this altruism involved subjecting the child to extra pain or distress and the parents in this situation did not always feel that their sacrifices were appreciated sufficiently. They wanted more gratitude and token gestures of appreciation.

When faced with the decision to participate, there was an almost universal desire to get as much information as possible, but those who were in a CT often complained that the information they had received was not easy to understand. Thus, they had to trust the doctors and nurses to guide them in their decision and it was common for parents who had entered their child in a CT to say that they had confidence in the staff and felt that it was a worthwhile study. They were often motivated by a desire to 'pay back' to the medical profession for help already received.

When we surveyed outpatients who had never been in a CT, we found that they were more hesitant at the prospect of participating. They did not feel any obligation to the clinical staff and indicated that there would have to be a positive relationship for them to agree to participate.

Most often, the child does not have much say in the decision and trusts that the parents have understood what the research involves. Thus, trust is a pivotal aspect of consent and it is important that families do not feel that this trust has been broken if the CT was not as they were led to expect. It was not always clear – even to the parents – what the CT would involve and it often came as a surprise that it was time-consuming or painful or that there were side effects. The child is at particular risk of understanding the least while suffering the most distress, and some of the older children reflected this when they said they would refuse if asked again.

Parents often saw the trial as an opportunity to get more information on their child's condition. They were eager to see the outcome of the study in total, but were not sure if there was such an opportunity or how they would receive the information. Other parents saw themselves as research partners in making medical progress and wanted to feel that their input was valued. This interest in the research was clearly a motivation for participating in further trials if asked again.

It is important to ensure that families understand the need for research and are respected for their valuable contribution to the improved safety of medicines for children.

6.2 The experience of patient organisations

6.2.1 Email survey: Patient organisations

The RESPECT project conducted an email survey to identify the views and perspectives of patient organisations (POs) on the level of participation in paediatric CTs and the reasons why children participate in CTs, why they do not participate and what can be done by POs to answer their needs and increase participation in and quality of paediatric CTs. (See also **Appendix 1b**.)

Thirty-six POs and 48 further organisations were contacted; 11 organisations responded to the questionnaire. Among the respondents, six POs reported having experience in paediatric CTs while five POs did not have this specific experience.

The survey aimed to explore critical aspects of the levels of participation in CTs and to highlight positive examples and best practices. These are the specific aspects investigated:
- the extent of paediatric CT participation per disease;
- the reasons why paediatric patients and families decide to take part in CTs;
- the specific barriers to participation;
- good practices and motivating factors;
- informing potential participants;
- the role of patient organisations.

Results

Extent of paediatric CT participation:
The results showed a lack of knowledge concerning paediatric CTs. There were no specific figures of paediatric CT per disease available.

Patients' needs: WHY patients DO participate in CTs
According to the experience of the POs responding to the survey, participants in CTs are mainly motivated by their direct interest in receiving new treatments. Sometimes the idea of helping other children with similar diseases is also a motivator. In certain cases, they also feel more confident in taking drugs that are under development than licensed drugs that have not been tested on children. The decision made by parents to improve the condition of their child is also one of the reasons that contribute to the participation of children in CTs.

Patients' fears: WHY patients DO NOT participate in CTs:
The analysis of the answers provided by POs, sometimes citing direct responses from parents and children involved in CTs, indicate four main types of barriers to participation:
- emotional barriers;
- ethics and transparency of information;
- practical barriers;
- the relationship with physicians and other entities.

The emotional barriers concern fears of the parents. Parents are afraid that their child might not understand the process. They also fear that the treatment might not provide any direct benefit or that it could even worsen the situation. Finally, they are concerned with the invasiveness of the treatment and of health checks. These fears translate into a perception of risk and into safety concerns related to CTs.

Ethics and lack of transparent information constitute another group of barriers to participation in CTs. Parents are especially concerned with the possibility of complicated 'informed consent' procedures for children whenever communication is not implemented at the right level for the child to understand. According to POs, the lack of knowledge from the parents about the existence or on the importance of CTs is also an obstacle to participation.

The third group of barriers relates to practical aspects of CTs. Time-consuming treatments, extra visits to hospitals and an excessive waiting time before having results are considered reasons that reduce participation in CTs.

The fourth group of barriers is in the realm of the relationship with physicians and concerns the role played by institutions and POs. Parents are afraid that they will not receive adequate support from physicians and that the legal system lacks regulations to ensure trials are safe. Among the POs surveyed, the absence of training for patient organisations might also constitute a barrier to participation.

Good practices and what should be done

Informing potential participants
The results of the survey highlight a need for a more transparent and structured flow of information by involving in the process physicians, nurses and patients' organisations.

Two key concepts emerged from the survey: cooperation and trust. Better cooperation among stakeholders involved in CTs will provide tools to parents and children to be actively involved, informed and supported. *To know* will trigger mechanisms of trust. It is helpful if the person informing parents and children or introducing them to the 'informant' is somebody they know or somebody they consider reliable, such as their GP. To reinforce the feeling of trust in parents and children, the involvement of medical associations, national health authorities (but not of the industry according to some interviewed) can also be relevant.

Strengthening the role of patient organisations
A guiding principle is that patients must be treated as partners in knowledge rather than recipient only of health care treatments, therefore the role of POs needs to be shaped accordingly.

POs should be sources of unbiased and reliable information to guarantee transparency in the CT process to parents and children. In particular, they need to stand on the side of children and design their work as intermediaries, facilitating children's input as well.

POs should also be responsible in promoting ethics and principles through formal guidelines at the international level. To safeguard that the conduct of the CT is in line with these principles and that it is beneficial to the patient, POs can be involved in pre-study meetings.

They should also be in charge of disseminating available information about existing trials, the value of participating in it and sharing information with other POs when the trials are in their same disease area.

On the quality of the information disseminated, POs must opt for a 'family-friendly' language and methods. Focus groups, studies of child and parent attitudes are useful tools in ensuring that their input is included in CT design and implementation and to ensure that parents and children can truly provide informed consent.

Finally, POs should provide emotional support to parents and practical help. POs should play a role in facilitating logistic problems and reducing obstacles (e.g. by guaranteeing access to transportation when the child is requested to go often to hospital, or by helping to fill in forms).

Responsible role of Institutions:
A solid legislation framework is needed. Regulations and legislation will provide a more organised structure to rely on and will allow the development of a family-friendly CT system.

Below are some aspects from the survey that emerged as 'future landscapes' to be promoted:
- Work to develop a system in which true informed consent by families - including by the children themselves - becomes possible;
- Parents' opinions must be integrated during the trial;
- The creation of an internationally agreed principles charter must be designed and implemented. The Eurordis Charter on CTS for rare diseases can be used as a model;

Conclusions from PO email survey

Parent- and child-friendly CTs are needed to increase participation. Patient organisations are the key group to produce the change by organising themselves to empower patients involved in CTs and adopt a child-input perspective.

For this to happen, transparency, cooperation, education and training need to be further developed at all stakeholder levels. The final expected result will concern the involvement of patients in CTS as partners in knowledge and in the development of true informed consent by families, including by the children themselves where possible.

Physicians and nurses need to develop a family-friendly language and communication strategy, while GPs - who already have a trust-based relationship with their patients - are also expected to play a major role by being the first contact among patients and doctors involved in the CT.

A solid and reliable legal framework that prescribes international standards and guidelines will provide the political tools for all stakeholders to cooperate better but especially for patient organisations to take the lead in empowering children and motivating them to take part in CTs, by reducing their fears and concerns.

6.2.2   Online survey: Patient organisations

Introduction

This online survey focused more on the way patient organisations (POs) operate in the field of paediatric CTs. (See also **Appendix 1b**.) The results of the survey provide information on three main points: firstly, the type of questions parents of children involved in CT ask POs, when asked at all; secondly, why patients DO and why DO NOT participate in CTs and thirdly, what kind of good practices are already being done and the role of POs at present and for the future.

This survey is based on a questionnaire translated into all languages of the project consortium and conducted online. Nineteen responses were collected; below are the figures according to language/country:
- English: 2 replies
- Swedish: 7 replies
- German: 5 replies
- French: 1 reply
- Slovenian: 1 reply
- Greek: 1 reply
- Polish: 2 replies

The questionnaire targeted patient organisations involved in different areas of diseases, among the respondents there were organisations involved in pathologies such as asthma, diabetes, kidney issues, lupus, allergies, Thalassaemia, AMD, haemophilia, cystic fibrosis, Addison, child heart diseases, young rheumatic, Ehlers-Danlos syndrome, epilepsy, mitochondrial disorders, adrenoleukodystrophy, Duchenne muscular dystrophy and some unspecified self-help organisations.

The POs that participated in the survey were asked to provide information on their experience of paediatric CTs and specifically to address the issues mentioned above-.

Results

Questions to POs
The survey aimed to establish what kind of questions parents ask POs to better evaluate what role they (the parents) can play. The results showed that parents do not usually ask questions about CTs directly to POs, but it is more likely that parents tend to enquire with doctors or healthcare professionals involved in the CT. In case of questions asked directly to POs, these helped to understand parents' concerns and limits to participation in CTs.

Parents' queries about CTs

Several POs received questions about which studies are ongoing in their specific disease area in order to find out whether there are specific treatments being tested for children. This is seen especially with parents of children with severe and usually debilitating diseases or heart disease. In this last case, more information is often requested by parents about cardiac research, in the treatment of pulmonary arterial hypertension, research on anticoagulant medicines or on artificial pacemakers. Some POs registered questions linked with safety and efficacy concerns about the risks involved

Why patients DO participate in CTs

According to the experience of the POs that participated in the survey, parents agree to their child being involved in a CT mainly because they would like immediate benefits from a new treatment, access to new generation of drugs or if they want to ask for an early introduction to these. In some cases parents feel a sense of gratitude for the possibility of accessing new treatments and they are keener in having their child participate.

Why patients DO NOT participate in CTs

On the other hand, parents who are not willing to let their children participate in CTs are mainly concerned about risks and side effects. In certain disease areas, parents are more worried for girls because of possible fertility issues in the future. In some cases, logistical problems such as lack of time can be a barrier to participation, especially if the CT requires more visits to hospital to receive the treatments. Parents might be less in favour of invasive CTs but more prone when the trials are part of routine examinations.

These barriers to participation might be the consequence of a general lack of trust in physicians or in the scientific sector. According to one of the respondents, a major role is played by public media, which tend to create a dichotomy between the 'good' (alternative medicines, new age, chemical-free) and the 'bad' (conventional medicine, drugs). At the same time, scientific magazines that could provide more scientifically reliable articles are not read and not so accessible to the general public on a wide scale, creating a gap in knowledge.

Good practices

What should be done

The aim of good practices is to increase children's participation in CTs and ensure that this is a safe and empowering experience for the child.

Convincing parents of the usefulness/need of the CT, to better inform them, and to increase their interest to cooperate are the objectives of good practices. This can be achieved by educational activities, individually and in groups, such as by organising regular meetings. POs should provide a good level of expertise and structure during these meetings, which can be also organised in order to target children directly. A risk factor in focus groups may be the influence of one parent over the group. Indeed, among the respondents to the survey one PO gave as an example the case in which a parent who was especially negative about a CT could undermine their trust-building programme or, on the other hand when the good approach of one parent can enhance positive emulation.

Role of patient organisations

Participants in the survey were asked to describe what is being done already in their POs and what can be improved.

Among the responding POs, some are already quite dynamic in activating mechanisms to increase participation in paediatric CTs. The majority consistently disseminate information through their internal newsletters or magazines to members in letters or articles. The second choice is to liaise with CT projects, while the third choice is to get involved directly in campaigning and lobbying activities, sometimes at the EU level as well.
One of the respondents described in detail its own strategy, which consists of regular meetings, a specific phone line to share problems at national level, lectures and support groups, publication of pamphlets to target practical and daily needs. This organisation also works with universities by mentoring and co-mentoring graduate and postgraduate papers, financing research, promoting postgraduate courses ad hoc. Finally, this PO is also active in providing logistical support to patients who need to travel abroad to get surgical treatments.

Among proposals to improve the role of patient organisations, what emerged is that POs ask for a more active and recognised position as an intermediary in CTs between patients and professionals.

POs especially ask to be involved from the beginning in a CT, by helping to recruit participants and presenting them the information as first interlocutor; in this way they can act as a resource both for families and researchers. They further ask to be responsible for developing ethical guidelines and to advocate and campaign for regulations.

POs want to play their role of intermediaries among the researchers and patients through platforms that involve all stakeholders in CTs and they want to be the first to disseminate information to other organisations and to patients.

Finally, POs were asked to highlight critical aspects or their specific needs according to their area of research. These are the main findings:
- Research into a rare disease area is less profitable, therefore some diseases are neglected
- To improve education of staff participating in clinical research provides an important source of income
- There is a risk of sponsors and investigators having vested interests in recruiting a patient for a CT of a test drug when it is not necessarily in that patient's best interest to switch from their current treatment, if it is relatively effective. There should be an independent assessment of such decisions, and the test drug should be compared against the existing treatment, not just against a placebo.

Conclusions from PO online survey

Patient organisations are ready to be active players in managing the relationship between paediatric patients and the research sector to improve participation in CTs and to make the experience more empowering for children.

To achieve results through good practices, POs ask to be formally recognised as the intermediary among patients and professionals and to act within a common legal framework. They want to be involved all along the process of CTs, starting from recruiting the participant, though information activities and disseminating the results.

Reinforcing the role of POs will increase the level of trust towards the research sector. Indeed, both of the surveys conducted by EPF highlighted that parents tend to mistrust based on their lack of – or limited access to – information.

This second survey stressed an additional aspect: the role of the media in creating fallacious perceptions. General media tends to emphasise the importance of natural remedies, creating a negative perception of traditional medicine. This can bias the approach of parents considering involving their children in CTs. At the same time, scientific magazines with more accurate information are not so accessible at the public level.

POs can thus be expected to reduce information gaps at the level of parents involved in CTs through education and training, but also at public media level, by pursuing and reinforcing their activities of information dissemination.

6.3   The experience of CT staff

6.3.1   Focus group with German clinical research staff

RESPECT conducted a focus group with German researchers and clinicians to explore their concerns about the difficulty of recruiting children to studies that imply some risk for the child.

Themes that emerged

Good Clinical Practice
- They all give information about the study to the parents and children, but the whole process is not standardised. They also explain the risks and benefits of participating
- Standardised consent documents (often provided by the sponsor) are used.
- To protect participants, the study group makes clear that the participants have the right to withdraw from the study at any time.
- They offer no special legal or psychological advice.
- They reported that CTs with children do need more time than CTs with adults.
- The participants get information about their health status, but not about the global research results of the trial; the sponsor will not disclose the results

Consent and assent
- The age of the child who is asked to participate (assent) is a problem: sometimes the children are so well informed that even a 5-year-old is capable of stating if he or she wants to participate or not. It is difficult to say where to draw this line.

- On the other hand, everybody from the study group agreed that if the child has a life-threatening disease any refusal from the children should be ignored even if the assent is very important.

Motives for the child to participate
- The study groups were in agreement that, for the older children, the money they receive is the most important motive. The parents identified a mixture of getting the latest medical care and the feeling that they wanted to do everything possible to help the child.
- Concerning the level of knowledge parents and children do have about medical research, they agree that most people they spoke with fear being treated as a 'guinea pig' - they stressed that this is an outdated idea of medical research. On the other hand it depends strongly on the diagnosis: parents and children with serious diagnosis know better about medical research because of personal research about the diagnosis.

Barriers to CTs with children
- - The clinicians expressed problems with participating by design - parents are more likely to refuse participation in studies with a placebo wing.
- - They sometimes think that panel research will be better than CTs.

6.3.2 Focus group with Swedish clinical research staff (Team A)

RESPECT ran a focus group with Swedish nurses involved in a CT. The discussion material consisted of patient statements drawn from our earlier literature search and case studies indicating why they had participated in a CT, as well as additional statements suggested from the literature review indicating why a patient might refuse to participate.

Themes that emerged

General
We explored which of the statements they believed their patients had expressed and whether there were additional opinions reported by patients.

It was much easier for the nurses to remember patients' reasons for participation in a CT than reasons against participation, largely because it is extremely rare for patients attending this clinic to refuse to participate. (The patients and parents we have interviewed in our case studies are full of praise for these nurses and seem happy to get more attention from them by being in a trial.)

Motives the children and/or their parents have expressed for participating
The nurses confirmed that the following reasons were sometimes or often given:
- The study could lead to improving other children's health.
- The research could help me/my child personally.
- It is not painful or unpleasant.
- I/we do not mind the time it takes.
- I/we have no problems travelling to the hospital.
- It is better than being at school / at home / at work.

This suggests that the families consider their participation to have no real disadvantages while having the advantages of potential benefit to their child's health and that of other children. Of course, we cannot rule out that they only make positive comments to the nurses and privately have some worries but, nevertheless, we know that they willingly agree to participate and continue for the duration of the trial.

The nurses also commonly heard the following comments:
- I want to receive a report on the research results at the end of the study.
- I/my child would be willing to participate in further research.
- I would like to be a researcher / doctor / nurse.

This suggests that the families also consider themselves active participants in the research (not just passive patients) and feel entitled to know the findings at the end of the study. It is not clear whether any of the families are given a study report of any kind.

Motives the children and/or their parents have expressed for refusing
As stated above, this is a rare scenario, so there was not much to say. However, the nurses did recognise the following statements from parents:
- I do not want to put my child through unnecessary procedures.
- It would be painful or unpleasant.
- I was worried that my child would be put in a control group that does not get any treatment.
- It would involve too much of our time.
- It is inconvenient to travel to the testing location.

They reported that pain and distress to the child do get mentioned frequently by both parents and children in connection with having to undergo blood tests and injections. The children are often afraid of needles and complain that it hurts. Several parents have said that they do not want their child to participate in future trials if it involves more needles. If they are coming to the hospital anyway for tests then it might be acceptable.

6.3.3 Focus group with Swedish clinical research staff (Team B)

The clinical staff reported that, because their patients have a serious chronic disorder, they build up a strong relationship with them over many years, which makes it easier to encourage them to be in a CT. The team staff reported low dropout rates in their trials, probably because of this strong relationship. They discussed how much harder this would be if they were dealing with, for example, cancer patients who would have recently got a diagnosis and be coming to a clinic where the staff did not know them. It would be hard to establish trust quickly and their acute condition would make them less willing. Parents would find it tough to make such a decision in this situation.

The doctors present stated that they want what is best for their patients and would not enter them in a trial unless they felt it would help them.

The staff members explain what the trial is about verbally, in addition to the written information, and answer any questions the family may have. Parents are quite knowledgeable, especially when they have been in several trials, and it is not clear if specific education would help them. The children are not so aware.

The only risk is that families get 'study fatigue' and do not want to be in yet another trial. Then it is the staff's job to explain how important it is to take part and contribute to research.

They also reported that children themselves may not want to participate in a trial because of the blood tests (fear of needles), but that the staff then encourage them to be 'brave and strong'.

One nurse reported that some healthy children were recruited to a trial involving bowel investigations (which she would have refused to volunteer for herself). Surprisingly, they were keen to participate and did not regret their decision once the trial was underway. They felt that they had a special status. (It has been mentioned by Slovenian and Swedish doctors that it helps to make the patient feel that they have 'VIP' status if they are in a trial, even though this would not really be true.)

When asked if they had any patients spontaneously asking to be in a trial, most did not think that this happens, but one nurse said that she had one such patient. It is more usual that patients respond to a request from the doctor. (It may be that most patients here are already in a trial.)

6.3.4 Interviews and survey with paediatricians

Background

This part of the RESPECT project aimed to explore how paediatricians approach the task of recruiting children and their parents to CTs.

Data collection took place in Nov-Dec 2009. There were four interviews with professors of paediatrics in Sweden, Italy, Germany, and the Netherlands. The same questions in the form of a survey were distributed to paediatricians in Slovenia and we received ten responses. These respondents had considerable experience of CTs, recruiting on average 85 participants each (ranging from 10 to 300). For more details on these results, see **Appendix 1c**.

Themes that emerged

Barriers to participation
When asked about the timing and their general approach, several of the respondents commented that it is particularly hard to raise the issue of participation while the family is stressed. Often this is because of the shock of just having received a severe diagnosis or because they only have a short time to think about the request to participate. One paediatrician reported that he sleeps

badly when he knows he will have to approach a parent for consent in an acute situation (such as taking a blood sample before and after bypass surgery); they need more time to decide and a good relationship of trust with the staff.

Parents do not want any extra distress for their child, particularly when the child is very small, or has a devastating disease or even mental or motor disabilities, and the CT protocol includes invasive or semi-invasive procedures. They are also afraid of infection or side effects,

They do not like to think of their child as 'guinea pig' and dislike being assigned to different treatment arms (especially in double blind randomisation). This is because they assume there is a personal disadvantage if they miss out on the test drug. It is thus important to explain to the family the novelty of the new treatment and the fact that they will be able to receive the new treatment after the trial if it proves to be effective (regardless of which arm of the study the child was in). They considered the ideal situation to be when a separate appointment is made with the family, meeting in a more comfortable room (not behind a desk).

A common problem that families report to them is the inconvenience of participation (time lost and the logistics of getting to the trial site). The paediatricians were often frustrated that they could not offer more logistical support.

Doctors themselves feel less motivated to join a CT when the workload will be high with too many complicated, formal procedures.

In some cases, families are reluctant to make the long-term commitment that participation involves. If they have participated in many trials, they may show 'CT fatigue' and a loss of hope in the promise of new treatments.

Families' motivations to accept
The expectation of better treatment motivates both the families and the paediatrician. Indeed, the paediatricians commonly reported that they emphasise the extra monitoring and potentially better treatment when encouraging families to participate.

As a consequence, a comment was made that some parents may feel that they will not get full and appropriate treatment unless they agree to participate in the CT.

The personal relationship with the doctor was considered to have an impact, with the child and the parents wanting to follow the doctor's wishes. In return, the paediatricians were concerned to reduce inconvenience & pain as far as possible and wanted protocols to minimise the number of blood tests the child would undergo.

Explaining CTs
When asked about what families understand about clinical research and whether it is hard to explain about the CT, many of the paediatricians reported that the parents' level of knowledge varies; furthermore, children understand even less and can be inattentive. These paediatricians gave vastly different responses when asked how old a child needs to be to give their assent (ranging from 4 to 18 years of age).

Particularly problematic are situations where the parent will consent, but the child will not give assent (especially if he or she is rather small); children do not see the necessity for the study.

On the question of explaining risks & benefits, they stressed the importance of being honest, as you would with your own child, with explanations appropriate to the child's age. Listening and responding to the family's questions was considered important. These subtle skills are not available in the ethics committee guidelines.

Payback to participants
More than half of the respondents reported that they give the family information on the results of the study, but in several cases this was only on request. One paediatrician suggested that knowledge is something they could offer when encouraging participation, because the interested parents and children will learn about the research by participating.

Interestingly, some of the respondents mentioned that patients would like to see more gratitude from the staff or the sponsor, probably reinforced by token gestures (gifts or treats, such as a meal) for the children.

6.3.5 Recruiting patients: discussion with experienced paediatricians

In January 2010, we held a seminar with the senior paediatricians among the RESPECT project partners, to find out more about their experience in relation to the interview and survey responses we had gathered from other paediatricians. They gave us the following insights.

Barriers to participation
The parents who are most resistant to invitations to enter their child in CTs are the ones for whom the existing treatment is working well and the CT concerns testing different doses or oral versus intravenous administration. They do not want to change anything, so recruitment will be a problem and the CTs will probably have to reduce the sample size required for significance (as they do now for orphan diseases). It may even be necessary to recruit from more countries. Often around half of those asked to participate will refuse. One suggestion was that there should be campaigns (appeals) to the public to raise awareness of CTs and increase the likelihood of participation.

If the parents have no established relationship with the doctor (for example, a mother approached when she has just delivered), only about 20% will agree to let their child participate. They are usually the more educated mothers who feel research is important and personal benefit to the child is likely. The other 80% do often come round to the idea later and it is very rare for families to withdraw once they are in a trial. If their child has a chronic disease, they are more likely to participate for altruistic reasons; they feel that they will see reciprocal benefit in the long run.

In the case of chronic diseases, the clinicians already know the patients and may ask them to be in many trials. Indeed, they avoid inviting new patients to participate and wait until they know them better. In any case they would always contact the patient's primary care physician for background information (medical history and also previous compliance to their medical regime). The patient's physician may have little experience of randomised CTs or alternatively have been involved in many trials before. He or she may be asked to join someone else's CT as a satellite trial centre but an alternative is to send the patient(s) to the main trial centre instead. This may be better for the patient in terms of expert monitoring. It means that the patient effectively receives a second opinion on their diagnosis and prognosis, which the primary physician may see as a benefit or (possibly) a threat.

Exclusion
Immigrants tend not to get included in CTs. There is an assumption they will not understand the instructions because of low education, but this may be an assumption by medical staff. We need to be more inclusive and provide cultural mediation, not just translation. There is a European Commission project called European Standards on Confidentiality and Privacy in Healthcare among Vulnerable Patient Populations (EuroSOCAP) that is producing guidelines on addressing patients in their strengths instead of focusing on their weaknesses.

In the case of HIV (in which the child contracts their condition from their mother), it has been observed that some mothers refuse to let their child participate because they themselves had a bad experience (such as a rash) with the drug and do not want the child to risk this. Since adherence is important, the clinician will not enter these patients in a CT of a drug they are unlikely to take.

Spontaneous requests
If the patient is on a standard drug and it is not helping, the parents are glad to try something new. In fact, they consistently ask spontaneously to be included in any trials that may be started, especially if their child has a fatal disease. Many parents spontaneously seek information about their child's condition on the internet.

Patients who are more empowered will want to find a CT that suits them. It is possible – at least in USA and Sweden – to respond to an advert in the press or radio recruiting CT participants, but in other countries, these spontaneous applications by patients may not be allowed.

Conclusions from survey and interviews with CT staff and paediatricians

These responses raise the question of whether the existing Good Clinical Practice guidelines are enough. Just ticking informed consent checklists may not be a guarantee of true informed consent. We cannot be sure whether parents and children have really understood what they are being asked to do or whether they consent instead because they trust the doctor, the nurse or the researcher to do what is in their best interests. This leaves families in a vulnerable position.

There is a risk that some adults (among both clinicians and parents) do not consider the child's opinion to be valid and do not communicate directly with the child. It is important to gain the family's respect and trust by being honest - as one would with one's own child; the clinical staff must give and take feedback before, during and after the trial;

The responses highlight the importance of clinical staff respecting their patients' needs in order to increase willingness and motivation to participate in a CT. It is important to listen to the family's concerns; wherever possible, the clinical staff should strive to reduce distress for the child and keep inconvenience for the family to a minimum

Physicians are in a unique position to inform trial sponsors about the child's unmet medical needs and to influence which trials are conducted, but it was not clear whether they use this influence; however, they do sometimes emphasise to sponsors that they prefer to avoid too many blood tests on their young patients.

It is important to ensure that families understand the need for research and are respected for their valuable contribution to CTs; randomisation must be clearly explained and the clinical staff must show appreciation, acknowledging that the child is a 'medical hero'.

6.4 The experience of CT networks

6.4.1 CT networks: involvement of paediatric patients and their parents

Survey findings

Answers were collected from eight of the twelve networks contacted. For more details on the survey results, see **Appendix 1d**.
The participating CT networks were:
  CICP – French Network of Paediatric Clinical Investigations Centres
  FINPEDMED - Finnish Investigators Network for Paediatric Medicines
  PENTA - Paediatric European Network for the treatment of AIDS
  BPCNR – Belgian Paediatric Clinical Research Network
  PRINTO – Paediatric Rheumatology International Trials Organisation
  ECFS – European Clinical Trials Network
  MCRN - NIHR Medicines for Children Research Network
  CVBF – Consorzio per Valutazioni Biologiche e Farmacologiche

Our consultation shows that only three out of the eight paediatric CT networks participating in the survey systematically involve patients and/or patient organisations (POs) in their clinical research. Two of these networks are disease oriented and fall in a very specific 'rare diseases' category, while the third is a generic network facilitating the development of medicines that are both safe and effective in the treatment of children.

One network highlighted the fact that the direct participation of patients in the planning stage of the clinical research depends on the type of study, and in particular on the investigated disease: if there is a strong patient organisation, it is more likely that their input is sought from the early stages of the research.

Recruitment is usually carried out within the network's members and/or participating centres; if the number of patients recruited through the network is not sufficient, specialists and/or POs (in the case of rare diseases) are contacted; only occasionally the CT is publicised through advertisements.

Feedback is systematically given only by one of the networks, while usually it is encouraged, but not always attainable. The amount of information given to patients depends on the Sponsor, but usually data relate only to the general outcome of the trials, while personal information are typically not given.

Examples of best practice are:

- A national template for providing information on a CT to paediatric patients of all age groups and templates for informed consent in all age groups. The network has also developed picture cards to use when providing information on a CT for children.
- Youth groups that provide feedback on their health status and their medical and social care.
- Active involvement of young people and families in the design and delivery of CTs via a young persons' advisory group, or topic-specific focus groups.

Conclusions from the CT networks survey

The following conclusions can be drawn from the results of our survey: direct involvement of patients and POs is still not in the current practice of most paediatric CT networks, and it is necessary to increase awareness on the subject. Some networks are very active and they can set an example for networks that need guidance on how to involve the public in their CTs.

It might be useful to draft and circulate recommendations targeted at families and POs to encourage their involvement in CTs.

6.4.2 CT networks: involvement of public stakeholders

Background: The European network of paediatric research (Enpr-EMA)

The European Paediatric Regulation posed the legal basis for the development of the "European network of existing national and European networks, investigators and centres with specific expertise in the performance of studies in the paediatric population".

The European Medicines Agency (EMA) was appointed the responsibility to set up such a network and in May 2010, the recognition criteria requirements to become member of the Network were agreed on by participants from 38 national research networks and CT centres and the European Medicines Agency.

CT networks interested in joining the network were invited to complete a self-assessment form (to be updated annually). A total of 33 networks submitted self-assessment forms to the European Medicines Agency: eighteen are now officially members of the European network of paediatric research (Enpr-EMA); one is, at the time of writing, undergoing clarification and fourteen do not qualify for membership.

Recognition criteria for self-assessment

The self-assessment form contained the following six criteria that networks should fulfil to be recognised as a member of the Enpr-EMA:

- Criterion 1: Research experience and ability.
- Criterion 2: Network organisation and processes.
- Criterion 3: Scientific competencies and capacity to provide expert advice.
- Criterion 4: Quality management.
- Criterion 5: Training and educational capacity to build competences.
- Criterion 6: Public involvement.

The RESPECT partner CVBF analysed the responses to **Criterion 6** to find best practice examples of family or patient organisation involvement. For more details on this analysis, see **Appendix 1d**.

Within Criterion 6, the minimum requirement was involvement of the public in at least one of the following three component items:

6.1 Involvement of patients, parents or their organisations in the protocol design.
6.2 Involvement of patients, parents or their organisations in creating the protocol information package.
6.3 Involvement of patients, parents or their organisations in the prioritisation of needs for CTs in children.

Results: Involvement of families or their organisations

Almost 85% of the CT networks submitting applications involve patients, parents or their organisations in at least one of the activities included in Criterion 6 (Public involvement).

In particular, 54.5% include the public in protocol design, 51.5% in the creation of protocol information packages, and 57.6% in the prioritisation of needs for CTs in children.
Moreover, 27.3% of these networks involve patients, parents or their organisations in all three criteria, 24.2% in two of the three criteria, 33.3% in just one criterion and 15.2% do not involve the public at all.

When taking into account the two most represented categories separately, we see that almost 67% of member networks involve patients, parents or their organisations in protocol design and in the creation of protocol information packages, while 72.2% include them in the prioritisation of needs for CTs in children.

Moreover, around 35.7% of networks currently *not* qualifying for membership at Enpr-EMA declared that they involve the public in the protocol design and the creation of protocol information packages, while almost 43% involve them in the prioritisation of needs.

Conclusions on the involvement of families or their organisations in Enpr-EMA

The inclusion of patients, parents or their organisations in the network's activities as one of the qualifying criteria for membership in Enpr-EMA is just one of many examples within the European Medicines Agency, which includes PO representatives in their various committees and working groups.

It is sometimes assumed that involving families in making the informed consent material clearer is the closest patients, families and/or POs can get to involvement in the design of CTs, but this analysis shows that much greater involvement is possible and is already practised by these member networks to some extent.

The fact that those networks not qualifying as members of Enpr-EMA are also those that apparently have weaker links with patients is a fact that should not be taken lightly, especially if compared with the very different approach employed by Enpr-EMA member networks that, in contrast, more systematically involve patients and their representatives.

There are many initiatives aimed at promoting and encouraging patient and public involvement in clinical research and many examples of how to make these initiatives successful. These networks prove that the involvement of the public does work.

Allowing patients to have a direct input in the design and execution of the trial, as well as in the prioritisation of needs, will motivate their participation. In addition, a closer cooperation between researchers and children and their representatives as active research partners enriches our understanding of both the medical condition and the outcomes.

6.5 The experience of ethics committees

6.5.1 Survey on the involvement of European ethics committees in paediatric research

The CT-Directive introduced a number of measures to harmonise the ethical review of CTs and facilitate clinical research. It required Member States to legally establish ethics committees, including obligations and specifications, formal procedures and timelines, composition and competencies. Specific provisions were also adopted for reviewing CT protocols including children. However, due to the nature and legal force of a Directive, Member States had some flexibility in implementing its provisions in their national legislation. Thus, ethical review procedures and the amount and quality of publicly available information vary significantly among European countries.

To evaluate the impact of the new European paediatric regulatory framework on the activities of ethics committees charged with reviewing paediatric research protocols, the TEDDY Network of Excellence and RESPECT set up an inventory of ethics committees existing in Europe and conducted a survey among them on their approach to paediatric trials. Replies were gathered from a total of 154 ethics committees (18.2%) operating in 22 countries; with a response rate below 10%, in 4 countries (Spain, Finland, Germany, UK) but exceeding 30% in 12 countries. For more details on the survey results, see **Appendix 1e**.

Themes that emerged

Ethics committees' knowledge of the European paediatric regulatory framework

Our results demonstrate that a gap exists between the current regulatory framework and ethics committees' awareness, knowledge and understanding of the major issues related to paediatric clinical research; only 14% of 139 ethics committees had discussed and analysed the most important European legal instruments devoted to paediatric research. That could explain the lower response rate (73 committees) answering the optional questions related to more specific issues.

Impact of the European Paediatric Regulation and European Ethical Recommendations

Overall, ethics committees recognised, as possible effects of the new European paediatric regulatory framework, the increased involvement of children in clinical research and, thus, an increase in the number of medicines tailored for children, as well as better-designed paediatric trials and more multicentre paediatric clinical studies.

When asked about the influences of the new regulatory framework on their work, around two-thirds of the 73 respondents reported no impact or low impact from the Paediatric Regulation or the European Ethical Recommendations and under 10% acknowledged a high impact.

This low impact was particularly true of ethics committees operating in EU-15 Member States (Belgium, France, Germany, Ireland, Italy, Luxembourg, Portugal, Spain, Sweden, and The Netherlands). In contrast, one-third of respondents in new EU Member States (Cyprus, Czech Republic, Estonia, Latvia, Malta, Poland) declared a high impact of the Paediatric Regulation and most acknowledged either high or sufficient impact of the European Ethical Recommendations. These data suggest that ethics committees in the new EU Member States are more actively involved in efforts for integration and harmonisation towards EU research and health norms and systems than EU-15 ethics committees.

The major influences recognised by ethics committees were: the creation of new rules for reviewing paediatric protocols and sometimes changes in their own organisation; increased quality and number of paediatric protocols and especially the increased time needed to review these protocols. Lesser effects included increased attention to paediatric protocols; increased facility to carry out paediatric trials; and the necessity to specify ethical requirements. It was also underlined that it is difficult to adapt information to parents and children in accordance with the new requirements.

Main issues to be dealt with by ethics committees

Looking at the opinions given on the major issues to be dealt with under the regulatory framework, about half of our sample identified the increased need for additional expertise to evaluate paediatric protocols and for measures to minimise pain, distress and fear of children. It was stressed that there is still a lack of knowledge regarding the risks and burdens that are acceptable for children in different age groups. Complexity in evaluating inclusion/exclusion criteria, risk/benefit balance and consent/assent procedures were also highlighted as main concerns.

Training and networking for ethics committees
Only 30% percent of the 73 respondents indicated that they had participated in initiatives in the field of paediatric research and those who did mainly took part in conferences and, to a lesser extent, training activities. Moreover, a significant number of ethics committees operating in Europe showed interest in initiatives related to paediatric research, preferring means such as training at national and local level and networking among ethics committees. Debates and conferences (at the national level) and educational initiatives supported by European institutions were also of interest. Three-quarters of those interested in networking belong to the EU-15, while the remainder are established in new Member States (Cyprus, Czech Republic, Estonia, Latvia, Malta, Poland).

Conclusions from the ethics committee survey

This survey demonstrated that there is a lack of knowledge of the European paediatric regulatory framework among ethics committees, and that their awareness of ethical issues related to paediatric research is limited, reflecting their low level of involvement in paediatric research, especially in terms of training, education and other similar activities.

Given that ethics committees are one of the most important actors in guaranteeing the safety, rights and well-being of children involved in clinical research, it is of primary importance to increase their competence and their involvement in paediatric research, and to promote the implementation of the European Ethical Recommendations at the local level. In this context, training and education in the field of ethics of paediatric clinical research should be an important objective.

Networking may be a fundamental tool to enhance collaboration and experiences and information exchange. It should be particularly important to promote these initiatives in the new Member States, where the number of CTs is increasing.

One possible relevant result of networking could be the development of a comprehensive guide practically addressing paediatric ethical issues in accordance with all the relevant international and European ethical and legal sources. This guide, chaired at the EMA level, should address all those specific ethical issues related to paediatrics: information/authorisation-assent process, paediatric expertise of ethics committees in charge of reviewing paediatric protocols (including training and education of the members of the ethics committees), use of placebo, compensation for damage, as well as other specific aspects to be considered in reviewing paediatric protocols.

6.5.2 Swedish Central Ethical Review Board interview

Background: the structure of Swedish ethics committees

In Sweden there is one Central Ethical Review Board, which was founded in 2004, and six regional boards, which are situated at the Universities of Gothenburg, Linköping, Lund, Umeå and Uppsala and at the Karolinska Institute in Stockholm.

These are independent authorities, divided into two or more sections that make decisions on behalf of the regional board. Each section is headed by a chairperson who is a judge or has been one. The sections have ten members with scientific qualifications and five members representing the general public. It is important that every application should be processed by members who have sufficient expert knowledge. The scientific members are therefore highly qualified. All members and their substitutes are appointed by the government. Each of the sections is expected to have 10 to12 meetings annually.

Within each section, a scientific secretary is appointed from among the scientific members. Together with the chairperson of the sections, the scientific secretaries are responsible for processing cases and dealing with them.

Interview responses

In 2009, RESPECT interviewed the scientific secretary of the Central Ethical Review Board.

The respondent reported that the regional boards reviewed a combined total of 1125 applications for CTs in the period 2005-2007, but these figures are not divided into paediatric applications versus other applications. The respondent confirmed that a paediatrician is a member of the committee and is always involved in paediatric application decisions, and also that the ethical review of paediatric research is preceded by a scientific review.

When asked which documents the Central Ethical Review Board refers to in its review of paediatric research, the respondent cited four statutes concerning the ethical vetting of research on humans but did not refer to the European Paediatric Regulation (EC) 1901/2006 or the European Ethical considerations for CTs on medicinal products conducted with the paediatric population (European Commission, 2008).

The respondent could confirm that the committees never consulted an external patient organisation on an application for paediatric research.

Conclusions from the Swedish interview

This interview confirmed the picture of a lack of knowledge among ethics committees of the European paediatric regulatory framework. It also reflects the closed structure of ethics committees and their reluctance to include parties who could contribute to their work.

6.6 The experience of sponsors

6.6.1 Pharmaceutical industry interviews

RESPECT conducted phone interviews with senior managers in the area of protocol feasibility and patient enrolment within both small and large multinational pharmaceutical companies.

Themes that emerged

Transparency
The current moves towards increased transparency throughout the biotechnology and pharmaceutical industries regarding drug-development information are increasingly being accepted but companies vary in how they interpret this.

The two larger companies that responded represented best practice by posting information about on-going and completed CTs on their website. They do not give patients the results about the CT while it is still in progress but, when the trial is completed, a detailed report of the results is published on their website.

Information to participants
Since the fear of something unknown is the most frequent reason the parents express when they refuse to enter their child in a CT, some sponsors attempt to expand parents' knowledge by providing in-depth information material about the products they are developing and what the CT will involve, for the investigator to give to the parents of participating – or prospectively recruited – paediatric patients. They want to ensure that physicians and patients have access to all relevant information.

One interviewee stressed that they strive to find the best-qualified and fully engaged investigators with a broad spectrum of knowledge and strong commitment. They consider these qualities in a physician to be extremely important in order to assure the patients' and their parents' best interests.

Willingness to participate
Several of the companies we contacted develop drugs targeting rare diseases. They acknowledged that, because of this, they do not usually have problems recruiting paediatric patients. In the case of rare diseases, there might be no existing medicines, or only 'good but not great' medicines that the parents assume could be substituted by new, more beneficial drugs provided through CTs. Furthermore, the interviewees indicated that many of these families, after the child has participated in a trial, report that they would do it again if asked; the inconvenience (such as time off school and work) is not a major problem to them, since they will gladly go to great lengths to help towards finding a cure for their child's disease.

In the event that these companies do not get enough recruits to continue the CT, they try to make the reluctant parents understand the beneficial input they would make by entering their child in the study.

Education

The improvement of public awareness about clinical research was stressed by one interviewee. This large, multinational company works with non-profit organisations and the media to broadcast a positive message about clinical research. They support events such as the *AWARE for All* Clinical Research Education Days, live webcasts run by the Center for Information and Study on Clinical Research Participation (CISCRP), USA. The aim is to educate the public and widen knowledge about CTs and the positive aim of clinical research.

Patient organisation involvement

POs (usually for orphan diseases) provide pharmaceutical companies with lists of their members' unmet needs for treatment. One respondent confirmed that the company's R&D department consults such lists.

One company reported actively consulting POs when designing CTs, for example to seek their opinions in the selection of which drugs to test, whereas other companies merely expressed an 'open attitude' to strengthening their relationship with POs. One respondent representing a larger company was sceptical about this possibility, as it would imply creating policies for guidance and an understanding of what the company's role should be. They have never received any suggestions or other involvement of POs.

A company providing regulatory advice on Paediatric Investigation Plan (PIP) submissions reported that there has never been a situation in which a PO requested access or input into a PIP; if that should happen, they would have to get approval from the pharmaceutical company.

At the other extreme, a respondent representing another large pharmaceutical company had an interesting case study illustrating the attitude of the company in general to relationships with patients groups:
A few years ago they acquired two smaller pharmaceutical companies with a lot of experience of oncology trials, which this company lacked. Thus, they decided to consult with all the different stakeholders, from top leaders in oncology, economists to patient groups for both common and rare cancers. They wanted to find out what are the current big issues in cancer research and standards of care. The patient groups gave feedback about their wishes, which was new and unexpected for the company:

1. a desire to get more information about what research is in the pipeline of pharmaceutical companies;
2. hopes for improvements in the experience of patients participating in CTs;
3. interest in involvement in protocol design

This company has now created a board to look at a way forward to address such issues and it includes a patient group representative. The board recognises there is a role for patient involvement but that it needs to be carefully designed. It requires that the people who are given this role be knowledgeable, and it requires there to be assurances to researchers that there will not be too much interference or multi-source input delaying the research process (which, the interviewee felt, is already painfully slow).

Regulatory issues

The Paediatric Regulation amendment (EC) 1902/2006 (European Parliament, 2006b) brings the obligation to conduct a paediatric CT unless a waiver is obtained. A paediatric investigation plan (PIP) has to be submitted to the Paediatric Committee once adult pharmacokinetic data are available.

The paediatric needs assessment lists compiled by the EMA-PEG group did not actually address unmet needs for treatment but rather a 'top-down' assessment of which existing drugs urgently need efficacy/safety studies for paediatric authorisation and labelling. The assessment procedure explicitly excluded the identification of priorities with these lists. One interviewee pointed out that the increased number of CTs required by the Paediatric Regulation also diverts resources from adult CTs, and some of these paediatric trials would otherwise qualify as low priority.

Inclusion of patient-reported outcome measures in the protocol

Many pharmaceutical companies include quality of life as an endpoint (outcome measure) in their CTs; indeed, this is necessary in many EU Member States in order to get reimbursement from their customers. For example, the UK National Health Service is more likely to buy a company's medicinal product if they can show that they have followed the NICE guidelines on health technology appraisal, which includes a criterion of documented improved health-related quality of life for patients using the test drug. This requires the development of patient-reported outcome measures.

Reducing the burden on paediatric participants

Although equipoise is the basis for all CTs, one interviewee commented that the sponsor would generally be relatively confident already that their test drug is likely to be an improvement on the standard care, based on the results of trials in adults, and the fact that in many cases there are no tested paediatric medicines already available for the condition in question (in which case, an increased burden is acceptable in relation to the burden of taking drugs not tested on children).

One interviewee mentioned the emerging use of adaptive design methodologies, in which patients can be switched to another arm in the course of the CT if they were assigned to an arm (e.g. a particular dose) that is proving ineffective. This involves the intervention of a data monitoring committee to unblind the study. The CT may include interim analysis, whereby early assessment may be made, although some health authorities and ethics committees are not in favour of this.

The interviewees were asked about pharmacokinetic/ pharmacodynamic (pk/pd) modelling and simulation and they indicated that their companies increasingly use these techniques. If this type of simulation is run, the number of patients entered in a pk/pd CT could often be reduced to around 50 children, relieving the burden on individual sick children and on the CT team recruiting participants to the trial.

Conclusions from the pharmaceutical industry interviews

It should be pointed out that pharmaceutical companies lacking a strong patient focus were less likely to agree to be interviewed and it was generally difficult to make contact even with companies who appeared to have admirable practices, judging from the materials they made available in the public domain, because of standard corporate policies about protecting company-confidential information.

Our interviews gave a snapshot of pharmaceutical companies with a commitment to facilitating patients' participation in paediatric CTs. They are aware of the importance of keeping families informed and reducing the burden for the child, but they still have to improve their contacts with patient organisations, for example in allowing them to contribute by reviewing the CT protocols.

6.7 Main conclusions from the reported experiences

Many of the parents we interviewed saw the trial as a way to get the latest and best medicine for their child (thus misunderstanding the principle of equipoise that is fundamental to CTs). Both children and parents were surprised to find that some of the procedures were painful, illustrating that this information had not been conveyed to them effectively.

Paediatricians reported that parents did not always understand the difference between CTs and regular treatment. They felt that many parents did not see the importance of medical research and did not always have an altruistic attitude. Longer-term participants were thought to no longer be able to identify differences between their normal treatment and the CT.

When faced with the decision to participate, families identified a need to trust the doctors and nurses as a motivation for participation.

However, other parents saw themselves as research partners in the trial and wanted to feel that their input was valued, although they did not always feel that their contribution was appreciated sufficiently. They wanted to receive the study results but several paediatricians confirmed that they do not inform parents about the results unless specifically asked.

Several patient organisations reported that they were ill equipped to give input on which trials and which outcomes have the highest priority for their members. This is something that could be improved through surveys of their members as a basis for contact with pharmaceutical companies.

We found good examples of CTs where patients felt empowered to make valuable contributions. We also found patient organisations giving input into trial design and protocols, helping to define outcome measures and to recruit trial participants, as well as pharmaceutical companies making their trial results accessible to all via their website.

It is important to ensure that families understand the need for research and are respected for their valuable contribution to the improved safety of medicines for children.

PART III

7 Empowering children in clinical trials

7.1 How can children be better mobilised and empowered?

The RESPECT project is based on the idea that, by increasing empowerment, it is possible to increase the level of participation of children in CTs. The objective of the RESPECT project is that all children participating in CT research should feel that they contribute to the research in a meaningful way and that they are a part of the research team and not just an object to be studied.

Attempts to motivate children to participate in CTs can be described in terms of social learning theory. The premise of the social learning theory states that new behaviours are learned either by modelling the behaviour of others or by direct experience. Social learning theory focuses on the important roles played by vicarious, symbolic, and self-regulatory processes in psychological functioning.

Therefore, attempts to increase participation have focused on the importance of good role models. Indeed, in the USA, websites exist where videos of children who have participated in CTs describe the positive aspects of participation, such as the NHLBI/NIH website. Children are more likely to respond to getting information presented in a child-friendly way. Thus, the idea of a *medical hero* as someone to look up to becomes one way to encourage recruitment. In order to participate there are certain, often unspoken, needs that the family expects to be met in order that they participate.

Participation in CTs as a subject of the research has historically been something that is the opposite of autonomy and empowerment. However, there is increasing evidence to suggest that empowerment in health care provides better results because the patient is in better control of their health care and follows the treatment regimen more carefully. If this can be transferred into the realm of CT participation, there would be enormous benefits to research. Of course, many aspects of the research will be determined by the need to follow a scientific protocol that may be determined long before any patient is contacted. However, the importance of CT participant empowerment in key areas cannot be underestimated. Most importantly, we need to address and respect patients in their capacity to understand, not in their weaknesses, especially children. All too often we focus on the weakness of patients. However, patients are repeatedly telling us that they want to be addressed in their strengths, their very real capacities and not to be treated as research objects. Patients are in a unique position as experts on themselves and therefore their full cooperation is vital. Unfortunately, even when efforts are made to include patient participation in health research, there is a risk of *tokenism*; in a recent observational study of a dialogue meeting between experts, adult patients and patient representatives to develop a joint research agenda, exclusion mechanisms were evident. For example, the experts used technical language and sometimes sidelined issues raised by patients or their representatives as not relevant (Elberse et al., 2010). The risks of tokenism are even greater when children are involved.

Figure 6 illustrates how children and their representatives could be involved in the CT process. Greater empowerment can help people to feel more in control of the situation and more able or willing to participate. It can also improve the retention of participants within the study, greater compliance with the protocol and, ultimately, benefit the scientific outcome.

Figure 6: Potential levels of involvement for children and their representatives

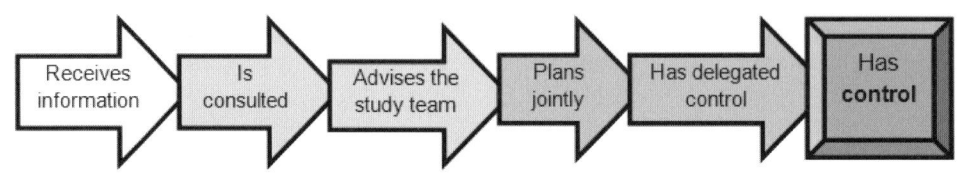

Receives information → Is consulted → Advises the study team → Plans jointly → Has delegated control → **Has control**

Some researchers attribute problems with recruitment and compliance in part to the way trials are organised and to a lack of respect for the patient. These factors must change if the number of CT participants is to increase and compliance to improve. In many CTs, key decisions about the protocol are made with no input from patients or patient groups.

The RESPECT project has shown that the experience of the CT is discussed with more confidence where the family has greater involvement and control over their participation. The more parents and children become members of the team, the better their experience is of their participation. Unfortunately, in the majority of trials carried out in Europe, the most information or involvement that the patient can expect to be provided with during the trial is information on how the recruitment is going and how many patients are in the trial.

Information and involvement in the CT is generally restricted to the information sheet and verbal explanation at the start of the trial. The patient is initially given information about why the trial will take place and how the trial will be carried out and asked to sign an informed consent form to show that this information is understood. However, the informed consent form does not give the patient any further responsibilities for the research. There is no reciprocal obligation on behalf of the researchers to provide information to the patient. If the children or their representatives are to become research partners then they must be given a greater role in the CT, either in the development of the procedures or provision of results. Examples of highly involved patient groups can be found; for example, HIV adults generally have a substantial involvement in the trial design itself.

RESPECT also found that not all families wanted this kind of involvement in the research and were happy with the absence of responsibility. In some cases it was found that both parents and children wanted the doctor to 'carry the burden' of the responsibility for them. It is therefore, important to be sensitive to how much the patient wants to be involved in the research. How then can we build patient empowerment and control into the CT process without burdening those families who do not want this responsibility?

First we have to understand what is meant by 'empowerment', the reasons children and families have for participation in CTs and potential modifying factors.

7.2 Definitions of empowerment

Empowerment is a complex concept that has been used in different disciplines, and the definition can vary depending on the context. Empowerment is a central element of the RESPECT project and here we distinguish two concepts: firstly, patient empowerment *at the individual level* and secondly, the empowerment of CT participants *on a collective basis*. These two concepts are defined differently.

Empowerment has been defined as '*a social process of recognising, promoting, and enhancing people's abilities to meet their own needs, solve their own problems, and mobilise necessary resources to take control of their own lives*' (Jones & Meleis, 1993). In this definition, patient empowerment is an individual process of asserting control over factors that affect the personal health of the individual. Empowerment requires that the individual should take control over personal health choices and choices among the options provided by their physician (Funnell et al, 1991).

An alternative definition of empowerment is '*a process, a mechanism by which people, organisations, and communities gain mastery over their affairs*' (Rappaport 1987). This second concept focuses on the community or group rather than on the individual.

The first concept is illustrated by the example of a patient who decides to participate in a CT in the belief that there will be a personal benefit from participation. In contrast, a person who joins a CT in order to make an active contribution to the benefit of the community of patients sharing the same medical condition exemplifies the second concept. This kind of participant does not expect to decide, for example, which arm of a randomised CT to join. The individual gives up certain freedoms in order to participate in the trial but is still empowered through this contribution to the community of patients. Individuals showing this kind of solidarity are also much less likely to drop out of the CT or deviate in their compliance to the protocol because of a lack of personal improvement in health.

In order to understand which aspects of these empowerment concepts are most applicable in the real world of paediatric CTs, the RESPECT project explored the reasons behind children's participation in CTs. These reasons, however, need to be placed in the real-life situation of affected families and therefore the factors that influence or modify those reasons were also explored.

7.3 The gap between the researcher and the family

The RESPECT project has identified the needs of the child and parent on one side and concerns of the CT professionals on the other We have identified a set of issues that were generated by the case study interviews with children participating in CTs and from the literature, and we looked at the modifying factors that influence their needs. Our model of the CT landscape is that these needs represent a gap between the child and parent on one side and the clinician and sponsor on the other (see Figure 7).

Figure 7: Synapse model of the CT landscape

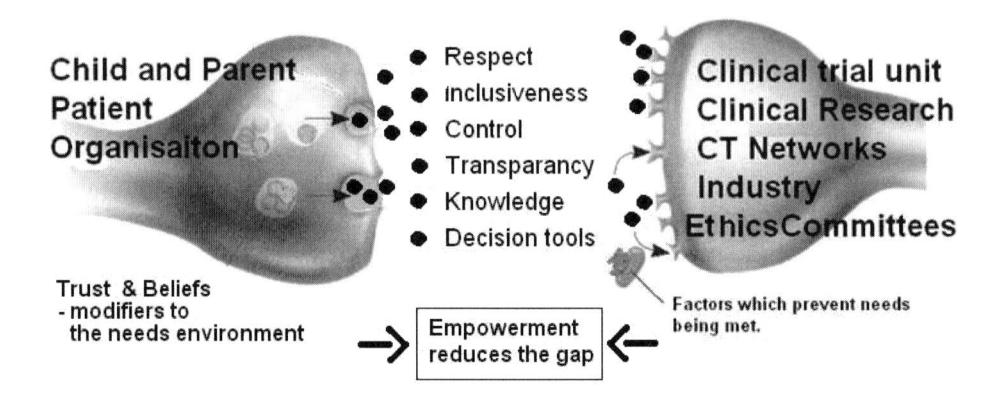

This gap between the researchers and the family can influence the decision about participation. It is proposed that the family's needs are modified by aspects of their relationship to the clinical research, for example, whether the child and the parents believe in the necessity of the research and whether they trust the doctor requesting their participation in a particular CT. If they are aware that medical research takes place, then they may have formed a positive or negative attitude to medical research in general that will influence their views on any specific trial. The parents may themselves feel that their child has medical needs that are not being met by the current medication and that new drugs are needed, which will influence their attitude to CTs.

Once asked if their child will participate in a CT, the parents' primary judgement is whether they trust that their child will benefit and be safe. In many cases, the information provided is too complex and therefore trust is focused on the doctor alone. If the parents trust neither the doctor nor the health system, they will not participate in a CT.

Through satisfying these needs it is possible to close this gap. Satisfaction of these needs is achieved by empowering the child and the family to take greater responsibility in the research and, in effect, to become a partner in the research, respected for their valuable contribution to the improved safety of medicines for children. This creates a climate of mutual respect, fostering collaboration on both sides in clinical research.

7.4 Reasons for participation

7.4.1 Children's perspectives

The RESPECT case studies illustrated that the children often reported not having had a choice in the decision to participate or not. However, many children also thought that it was fair that they should participate and contribute to the wellness of other children who had perhaps contributed in a similar way to their health care. A different emphasis is found in the literature, where children – particular those suffering from severe illnesses like cancer – often report motivations such as "To get help for my problem", "To find out what is bothering me" (Broome et al 2001, Varma et al. 2008, Wagner et al. 2006, Brody et al. 2005). Other, less frequently given, reasons for participation were: "To help other people with problems" (Varma et al. 2008, Dolan et al. 2008, Wagner et al. 2006), "My doctor told me to be in the study" (Varma et al. 2008, Wagner et al 2006), or "My parents told me to be in the study" (Wagner et al 2006). Unguru, Sill and Kamani (2010) showed that more children with cancer enrolled in trials to help other children with cancer (27 of 37 [73%]), than to get personal benefit from the trial (22 of 37 [60%]).

7.4.2 Parents' perspectives

From RESPECT interviews and case studies, we identified two main reasons for participation:

1) Families think that they will get something out of participation, such as better health care or a drug that is not otherwise available.

2) They feel obliged or bound to the doctor to the extent that they cannot refuse or they want (or explain it to themselves that they want) to pay back or make a contribution for all the help they have received from the medical profession.

In the literature, we find that parents of ill children give reasons for participating that include health-related benefits such as receiving treatment for the child and learning about the disease (Chantler et al. 2007, Tait et al. 2004, Wagner et al. 2006, Stuijvenberg et al. 1998, Hoehn et al 2005, Rothmier et al. 2003, Pletsch & Stevens 2001, Zupancic et al. 1997). Less frequently cited reasons were dissatisfaction with prior treatment and financial reimbursement (Wagner et al 2006). Other studies confirmed this, but stressed motives such as contribution to science and the benefit to other children (Chantler et al 2007, Hayman et al 2001, Sammons et al 2007, Wagner et al 2006, Hoehn et al 2005). As in the RESPECT case studies, it was found that parents also feel a sense of obligation associated with the fact that their children were benefiting from previous clinical research (Eiser et al 2005).

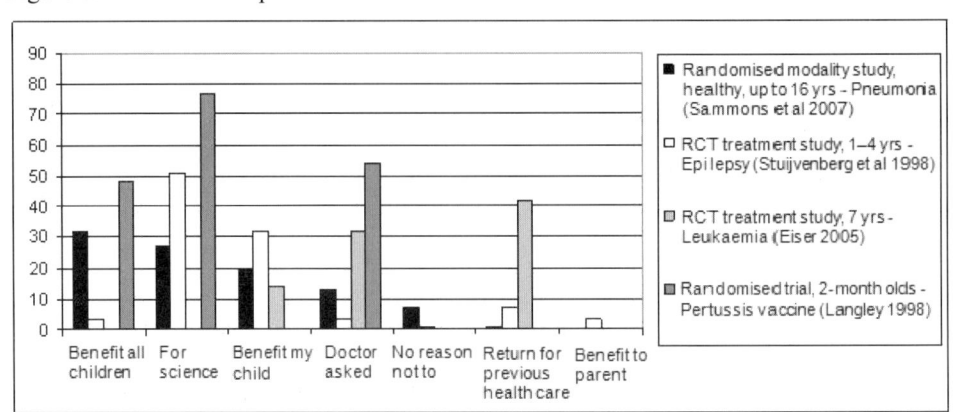

Figure 8: Influences on parents' decisions

Legend:
- Randomised modality study, healthy, up to 16 yrs - Pneumonia (Sammons et al 2007)
- RCT treatment study, 1–4 yrs - Epilepsy (Stuijvenberg et al 1998)
- RCT treatment study, 7 yrs - Leukaemia (Eiser 2005)
- Randomised trial, 2-month olds - Pertussis vaccine (Langley 1998)

Categories: Benefit all children; For science; Benefit my child; Doctor asked; No reason not to; Return for previous health care; Benefit to parent

Figure 8 illustrates the variation in the literature; some studies found that contribution to science was the most influential factor, while one reported that a sense of obligation for previous health care was highest and another found that benefiting all children was the highest cited motivator. Reasons depend on the type of condition and health status. Among other perceived benefits were: an offer of hope (Snowdon et al 2006, Caldwell et al 2003); the belief that the RCT guarantees receiving the most advanced treatment available for their child (Levi et al 2000, Caldwell et al 2003, Eiser et al 2005); the belief that participation in a RCT improves survival rates (Eiser et al 2005); the belief that participation in a RCT will result in a higher level of attention from medical staff (Levi et al 2000, Eiser et al 2005); as well as the possibility to meet others in the same position (Caldwell et al 2003).

The research carried out by the RESPECT project has found that there are many reasons for participation in a CT and the reasons depend upon the situation of the child, type of medical condition and the relationship with their health care provider and CT team. The guiding principle for any family entering a CT is to do the best for their child. Reasons for participation can be divided into medical, social obligation and psychological reasons.

There are also other reasons for participation that families may not always articulate as a need but from which they can benefit. If these are not an identified need prior to participation then they are often cited as an advantage to participation. The patient needs form a hierarchy, with the need for safety as the basic requirement, followed by the need to obtain direct health benefits. These are the basic requirements; if they are fulfilled, the patient will focus more on other higher-order needs. In our discussions with CT participants, the most frequent need expressed once the basic needs were satisfied was a need to complete the social contract, in other words to pay back for health care received. Once the family had started participation then further needs emerged, related to personal recognition and the feeling that they were contributing in their own right. This hierarchy follows Maslow's hierarchy of needs (Maslow, 1943), with the highest need being that of self-actualisation. In the context of CTs, this hierarchy is modified in Figure 9.

Figure 9: The CT participant's hierarchy of needs

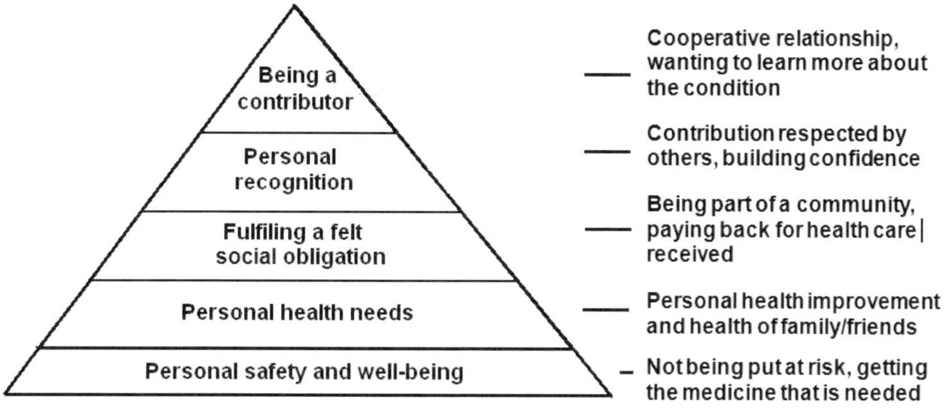

- Being a contributor — Cooperative relationship, wanting to learn more about the condition
- Personal recognition — Contribution respected by others, building confidence
- Fulfiling a felt social obligation — Being part of a community, paying back for health care received
- Personal health needs — Personal health improvement and health of family/friends
- Personal safety and well-being — Not being put at risk, getting the medicine that is needed

Below we look at some of the reasons for participation that have been identified through the RESPECT project.

7.4.3 Personal health needs

Monitoring and specialist care
The parents may feel the need for further health care for their child and believe that participation in a trial will gain them more attention from the doctor and medical staff. They expect the benefits to outweigh the risks.

Medical benefit to the child
In some cases, the feeling is that the CT is a better option than continuing with the current treatment. Families may feel that they have been presented with an opportunity to receive a medicine that would not otherwise be available to the child at all, as is the case with growth hormone treatment for idiopathic short stature; alternatively it is an opportunity to receive medicine that would not be available for some years within the health care system. In our case study interviews of Swedish children in a CT, some parents stated that they were happy for their child to participate, even if there was the possibility of being in the control arm, because this would give them a two-to-one chance of receiving the new drug that would not otherwise be available to them in the short term. Thus, families and children see their participation as leading to improved health or a cure for the child. Purely from the scientific principle of equipoise in CTs, this is a misunderstanding of the trial process. Nevertheless, better medication – or indeed a cure – is what some families think they will get and, the more severe the condition and the worse the current treatment, the more likely they are to participate.

7.4.4 Social obligation

There are several reasons why parents may feel a social obligation to participate in a CT. Firstly, and what is often mentioned, is that the family wishes to pay back the health care system for providing health care for the child previously. In the RESPECT case study interviews, a number of families were willing to participate in the research because their child had been ill previously and they had received so much help that they felt that they had been unable to thank their health care staff adequately for the personal attention their child had received.

Apart from this feeling of personal gratitude, families are often willing to enrol their child out of a feeling of obligation to improve the health care of other sick children. Families feel a duty to participate in the production of advances in healthcare, to which others have previously contributed and from which they have been the beneficiary without any contribution on their part. It is a way to balance the books. However, this is not done without requirements from the family's side. They are willing to contribute but not willing to participate in pointless research. Once the decision to participate has been made, there is a need to feel that one is part of a group contributing to trial, although the importance of feeling that you are a part of a group is no doubt different in different countries.

There are different layers of group membership to which the family sees itself belonging, as shown in Figure 10.

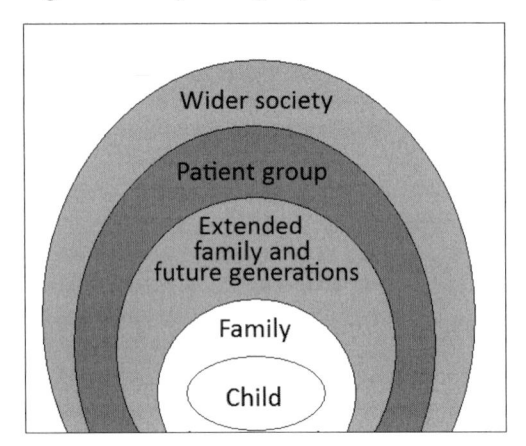

Figure 10: Layers of group membership.

The first obligation is to siblings and the immediate family. But, depending on the salience of the relationship with others, this membership can be extended to other members of the family such as cousins and their children and also to future generations. The parents can also feel that their child is a member of a wider community. The next layer is the patient group to which the child belongs. This may be more obvious where the illness is severe and the family is put into a position of meeting other families and children with the same condition. The sense of belonging to a patient group is an important element explaining why families with some conditions are more willing to participate in CTs than others.

7.4.5   Contribution to health care of others or extended family

The research must have a value for the patient group that they belong to or be seen as useful to future generations of that group or indeed useful to future family members, that is, their children's children.

The final layer is the wider society; here the sense of belonging to the wider society is different within communities and between communities. In some societies, a sense of belonging is encouraged and in others a sense of self-interest is seen as being more important. At the highest level of social obligation, where an emotional bond is less likely to exist, there are many different issues that influence participation. One of these is the level of knowledge about how science works and the necessity to create evidence-based medicine and how to achieve this.

A feeling of solidarity with others in our society is seen as a positive thing and something that parents wish to teach their children. Participation in a CT is an example of this solidarity. In one RESPECT case study, a parent said that the reason she enrolled her child in the CT was to teach the child the importance of making a contribution to society.

It would appear that people are more willing to participate in CTs for vaccines where the benefit is to the wider society; there is a more obvious benefit to the individual if the disease does not spread. The fewer people who have the disease, the less likely it is that a child will contract it from others. Viruses and the effects of a virus on a community, for example a school, are likely to have been experienced by all parents. Therefore, participating is seen as a good thing, almost like insurance. A good example of this is blood donation, in which the individual benefits from being a part of a much wider community.

7.4.6   Contributing to research: the need to know more about the condition

A major reason for participation was the need to know more about the condition. Through participation, the parents believed that they would learn more about the condition. According to learning theory, it is only through doing that people learn and many parents expressed the need to feel that they understood the condition better; consenting to their child's participation offered them the opportunity to learn more about the condition.

7.5   Factors that modify the reasons for participation

Regardless of what reasons are given for participation, there are still certain aspects of the trial and the situation that in the end determine if participation takes place.

7.5.1   Trust in the doctor

In order for participation in a CT to take place there is a need for the child and the parents to trust the physician. The parent and child need to know that the doctor knows best. Part of this includes the belief that health professionals would not use the child as a guinea pig, that the doctor would be honest with them about their child's condition and about the risks and benefits of participation. The family has to know that the doctor asking them to participate knows best and is trustworthy.

One unspoken need of participants is not to be put in unnecessary danger. According to the findings of Leach et al. (1999), just over half (53%) of the parents of children participating in a vaccine trial were aware that there could be side effects. Kass et al. (1996) reported that outpatients in their sample were so trusting of their hospital, physician and the research that they believed that no harm could be done to them. This high level of trust in doctors was illustrated in a study by Singhal et al (2002), in which almost a third of parents of newborn babies were willing to enroll their child in a study involving moderate risk and having no direct benefit.

7.5.2 Fear of missing out on what is best for the child

A number of studies indicate that the majority of parents entering their child into a trial believe that the new medication will be of benefit to their child. In one study, just under two thirds of parents (62%) believed that there would be an advantage to their child if they took part in the study (Sammons et 2007).

Parents are frequently unhappy with the randomisation process, fearing that their child will not be in the intervention group and that randomisation will delay the treatment start. This illustrates the common therapeutic misconception about CTs (see **2.3 *The therapeutic misconception***).

7.5.3 Ease of participation

The RESPECT project interviews showed that parents were less willing to participate where the costs to them were perceived to be too high. This does not only apply to financial costs due to extra travel for the family but also to child care, time from paid work and other missed activities. For example, there are missed opportunities for travel, holidays, participation in sports and leisure activities. How these costs are perceived will be different for each family. Also relevant were logistical reasons, such as being able to attend a nearby clinic or combining clinic visits for CT monitoring with regular appointments for the child's medical check-ups and treatment, so that participation will not cause much additional inconvenience (Caldwell et al 2003; Varma et al 2008, Dolan et al 2008; Stuijvenberg et al 1998; Brody et al 2005). The more the process of participation is incorporated into the normal routine of the clinic, the easier it is to follow the protocol and the less likely it is that participants will drop out.

7.5.4 Acceptable risk

The judgement of acceptable risk is based on the concept of minimal risk. Minimal risk regulates the participation of children and adolescents in medical research and is used by the participant or family as a moderator of the importance of the research and the importance of their participation. If the research involves minimal risk then the family is more likely to agree to the child's participation. However, the concept of minimal risk is open to many definitions and these will vary between individual families. Even what is meant by minimal risk in the medical community is unclear (Wendler et al 2005). A frequently used definition of minimal risk takes into account the other risks in the child's environment that may be considered minimal, such that the risk is not greater than the harm or discomfort encountered in daily life or during the performance of routine physical or psychological examination or tests (US Department of Health and Human Services, 2009).

However, this is open to interpretation as to whose daily life is being used as the criterion: is it the daily life of the potential participants or of children in general? How the parents judge minimal risk is pivotal to the participation decision. Added to this is how the parents weigh in risks of unknown side effects of the experimental treatment, which will be based on the information they received about the trial but also on what they know about medical research in general (Caldwell et al 2003, Morris et al 2004).

Depending on the condition, the level of risk of participation needs to be matched with the potential benefits. The milder the condition, the less risk will be acceptable. The more severe the condition, or in the absence of an effective treatment, the more risk will be taken in an effort to 'find a cure'. The participant with a mild condition would expect no more risk to participation than the alternative of continuing with standard treatments. Understanding of risk and how risk levels are represented are also important factors affecting the willingness to participate in a CT. The family needs to know whether this is a study incurring minimal risk or a higher level of risk to the child. Each CT should therefore clearly define and convey the risk levels. A clear and precise definition of minimal risk will also help children and their parents to understand what is being asked of their participation.

The determination of risk levels is, however, fraught with problems. Apart from the repeated observation that experts tend to disagree on what is minimal risk (Janofsky & Starfield, 1981; Shah et al., 2004), clinical research pays very little attention to evaluating the child's (or parent's) understanding of risk, which is likely to differ considerably from the researcher's understanding. What may be classified as equivalent to the risks of daily life (relative risk) by the researcher may be considered a greater risk from the child's perspective.

7.5.5   Previous participation

Parents who had already participated in studies were willing to take part in future studies (Sammons et al 2007). The availability of the research results also plays an important role here. Parents declare that because of receiving research results they have acquired additional knowledge about the health state of their child (Fernandez et al 2009). Moreover, information about research results makes parents feel more like a partner than a research subject in medical research (Fernandez et al 2007, Snowdon et al 1998).

7.5.6   Need to be actively involved

There is a psychological need for the parents and the child to understand what is happening to them and the consequences of the medical condition. Participation in a CT can promise to be a way to find out more information and be involved more in the child's healthcare, which can otherwise feel remote.

7.5.7 Meaningful contribution

The RESPECT case studies show that people want to feel that their participation will make a meaningful contribution to medical research.

8 Action points for integrating children's needs

While there are many definitions of empowerment, all of these include, to varying degrees, the following four elements:

- **S**elf-determination
- **A**ccountability
- **C**ooperative relationship.
- **K**nowledge

These elements are discussed separately below, together with suggested action points and illustrations. However, these elements are closely intertwined and act in synergy; therefore, the model must be viewed as a whole. For example, although access to information about CTs or protocols is a necessary precondition for making a decision, families may feel more confident leaving it in the hands of professionally trained people whom they trust to make the right decision on their behalf. The lack of established mechanisms to offer a cooperative relationship and accountable performance means that families may not welcome active involvement because it involves more personal effort and time than they are able to commit.

Figure 11: The RESPECT project's SACK model of empowerment

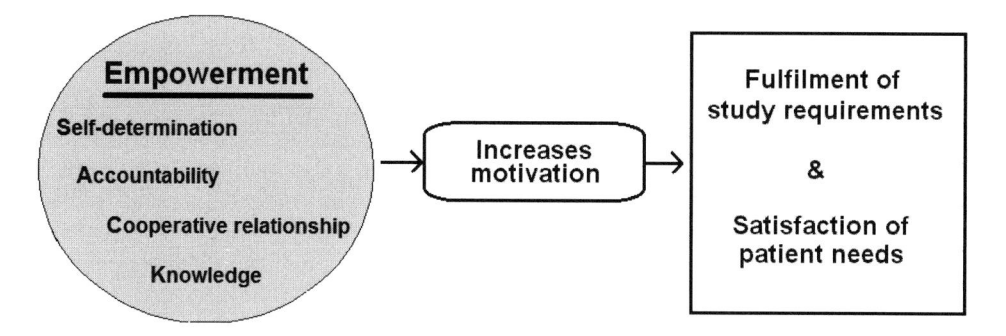

There is a balance between vulnerability and empowerment that is based on the motivations and needs of the participants. The empowerment model shown in Figure 11 illustrates the elements that tip that balance towards greater empowerment. The more the four elements described below are applied in practice, the more likely the participant will be empowered in the CT process.

8.1 Self-determination

An important principle is that it is not possible to empower another person without an active involvement from the person in question. In an empowerment process, power is not given, but is instead created by those in the weaker position. Self-determination is enabled through the possibility to participate and make one's own decisions, weigh risks versus benefits, negotiate and make choices. The parents and children themselves identify the benefits and barriers to participation. The involvement of children, parents and their representatives at the beginning and throughout the CT in planning and decision-making is important. An example of self-determination is the possibility of **self-referral to CTs**. There are barriers to self-referral, such as geographical catchment areas, access to medical journals and public awareness of ongoing trials, but the more these barriers are broken down, the more self-determination is possible.

Empowered individuals have access to the resources needed to strengthen their position in relation to those in a position of power. In the context of paediatric CTs, empowered children and parents should be able to influence all stages of the trial, have the status of co-researchers and receive all necessary information and support to assume responsibility for their desired contribution to medical research.

The right of all children to be heard and taken seriously constitutes one of the fundamental values of the Convention on the Rights of the Child, adopted by the UN General Assembly in 1989. Twenty years on, the UN Committee on the Rights of the Child presented a document outlining how to implement this right, based on the accumulated expertise and experience of governments, NGOs, community organisations, development agencies, and children themselves (United Nations Committee on the Rights of the Child, 2009). Important issues raised in the document can be applied to children's self-determination in CTs and are summarised below.

- Children's views have to be treated with respect and they should be provided with opportunities to initiate ideas and activities. This requires a preparedness to challenge assumptions about children's capacities,
- There should be information sharing and dialogue between children and adults based on mutual respect. This means avoiding tokenistic approaches, which limit children's expression of views, or which allow children to be heard, but fail to give their views due weight, or place children in situations where they are told what they can say.
- Adults working with children should acknowledge, respect and build on good examples of children's involvement and encourage the development of environments in which children can build and demonstrate capacities; they require capacity-building to strengthen their skills in, for example, awareness of their rights, organising meetings, dealing with the media, public speaking and advocacy. This requires a commitment to resources and training.
- Adults themselves need support, for example, with skills in listening, working jointly with children and engaging children effectively in accordance with their evolving capacities if they are to facilitate effectively children's involvement. Children can be involved as co-trainers and facilitators on how to promote effective collaboration with children.

8.1.1 Empowerment through being in control of the decisions

We want children to participate in CTs of their own free will and to be aware of the implications. Being empowered to decide is strongly related to how much information the family has. If the parents and children are confident that they have received enough information, then they will be empowered to make that decision independently and confident in their capability to decide. If they do not feel confident to make a decision based on the information they have, then they need firstly to demand that the information is provided in such a way that they can feel confident.

Secondly, the family needs to be in control of when the decision is made; they should not be pressurised into making a decision before they are ready. It is especially hard for children to feel confident that they have sufficient information to make the decision themselves and thus they defer to their parents. Many children report that they are minimally involved in the decision-making process and that they would welcome more involvement. However, tools to assist children's understanding would need to be made available in all CTs (Unguru, Sill & Kamani, 2010).

Our literature review (Wulf, Krasuska & Bullinger, 2012) showed that some parents want shared decision-making, whereas others prefer a paternalistic relationship in which the doctor decides on their behalf, so this has to be taken into account. It is not always useful to give a detailed medical background to the trial, although this should be available on request. It may be that a decision aid aimed at patient understanding would be more appropriate; this would help the children to decide whom to trust, but this still allows them to be treated more as equals in the decision process.

This decision situation is characterised by difficulty in identifying the best alternative and the scientific uncertainty surrounding benefits and risks; the parents need to make value judgements about potential benefits versus potential harm to their child. Because of equipoise, the test drug does not necessarily guarantee a positive benefit to the individual child, and parents must first understand the difference between research and treatment. Previous research has shown that children and parents do not understand what they have been told about the trial and many are confused about the difference between research and treatment (e.g. Unguru, Sill & Kamani, 2010).

Factors aggravating the difficulties families will face in making a decision about participation in a randomised CT are:
- lack of knowledge;
- unrealistic perceptions / expectations;
- unclear personal values;
- social pressure to choose an option;
- lack of support;
- lack of skills / self-confidence and
- lack of resources or access to resources.

Decision aids provide an opportunity to learn about CTs and form an opinion; they help the family to become aware of their attitudes, knowledge and emotions concerning participation and identify further information and support needs, as well as securing two-way communication with the clinical staff. The RESPECT project ran a pilot study to design a decision aid for children's participation in CTs. The preliminary version is described in **10.1 *Self-determination through decision aids*** and can be found in **Appendix 2**.

8.1.2 Empowerment through informed consent

Informed consent is of central ethical importance in CTs; it lies at the very basis of our understanding of what justifies experimenting on humans. The drive for informed consent is based on an implicit assumption that it will ensure that participation is based on an understanding of what will be involved. Children, being minors, do not usually provide consent but can only assent to the participation; it is the person with parental responsibility who is expected to understand the information. Unfortunately, as acknowledged at the 2012 annual conference of the European Forum for Good Clinical Practice, the current informed consent process does not always fulfil the purpose of ensuring that families are fully aware of what will be involved (Cressey, 2012). There is an increasing amount of material full of jargon to read and many parents may have little idea what they are actually signing up to. Cressey describes the process as "a box-ticking exercise focused more on offering legal protection to a trial's organiser than actually protecting patients". Signing the informed consent form should be a confirmation that the family *understands* the issues but more often it is merely an acknowledgement that the parent has been *informed* about what will be required of the child in the CT and *consents* to the child's participation.

Empowerment therefore comes through the processes and structures within the informed consent that are needed to ensure that everything is done to help the child to understand and that assent is justified. For empowerment to take place, we need to consider what practices hinder understanding, generate misunderstanding or confusion or tend towards deceit, be it intended or not. Empowering paediatric CT participants is closely linked to improving informed consent and assent practices. The challenge is to understand how children can express their will in a context of improved understanding. These practices begin with the protocol design, are part of the recruitment process, and run throughout CT participation to reporting of the research results. A return to an educational model may be needed. The educational process should aim to help children and parents develop a greater sense of control, becoming more competent in ensuring that they are given all the information they need to make their decision.

8.1.3 Empowerment through informed assent

In the RESPECT project, a major theme that emerged from the literature, the workshops and discussions was that the child must be respected as a person and should not be subjected to any pressure or improper influence to participate, as highlighted in the guideline document *Ethical considerations for clinical trials on medicinal products conducted with the paediatric population* (EC Directorate-General for Health and Consumers, 2008). Assent to participate should be built on information and knowledge as far as the child is capable. The concept of *informed assent* is therefore generated. The child, whilst being too young to give consent, can still be capable of understanding the aim of the research and the opportunities and the risks of the research, if these are explained in a child-friendly way.

Research has indicated that children between 7 and 18 years have a limited understanding of research (Unguru et al 2010) and that children younger than 9 years (O'Connor 2011) or 11 years (Tait et al. 2003; Ondrusek et al 1998) are not capable of understanding critical aspects of their participation, such as the freedom to withdraw from the CT. However, other research has demonstrated that even quite young children are capable of understanding the process of research they are being asked to participate in, as long as they are helped to understand with information materials aimed at their age group (Tait et al, 2007). It has also been shown that informed assent materials may be more likely to fulfil the aim of informing younger children if they are produced with the help of children themselves (Ford et al. 2007). Nevertheless, it should not be assumed that this is true in all cases; indeed, it may not always be desirable to confront children with making decisions they are not intellectually ready to make.

Structural changes
As a first stage in an empowerment process, the content, language and mode of communicating the information should be adapted to the child's capacity. This is already a requirement set out by all ethics committees when evaluating a new CT protocol but it is hard to measure whether comprehension has been achieved. The World Health Organisation Ethics Review Committee has produced templates for both parental informed consent forms and informed assent forms for children, containing advice on using non-technical language and example questions to elucidate understanding (available at http://www.who.int/rpc/research_ethics/informed_consent/en/). The assent form ends with a statement for the researcher to sign, confirming that he or she made every effort to ensure that the child understood what specific procedures would be carried out and gave the child an opportunity to ask questions about the study. This should be a standard requirement for all informed consent and assent forms, to make the researcher's responsibility more explicit. Unfortunately, the production of informed assent materials with the help of children themselves and in different formats (such as graphics) is not explored in these templates. A structural change to the assent process is required in order to ensure that guidance is available and that guidelines are adhered to.

8.1.4 Action points: mechanisms to generate self-determination

- ✓ Having access to information about ongoing and future trials and their inclusion criteria would allow patients to **identify the trials they wish to join**.

- ✓ As part of good clinical practice training, the **CT staff needs education about respect for participants** in order to facilitate the participants' empowerment. The role of children in the decision process has to be taken into account in order to involve them at a level that is appropriate for them.

- ✓ At the outset of a CT, the study team and the PO or patient representative should **define the type of psychological, informational and practical support children and parents need** in order to be in control and make informed decisions.

- ✓ Well-designed **decision aids**, targeting knowledge and feelings about medical research in general and the principles of randomised CTs in particular, should be developed to assist the family in making informed decisions

- ✓ The **informed consent should be treated as part of an education process** and not as an end in itself.

- ✓ It is important to open up **opportunities for children to acquire competencies and awareness** on critical issues related to CTs. Developmentally appropriate ways of presenting information should be developed that can be applied to all CTs.

- ✓ Tools to help the children explain their experience to their peers could be provided so that they have the **skills to control the information** that exists about them and their condition in their school or home environment.

8.2 Accountability and independent monitoring

Accountability refers to the ability to call members of the CT team to account, requiring that they be answerable for actions carried out during the trial. In this way, participants can be confident that the study is carried out in the way that was described to them, that they get the results that were promised and that good clinical practice is carried out. This is critical to the protection of the rights of the child. Accountability implies that there is an opportunity to advocate on behalf of the participant and this raises the possibility of the need for an independent ombudsman to be included within the CT process. The parent should be able to demand accountability through access to an advocate who is independent of the CT. Accountability can also be ensured through transparency of the CT process making it clear what decisions were made.

Independent monitoring or oversight of the CT process is needed in order to ensure that the participant has an opportunity to evaluate the experience of participating in a CT from the patient perspective. This can be undertaken by an independent body that provides for the possibility for advocacy on behalf of the participant. This is especially sensitive where children are concerned and it should be an important part of the CT process that the experience of the child participant is monitored.

The UN Committee on the Rights of the Child has made recommendations concerning accountability to children that can be applied to the paediatric CT context (United Nations Committee on the Rights of the Child, 2009). These are summarised below.

- A commitment to follow-up and evaluation is essential. For example, in any research or consultative process, children must be informed as to how their views have been interpreted and used and, where necessary, provided with the opportunity to challenge and influence the analysis of the findings.
- Children are entitled to receive clear feedback on how their participation has influenced any outcomes.
- Wherever appropriate, children should be given the opportunity to participate in follow-up processes or activities.
- Monitoring and evaluation of children's participation needs to be undertaken, where possible, with children themselves.

Monitoring gives the possibility to influence future studies (feeding back the families' acquired knowledge from participation), which can also be seen as a part of the empowerment process, namely, influence on future activities.

8.2.1 Empowerment through greater transparency

An important aspect of empowering patients in CTs is the increased transparency around clinical research, in particular the aspects outlined below.

The development of transparency within European regulatory authorities

A key element of the empowerment of patients in CTs is that the results of studies are made accessible. Transparency in clinical research has become a major focus, including in paediatric CTs.

In 2004, the European Commission and the European Medical Agency launched the EudraCT Clinical Trials Database established in article 11 of the Clinical Trial Directive 2001/20/EC. The database is used by national medicine regulatory authorities to enter CT data in advance of the study (methodology and hypotheses, inclusion criteria and outcome measures), updated information on recruitment during the trial and the outcomes when the study is completed. This was the first time paediatric CTs could be tracked at the European level. The EudraCT database contains information on approximately 30,000 CTs but is not openly accessible, even for patients who have themselves participated in one of the registered trials.

As a result of mounting public pressure regarding transparency in CTs and changes to the EU pharmaceutical legislation, the Clinical Trials Register (https://www.clinicaltrialsregister.eu/) was launched in March 2011 to provide the public with access to some of the information held in the EudraCT database.

Information that is not currently accessible but would be of special interest to patients and trial participants includes:
- the **results** of CTs;
- the **opinion document** from the relevant ethics committee;
- the **process for joining** any CT published on the website

The CT participant is not benefited by the non-publishing of results. If parents entered their child in the CT in order to increase their knowledge about a drug, then it would be appropriate if the study findings that resulted from their participation were made available to them if they wished.

The European pharmaceutical industry perspective on transparency

In 2011, the European Medicines Agency carried out a consultation on increased transparency and access to information included in companies' applications for marketing authorisation and concluded that a more efficient process would be achieved by redesigning the marketing authorisation dossier structure so that commercially confidential information and personal data could be removed more easily. The pharmaceutical industry has expressed support for this initiative whilst at the same time wanting to protect innovators from losing their advantage in the market. The difficulty for the industry is the timing of the disclosure of clinical test results, as they would prefer the information to be released after market authorisation has been granted. However, in relation to paediatric trials, the EMA has suggested that an overview of the PIP results should be published. The industry has indicated that this would reveal a company's development strategy and should therefore be considered confidential.

Where data is made available, there is a need to monitor how this data is accessed and interpreted. It would be a significant challenge to find practical ways to make the vast amount of data in a marketing authorisation dossier useful to the individual family, but the industry has put forward the idea of developing tools in collaboration with regulators and POs to make sure that data on CTs is provided in a way that is meaningful to patients and their families; this would be a significant contribution to the empowerment of paediatric patients

Transparency, responsibility and representation in ethical review practices
Before the 1950s, ethics committees did not exist in Europe or in other places. In the 1950s in some countries, physicians began to approach their colleagues informally for advice on ethical issues. This understanding of ethical review, as a discussion between a physician and a group of advisors remains a core role of ethics committees today and that is reflected in their closed culture, in which communication goes through the researcher in most instances. There is no direct contact with sponsors or participants in CTs and only limited transparency in some Member States.

Currently, the ethics committee is responsible for the protection of the participants in relation to the trial protocol. Once the committee has evaluated and approved the trial design, it issues an ethics committee approval. At this point, the committee's responsibility largely ends. It would be empowering for participants and their families to have the possibility to provide feedback on their experience to the trial sponsor and to the ethics committee. Although feedback is sometimes – formally or informally – provided to the research team, it is never solicited by the ethics committees and a mechanism for such feedback from CT participants could be an important area for development, empowering participants to take greater control over the process as a means to improve future decisions that affect them. Increased accountability and independent monitoring will put pressure on ethics committees to develop strategies for soliciting and dealing with participant feedback.

Greater transparency is likely to lead to greater demands for representation on ethics committees, putting pressure on committees to look at new ways of including representation or expanding the existing representation of patients. In a survey of ethics committee practices in ten European countries (Hernandez et al., 2009), only two, France and Germany, were required by law to have patient organisations represented on their committees. Three others had PO representation voluntarily and the remaining five did not include POs on their ethics committees, relying instead on non-professional members of the committee or professional members with experience from a PO.

A more radical idea is that a potential participant in the proposed trial should be included in the decision-making process, as this would be a closer representation of the patient group affected by the CT. A question to be answered is how greater transparency applies to vulnerable groups and, in the case of paediatric trials, how children can be included within an expanding transparency. Ethics committees will have to take a position on to what extent greater transparency will lead to changes in the structure of the committees and how transparency will be achieved. They will have to consider at which stage their decisions should be made transparent, to whom the information is transmitted and in what format.

Other considerations

An increased trend towards greater transparency will have an effect on the recruitment of patients. Transparency may lead to either an increase or decrease in participation, depending on how it is perceived by the potential participants. In either case, the ethics committee must take into consideration that the information they make available, and the way this information is presented, could affect recruitment to the trial. This implies greater professionalism and new ways of working for ethics committees.

Another consideration suggested by the RESPECT project is that there should be greater active involvement of patient groups in the CT process in general, including commenting on the protocol and participating in the production of the informed consent materials. Ethics committees will therefore need to develop strategies for responding to CT protocols that have been in part generated by the patients themselves.

It is important that the CT contribute to improving the child's wellbeing and functioning. The inclusion of outcomes that matter to the child are an important motivating factor for the family's decision to participate, and make it more likely that families will adhere to the protocol and attend all appointments. Therefore, in terms of patient empowerment, there should be a commitment by CT sponsors and investigators to develop patient-reported outcome (PRO) questionnaires for children who may be asked to participate in the CT.

8.2.2   Empowerment through patient-reported outcomes (PROs)

Patient-reported outcomes (PROs) are an important issue to be considered in the decision about whether or not to participate in CTs for children as well as their families. From the family's perspective, it is important that the CT contributes to receiving relevant support; in other words, the treatment should relate to the main issues associated with the health condition. If the outcomes of a CT are defined so that the patients see how these are related to their own wellbeing and functioning, the decision about participation might be easier. Therefore, in terms of patient empowerment, the inclusion of outcomes that matter are an important motivating factor for decision-making regarding participation.

The repeated assessment of quality of life, both of an individual patient in clinical care as well as a group of patients in a clinical study, helps identify the core areas of wellbeing and functioning over time. Health-related quality of life can also be used as an indicator with which the effect of treatments can be combined with health economic indices so that the patients' perceived benefit can be included in the overall benefit analysis.

Newer approaches to health-related quality of life assessment have combined patient expectations with quality of life. For example, if a child's problem relates to the experience of pain, the treatment expectation would be that treatment reduces the pain; therefore, the specific benefit of the treatment regarding the child's needs can be assessed.

Assessing patient-reported outcome can help to identify patient needs especially if included at the beginning of clinical studies or patient care process. It outlines where the patient stands in terms of wellbeing and functioning as compared to reference group data.

Definition of patient-reported outcomes
Patient-reported outcomes can be described as any report about feeling and functioning in relation to health and treatment as obtained from patients (Patrick, et al., 2007). The development and use of patient-reported outcomes has been accompanied by the FDA-Guidance, which was introduced in 2006, updated 2009 and is currently under further review (Erickson, Willke & Burke, 2009). While the PRO Guideline is related to assessing patient-reported outcomes such as health-related quality of life in adults, only a brief section refers to children. A new guidance for the validation of PRO tools for use in paediatric populations is to be published soon.

The term *patient-reported outcomes* has recently been defined to cover all aspects of self-reported wellbeing, functioning and evaluation of care. Thus, it also relates to patient satisfaction, the reporting of symptoms and side effects, the administration of treatment, as well as patient preferences and health-related quality of life. The concept of health-related quality of life is the one that has been most intensively researched as a PRO, both as regards adults and, increasingly, children and their families.

Challenges
Some of the major differences in assessing quality of life in children are related to the comprehension of language and cognitive development, which means that special consideration has be given to age-related items and the period of recall. The FDA has recommended age group ranges to observe differences in developmental states and to understand from which age younger children can respond in view of established criteria for validity.

Another question related to PROs for children is the role of the parental reports, previously called proxy reports. Parental reports have been recommended where children are too young to understand the questions or cannot respond themselves. Although parental reports are necessary they cannot be truly accurate to reflect the child's own view and therefore parental reports are seen as a supplementary source of information valuable for children of any age.

One aspect regarding the development of quality-of-life items for children relates to the more sensitive role of the environment in which the assessment takes place and the fact that aspects relevant to health-related quality of life may change in importance in relation to the context. For a child PRO instrument, the valid formation of the child's subjective quality-of-life concept and the generation of items are of great importance. One way to obtain their unique view is to conduct focus groups in which children are asked to respond in a group discussion to questions about health problems and activities associated with their condition. The focus groups have to be conducted in accordance with the age and other characteristics of the children.

A further issue to consider in developing a child PRO instrument is the use of developmental and age-based cut-offs, measuring when children are able to respond. It has been suggested that, very young children – pre-schoolers younger than five year of age – find it difficult to respond to questions about their quality of life. However, children ranging in age from five to seven are more able to respond if the questions are formulated and presented in an understandable way. Older children from eight to eleven have consistently been reported to be able to respond in a reliable and comprehensive manner to the questions and, from age twelve, most children are able to reflect upon their personal experience and comprehend questions regarding their health-related quality of life in an abstract way.

Finally, ethics in paediatric research is important in an international quality-of-life study. Participating countries and centres need to apply for and receive approval from the relevant ethics committee. Only after this can the study be started and patients recruited for focus groups, pilot and field-testing.

Guidelines for developing instruments
In recent quality-of-life research, the above-mentioned FDA procedures have been followed, including the use of focus groups for identification of relevant items and the underlying concept of health-related quality of life. This is followed by pilot testing of a preliminary item list with cognitive debriefing in order to understand how patients respond to the individual items and which items need to be changed. The next step is a field test, in which the questionnaire is given to patients in order to perform psychometric analysis of reliability, validity and also – if included in a longer-term study or in a CT – sensitivity.

For the validation of a PRO instrument for children, the main aspect is the content validity of such a paediatric tool, in other words, to what extent the instrument reflects important and relevant aspects of the concept that it intends to measure. Recent research shows that establishing content validity in young children is more difficult than in adolescents, who are able to include their experience in the development of a patient-reported outcome (Clarke & Eiser, 2004)..

Many of the currently available health-related quality of life instruments have been designed following these recommendations. However, in children, self-reported instruments accompanied by a parent-reported version are still rare. In children and adults, instrument assessment of quality of life can be differentiated into generic and condition-specific instruments. Generic instruments assess health-related quality of life independent of the health condition, while the condition-specific instrument focuses on the challenges of specific health states.

Creating, using and interpreting health-related quality of life measures
For a health-related quality of life instrument to address the patients' experiences, it is important that instrument development undergoes several steps that reflect patients' concerns and that the psychometric measurement properties are tested.

After developing a draft of the instrument – for example after having obtained relevant topics from patient or focus groups – it is important to make sure that children understand the content of the questions and can use the response scales appropriately. This step has been called *cognitive debriefing* and this can be conducted via individual interviews, or groups, going through the items of the pilot questionnaire, reporting their reaction to items and providing an opportunity for the children to suggest modifications. This step is especially important in children because it clarifies whether items are formulated appropriately, how the questions are understood, and whether they are formulated in a methodological and practical way.

After having formulated items and response scales and having tested them in cognitive debriefing, the next step is to assess the psychometric properties, especially reliability and validity in a larger patient sample.

Available instruments
Recent reviews of health-related quality of life assessment in children show that there is a large, slowly increasing number of validated instruments and cross-culturally applicable generic instruments available with which both the child's self-reported quality of life, as well as the parental report, can be assessed; however, with regard to condition-specific instruments, more development is needed.

Health-related quality of life instruments are increasingly used in paediatric CTs within the fields of oncology and allergy. However, a general reluctance to include such measurements in CTs has been voiced, especially self-report for children but also for parents. One reason is that, in order to ask children about their wellbeing and functioning, several ethical and informed consent procedures have to be observed. In addition, children may be overburdened by having to respond to questionnaires. Therefore, brief instruments have been developed that are easy to understand and easy to use. In addition, the parent's view of the child's quality of life has to be included, while bearing in mind that parental perception of the child's quality of life is not equal to the child's own view. In order to make CTs more relevant for children and parents, the use of health-related quality of life assessment, as well as measuring other PROs such as patient preferences and patient satisfaction, is highly recommended. In addition, if patients realise that the CT is about outcomes that matter to them, the subjective benefit of participation may stand out more clearly against potential barriers to participation. Therefore, in using generic measures for health-related quality of life or other PROs, it is highly recommended to identify the issues that are important to patients and parents in a given CT and to incorporate these areas into the psychosocial assessment.

8.2.3   Action points - methods to generate accountability

- ✓ Assign **responsibility for accountability** to the CT team, preferably to an individual member of the CT staff. The ethics committees could also require that this be done.

- ✓ Establish a policy that the CT staff will **meet individually with participants and parents to clarify their wishes** and agree on what is needed in order for them to achieve this. This agreement should be recorded in the documentation of the study.

- ✓ Establish **patient-reported outcomes and feedback from families on their experience** as integral to the CT, to be monitored during and after the trial. While PRO questionnaires may be the easiest method of providing feedback, other means may be more appropriate for children such as interview schedules. POs representing children can help to create avenues for the children and parents to give feedback on their experience of the CT.

- ✓ Each CT should schedule **regular follow-up sessions** to monitor the participants' experience.

8.3 Cooperative relationship

Engagement, acknowledgement, mutual respect, and active listening are essential components of a cooperative relationship. Although the clinicians may bring professional knowledge, the child and the family have unique perceptions and personal experience. This approach demands that the researchers and families collaborate as partners. In order for this to be achieved, mechanisms for mutual exchange need to be encouraged, in which valued input can be obtained and access given to the results. These mechanisms will only work if there is true representation of all stakeholders and transparency of their roles and the CT procedures. <u>Empowered individuals determine the extent of their cooperation with the CT staff.</u>

8.3.1 *Empowerment through setting the agenda: patient-identified needs (PINs)*

The standard source of information leading to a decision to proceed with the development cycle of a drug is the assessment of whether the proposed product has the potential to improve current treatment, which determines its potential viability on the market. However, a complementary approach is to gather, at an earlier stage, medical needs that have been identified by patients in relation to their health condition. This is the concept of patient-identified needs (PINs). <u>Empowered individuals select their own agenda.</u>

Patients, or their parents, often speak to their physician about problems with existing medication (such as undesirable side effects) or their need for a solution to a related issue. Thus, PIN information is already available to some extent. The physician can convey these comments to the pharmaceutical company representative who, in turn, can pass them on to a senior manager responsible for decisions about the feasibility of developing (or further developing) a drug to solve that problem.

If the channels of communication are developed, a PO can provide information about PINs directly to the pharmaceutical industry or contract research organisation. This can be a valuable source of information for the industry and a way in which the POs can provide the voice of the patient. This information should be made available for POs to monitor the uptake of requests from their members when reviewing CT protocols.

The PINs should also feed in to the PRO instrument development. Outcomes should be based on the needs of the patients, as identified before or at the start of the CT. (See **8.2.2 *Empowerment through patient-reported outcomes*.**)

In order for the PO or informal patient groups to create opportunities for dialogue, they will have to develop a set of advocacy skills that will be needed to influence the CT trial staff, pharmaceutical industry and health care policy. This would also give the PO an opportunity to be aware of future CTs and products that would be of benefit to their members and would help them to explain the importance of the product to their members and provide them with an opportunity to actively contribute to the recruitment.

8.3.2 Action points - methods to generate a cooperative relationship

- ✓ **Guidelines** would be necessary for researchers on patient involvement, patient rights & responsibilities.

- ✓ Training packages could be provided to researchers on **how to communicate** CT principles to children and parents.

- ✓ At the outset of a CT, the study team and the PO or patient representative should identify what the special contribution of children, parents and their representatives should be and how and where they can be involved most effectively. This should lead to the development of a **strategy for collaboration** between the researchers, the children, the parents and their representatives

- ✓ An actively involved, empowered PO can work with the pharmaceutical industry or CRO to **select the drug or treatment options that their members want to be trialled**.

- ✓ There should be a Europe-wide centralised database of PINs in order to monitor the uptake of patients' self-reported needs in CTs.

- ✓ The **PO can act as a mediator between researcher and the family** in the CT. Providing information about the trial to the parents and their child in a language that they understand and the PO can provide information from the participant perspective in a language that the researcher understands, for example through PROs.

- ✓ The families or POs could **provide input into the informed consent forms**. This would improve the information by making it closer to how the child thinks about the CT, thus enabling empowerment.

- ✓ Assessing the CT outcomes from the perspective of the participant is very important to the empowerment model. The CT researchers together with the PO could develop a strategy for monitoring and evaluating the trial from the perspective of children and parents, encouraging their involvement and empowerment within the trial. PRO or quality-of-life measures for children and parents could be provided so that they have the opportunity to **provide feedback whilst in the trial**. This may require an interview schedule for the study nurse so that feedback from the child becomes part of the reporting procedure of the trial.

- ✓ A further step towards empowerment would be for the family or the PO to have the opportunity to **modify or add to the CT protocol**. This would help it to understand what its members are being asked to participate in and provide an opportunity to actively contribute to the recruitment. For example the PO might suggest that PROs are included and the parents might propose changes to the scheduled visits so that they accommodate their child's needs.

- ✓ A **toolkit with key advocacy tools** for the representation of participants in CTs could be developed and made available to those POs who wish to develop their advocacy work. This toolkit would provide examples of how advocacy tools have been used and how they work in practice. POs without experience in paediatric CT research may require information concerning:
  - how to influence national policy on CTs in their country;
  - how to analyse legislation or policies that affect children in CTs;
  - how to work within the CT landscape and bring about change;
  - how to lobby for their members' needs (PINs) in the CT context;
  - how to produce documents that target specific areas of the CT landscape;
  - how to provide training and guidelines for children's participation in CTs;
  - how to demonstrate good practice.

8.4 Knowledge and understanding

It is assumed that, if the parent or the child has been informed and signs a consent form, this person has understood what was presented to them. However, individuals' perception of their own knowledge – especially in relation to such a complicated activity as a CT – needs to be established with more than a signature. For the parent and child to be fully knowledgeable, it is necessary to go beyond informed consent. Information thus has to be personalised and adapted to the individual's own needs. This relates to the informed consent process but also to the transparency of GCP requirements. <u>Empowered individuals select their own learning needs</u>.

The CT team needs to provide information and support for the involvement and empowerment of children, parents and their representatives and this is achieved through clear communication about the trial itself. This may include the provision of decision aids for the participants to assist in decision process; it may include providing a CT education package to the participants, either at the time of the trial or prior to the trial.

In a CT, the outcome is unknown by the very nature of the research. For the patient or PO, the way to increase the sense of control for the family and the child is to have an influence on the procedures of the CT. This would mean having access to decisions being made about what trials are carried out and what is included in the protocol and the outcomes to be measured. Even where there are large POs representing the patient group, they may still be disconnected from the clinic or research institution, and lack access to specific and critical information. It will be the clinic that has this knowledge and it is the clinic's responsibility to create access opportunities for the potential participants and their representatives.

A standardised risk assessment needs to be undertaken with every CT and a format for communicating this to the patients needs to be developed. This should be included in the content of the CT application dossier and for safety reporting. A simple categorisation of risk should be developed to help the participant understand the risks they are being asked to take. These risks include: physical risk from study treatments; the loss of individualised care; risk from non-therapeutic components of the research protocol; and the psychological impact of participation, particularly if the research may take place without informed consent in an emergency setting. The risks of research participation should be considered in comparison with the risk of non-participation; for example, the risks specific to research participation should be considered separately from the risks inherent in treatment of the potential research participant's underlying condition. Standardised rules would simplify the procedure and be easier for patients to understand. Risk judgement compared to normal clinical practice will be hard to standardise, given the probable differences in normal clinical practice carried out within Europe. This would need to be carefully assessed and studied.

8.4.1 Empowerment through access to information

Access to resources
Empowerment comes through patients access to resources (information, decision aids, etc.) to identify and solve problems related to their participation. This encompasses actions directed at strengthening the basic life skills and capacities of individuals.

While information leading to knowledge contributes to empowerment, the limitation of patients' knowledge is also a limitation on their decision-making capacity. In the case of CTs, there is very seldom a case where the patient is as well informed about the medical aspects of their condition as the doctor proposing participation in the CT; he or she is unlikely to be in a position to know as much and be able to judge the CT to the same extent as the doctor.

An effort to educate the parents about their child's condition and the process of the trial will not be welcomed by all, and indeed rejected by those who would rather not know or be put into a position of not understanding. They come to the doctor for advice because the doctor is the expert; they do not want to make the decision themselves and have the responsibility of possibly making the wrong decision.

Due to the nature of the trial, it may be undesirable for the patient to be fully informed. A randomised double-blind CT requires that the patient and even the doctor do not know which participant group has the active substance and which has the placebo. Participation requires that the patient accept this limited knowledge inherent in the design of such scientific experiments.

Education: beyond informed consent
The needs and motivations of paediatric patients and their parents identified in the RESPECT project were used as a foundation for pilot educational material to empower families in the future.

Focus groups with professionals and an extensive literature search were carried out to identify background material. Interviews with participants in CTs were carried out to explore motivations. Based on this evaluation, an education package was developed and piloted with staff and teenagers who also completed a questionnaire on their attitudes to CTs before and after the presentation of the educational material. The educational material was presented to secondary school pupils in two groups.

Questions parents considered before participation concerned: the informed consent process; the details of the CT process; the benefits their child would have from participation; and what was meant by certain technical terms such as 'standard treatment' and 'randomisation'. The main reasons for agreeing to participation were: receiving better treatment, additional medical oversight and access to medical staff. Safety risks were assumed to be minor. The teenagers in the educational session had no previous knowledge of CTs and their attitude was mostly neutral when given the first questionnaire. They were highly engaged by the material and discussed openly the ethical dilemma surrounding the consenting process. Several of the teenagers expressed a dislike of copious texts and felt that an education session would reduce this stress factor. In the follow-up questionnaire, the teenagers expressed increased positive attitudes towards paediatric research.

The educational material would make it easier to decide about potential participation in a CT. This pilot study indicates that the education material is an empowering tool that might decrease the frequency of withdrawal, increase compliance and develop a positive attitude toward future trial participation. The empowered individual has access to information resources.

Access to study results
A recurring theme in the RESPECT surveys was the request from participants to be given the results of the study in which they had participated. It is also shown in other research that patients want the results of CTs (Fernandez, et al 2009). However, participants rarely receive the research results (Partridge, et al 2004). Feedback of results should be conducted with care, especially where the participant has had less effective treatment or there has been a poor outcome (Partridge et al 2009). It is essential that the wants and needs of the participants are respected (Fernandez, Skedgel & Weijer 2004). Nevertheless, it is clear that in every phase III trial there should be a plan concerning how to share the results with the participants. The participants themselves should require this. Sharing results may facilitate communication between clinicians and participants, thus increasing patient satisfaction and ultimately greater public understanding of clinical research (Partridge & Winer 2009). The empowered individual has access to the study results.

8.4.2 Empowerment through understanding the risks.

The concept of risk that is generally provided in information about CTs is based on the principle of relative risk. In other words, the risk of participation is equivalent to the risk of some aspect of daily living for the participant. These comparisons are used to improve understanding but they are also used to determine whether the study involves minimal risk to the child or greater than minimal risk when evaluated as ethically acceptable by the CT approval process. However, it has been by argued by Westra, Wit, Sukhai and de Beaufort (2011) that a definition of minimal risk based on relative risk is flawed for the following reasons: 1) it is unclear if the comparative risk refers to the risk experienced by the average child or the risk experienced by the specific child being enrolled in the study; 2) comparison to daily *risks* experienced does not take into consideration the *benefits* of the activity undertaken, thus daily acceptable risks may be quite high but are compensated by other factors such as improved mobility, quality of life or 'learning experiences' as might be the case when riding a bike or riding a horse; 3) the impossibility of comparing research risk with risk in daily life, where discomfort and potential harm due to research participation are not related to personal needs.

In order to avoid these problems Westra and colleagues propose an alternative definition by evaluating individual *procedures within the CT* instead of treating the CT as a single activity

(Westra & de Beaufort, 2011) and distinguishing between the risks of *discomfort*, which concerns subjective and momentary experiences, and the risks of *harm*. They have furthermore incorporated different scales of risk likelihood into the definitions of discomfort and harm (Westra, Wit, Sukhai & de Beaufort, 2011). For the child and the family, this alternative definition can be used to increase empowerment by enhancing their ability to assess their level of acceptable risk. They can more easily distinguish between the different procedures; and see the difference between risks of discomfort and risks of harm. Added to this is the idea that acceptable risk may be higher if there are potential compensations to these risks, as is found in daily life.

8.4.3 Action points - methods to generate knowledge

- ✓ An **education programme** explaining what a CT is to potential participants and to participants in a CT should be developed. Go 'beyond informed consent' and emphasise the importance of knowledge in the CT process.

- ✓ In order to make the information for the children more salient to the child, the use of **child-to-child presentations** could be used. Children who have already participated in a CT could explain their experience of other children who are being asked to participate in a CT. The PENTA youth groups are one example of how this might work.

- ✓ In many cases it is the parent who has to take the responsibility of explaining and reminding the child why participation is important. There will always be some variation in the way that parents approach this task and therefore some **training for the parent in communicating the CT procedures**, which can be difficult concepts for the child, would be a step towards empowerment.

- ✓ Where information about trials is directed towards the patients, there should be **quality criteria that will distinguish information** about a trial from advertising. A Europe-wide code of practice may be required.

- ✓ **Decision tools** should have an interactive presentation at the level of the child's understanding. It will be necessary for example to define the meaning of randomisation and explain why it is important.

- ✓ Throughout the period of the CT, the child and the parents should be **aware that they are participating in an experiment and know what rights they have as a research participant**. Where CTs continue for an extended period, the difference between health care and CT participant can become blurred.

- ✓ **Research outcomes** should be made available to research participants via a dedicated website supervised by the sponsor or provided through the PO. Families want to see if their contribution has led to the drug being developed and it is not enough to inform them only when the results are published in scientific journals, which may never happen. The participant should still have the right to find out what happened in the trial.

9 Getting clinical outcomes that matter to children

How the clinical outcomes that matter to the patients are achieved is dependent upon collaboration between the various groups involved in CTs. In this chapter we illustrate a number of ways in which the different stakeholders can contribute to the development of empowerment.

9.1 Children and parents: role and recommendations

Empowerment cannot be forced onto a person; therefore, it is up to the parents of children and the children themselves ultimately to take power over the situation if this is what they want; this allows them to make demands on how the CT is planned and conducted.

9.1.1 Actively seeking trials

Families can search for CTs that may fit their own needs by consulting the EU Clinical Trials Register website (https://www.clinicaltrialsregister.eu/), which has only been available since 2011, as a result of mounting public pressure regarding transparency in CTs. It provides public access to the following information on each CT in Europe:

- the hypotheses being tested,
- methods used and protocol,
- outcome variables,
- criteria for acceptance as a participant in the trial and
- updated information on recruitment during the trial.

9.1.2 Getting treated as an individual

Empowered families should expect to be treated with respect and that their contribution to the research is valued. They should expect to be treated as individuals and not objects. The family and the child should expect the trial to be carried out with consideration to their convenience. After all, they are being asked to participate in something from which they may derive no direct benefit. The family should not expect the CT staff to bend to all their wishes but to listen to their suggestions. They should expect that procedures be organised within the limits of the CT to try to meet their wishes.

There should be opportunities for the child to express their own opinions and be listened to. Families should expect to be treated with respect and that their contribution to the research is valued. The child should not be treated as a guinea pig (object) but rather as an individual. The family and the child should expect the trial to be carried out with consideration for their convenience.

9.1.3 Getting treated as a member of a team

The child and parents are being asked to participate in a CT and they should see themselves as adopting a role that is more than just as a research subject, but closer to that of a team member. This new role should bring with it the expectation to be kept informed about the trial. Most families feel they have the most right to information on the results of their trial. The role of the parents is to negotiate with the research team at the outset which information will be available. Even where the child is not able to understand the results, they should have the right to be given some information about the results when the CT is ended.

Once the decision to participate has been made, the child should be acknowledged as part of a group contributing to the development of medicines for children. However, families have to be aware that certain aspects of a CT cannot be influenced. For example, in a randomised CT the child is assigned to the test drug or the standard treatment. The participant and the family give up certain freedoms in order to participate in the trial.

9.1.4 The need to make the right decision for the child

The parents' role is always to make the right decision for the child. This role still applies following agreement to participate in clinical research. The parents have the right to retract that decision at any time and to withdraw the child from the study. The family should therefore re-evaluate their decision at intervals. In this process, decision tools for clinical participation will not only be useful to make the initial decision to participate, but also to re-evaluate the decision and confirm that they have made the right choice. It should not be assumed that the child is too young to be informed about the CT; especially children with prior experience of CTs should expect to be able to give opinions and even counter sign the consent form themselves.

9.1.5 Need to avoid being overwhelmed

Parents with a sick child can easily feel overwhelmed by information concerning a CT. The parent and child have the right to evaluate the information at their own pace. Too much information or information that is difficult to understand will overwhelm anyone. It is acknowledged good practice to give patients time to consider their participation. In the RESPECT case studies, CT staff commented that they evaluated the capacity of the parents to take on the decision. There was a desire not to overburden stressed parents, for example by asking them to make several important decisions all at one time. The role of the empowered child and parent is therefore to take control of this information flow and not be steered by others. Parents should probe the doctor's knowledge; for example, they can ask questions about the kind of benefits and the possible risks associated with the drug being tested.

Parents should be able to demand information about the trial in non-scientific language if they have any doubts about what is being asked of their child. They can also request more time to make their decision and ask for an independent decision aid. Parents should have an opportunity to learn about CTs in general and form an opinion; parents and children should become aware of their attitudes, knowledge and emotions about medical research in general and about their child's participation in the specific trial in question, for example, how much risk is acceptable given their child's medical condition.

9.1.6 The doctor knows best

There is a qualitative difference between health care and CT participation. In health care, patients are willing to give over some control of their bodies to someone else who may recommend a change in treatment in the capacity of an expert; the doctor is, after all, the person with most expertise, who would only recommend a new treatment with proven efficacy in the patient's best interests. In many cases, this feeling that *the doctor knows best* is transferred to the CT context, where it is not in fact so clear that the doctor knows best. The reason for conducting the CT is usually that there is some doubt as to the efficacy and safety of a test drug compared to existing treatments.

The best interests of the individual child, which always have priority, are not the main focus of a CT, but rather the development of a drug that will help all children with the health problem in question. This has to be tested experimentally on many children, but often the new medication has been tested in adults prior to being tested on children; this makes the decision about participation in paediatric CTs closer to the health care situation and the doctor may use clinical experience to judge whether participating in the CT incurs an increased risk for the individual child over remaining on the current medication. The role of the empowered family is to probe this judgement and evaluate how much they trust the doctor to know the level of actual discomfort and risk to which the child will be subjected.

In many CTs, key decisions about the protocol are made with no input from families or patient groups. However, there are some patient panels, for example, run by larger CT networks, which provide an opportunity for parents and sometimes children themselves to have a say on research priorities, specific CT proposals and the clarity of the informed consent materials. In this way, children and parents can make a meaningful contribution to medical research.

9.1.7 Recommendations for children and parents

- ✓ Join or create a patient organisation that will represent children in CTs by lobbying pharmaceutical companies for the clinical research that matters most to children and parents.

- ✓ Seek out CTs that fit the child's needs.

- ✓ Request more information. It is up to the CT staff to present the information about the trial in a way that can be understood by everyone.

- ✓ Get the clinical research team to clearly distinguish the difference between research and treatment.

- ✓ Request time to read and consider the trial information, the child and parent should set the time frame for the decision.

- ✓ Negotiate with the research team at the outset to establish what information will be available after the CT.

- ✓ Make suggestions about how things could be better organised to make participation easier.

- ✓ Ask for a personal health report for the child at the end of the CT.

- ✓ Request a general report about the results of the research.

9.2 Patient organisations: role and recommendations

Empowerment comes through patient organisations representing the patient in different stages of the CT process and in making demands about the participation of patients. Although many CT units and CROs believe they are open to participation in decision-making, such participation is still closely controlled by the CT staff. True empowerment would encourage patients to voice conflicting opinions on important issues, which would yield more truthful and productive dialogue. It cannot be emphasised enough the importance of creating an environment of trust and providing training in reaching consensus. A major challenge for POs is the need to identify ways of building trusting relationships for CT involvement.

It should be noted that the added value of the involvement of POs in CTs will be apparent only if two prerequisites are fulfilled, namely **ethics** and **transparency.** While regulations framing CT practice guarantee the respect of ethics, the same cannot be said about ensuring transparency, which is crucial for the empowerment of children and their families and for POs to support effectively that empowerment.

9.2.1 Prior to the CT

Conveying members' needs and demands to decision-makers
One of the findings of the RESPECT PO survey is the often-neglected fact that many patients – especially those suffering from rare conditions – want more CTs to be carried out that could contribute to the improvement of their situation. This demand that there be further CTs should be explored. Similar discussion arose during the PO workshop, where the participants clearly expressed the crucial issue of finding appropriate mechanisms or channels for patients to be involved in identifying drug and treatment options to be trialled. As a result of the discussion, another essential role of POs was pointed out: being mediators between their members and researchers, passing on patients' ideas and needs to researchers and decision-makers. Thus, POs should advocate and push for CTs in under-researched conditions.

Ensuring a child-centred trial design
CT design and protocols are oriented towards specific scientific outcomes in order to answer questions concerning the action of new drugs. It is, however, very important – and currently not given enough consideration – that the protocol should take into account all aspects of the

everyday life of the child and the parents. For example, missing too many school lessons or working days can discourage participation, and minimising pain with an oral treatment rather than an injection can facilitate compliance. Moreover, the focus on outcomes should assess whether the outcomes are those desired by children themselves (such as lack of side effects) and aim at improved quality of life. Knowing very well the challenges encountered by their members, POs should be involved in the CT design and review of the protocol.

Generating patients' trust
Earning the trust of patients and their carers is the primary prerequisite to getting them to agree to participate in a CT. The willingness of children and their families to participate definitely increases if the POs recommend participation to their members. However, to vouch for CTs and to convince families, the POs would need to be convinced in the first place. To this end, they should be involved in every step of the process: planning, design, initiation of a particular CT, deriving conclusions and dissemination of the results. In addition to that, POs could provide guidelines to researchers on patient involvement, patients' rights and researchers' responsibilities towards patients that go beyond the ethics principles that researchers already have to respect. Another aspect is that POs could train researchers on how to communicate with children and parents.

Finding suitable patients
The involvement of POs will make it easier for researchers to find suitable candidates for CTs due to their huge potential in reaching patients. Advertising the CTs through POs will increase the number of families who have a positive attitude to participating. This is especially the case for families who do not regularly attend any of the CT clinics.

Obtaining true informed consent
POs should be involved in the development of the consent form to make sure it is presented in non-scientific language and in an age- and disease-appropriate way. Encouraging members to participate in CTs is also a matter of being able to communicate with them, to speak the language they understand and to provide the information they would seek regarding the relevance of CT and its possible outcomes. So, POs have a key role in supporting children and their families to fully understand informed consent and in providing decision aid tools that members can use to make their own informed choice.

9.2.2 During the CT

Supporting the patients
POs could play an advisory role to the families who are participating in a CT throughout the trial. A CT can lead to difficult emotional experiences and also practical difficulties; this is even more true for paediatric CTs. POs are in a privileged position to help families identify difficulties and possible improvements during the trial and convey them to the researchers. POs can help define the type of psychological, informational and practical support their members need to feel in control and empowered. Furthermore, they can develop a strategy for monitoring and evaluating within the CT from the perspective of children and for encouraging their involvement and empowerment.

Ensuring the patients are respected
Many children and their representatives continuously stress the importance of being treated as human beings during CTs, not as test subjects. Among the survey results, this issue presents itself as a very highly ranked reason for parents to refuse the participation of their child in CTs. Note that earning and keeping the trust of patients and carers is not only about promises on paper but an ongoing delicate process. Showing children respect will help them to feel good about their participation. In this regard, the POs could play a role in undertaking the safeguarding of their members. Moreover, the POs could be involved in the creation of a child-friendly atmosphere during the CTs and ensuring that the participants acquire the status of co-researchers instead of mere experimental subjects.

Intermediary for communication
For a number of reasons, patients may hesitate to give feedback on the CT in which they are participating. To encourage their input, the POs could develop a strategy for communication between the researchers, the children, the parents and their representatives, so that enough attention is paid to the children's quality of life. There are other possible ways to get feedback from as many participants as possible about the course of the trial, for instance setting up a website or an online forum.

9.2.3 After the CT

Assessment of results
POs should have a say with regard to the results of the study and be involved in the assessment of the process. The overall assessment by researchers should not be made solely based on quantitative data collected during the research, but also the experiences of participants in their daily lives throughout the CT should be taken into account. At this stage, the POs should act as mediators, communicating both parties' perspectives to one another. This is a must for the appropriate recognition and acknowledgement of the child's contribution.

Taking action for the well-being of patients
Participants attending our workshop felt strongly that if the test drug or treatment has been successful during the trial, the participants' treatment should not be interrupted but continued without waiting for the approval of European Medicines Agency. It would fall on the POs to take the lead to advocate for the treatment to continue.

Sharing outcomes and good practices
POs should be involved in disseminating the results of the study to participants and to their broader membership from a patient perspective and in a child-friendly format. There is also a need for alliance between POs to share experience, knowledge and good practices concerning past and ongoing CTs. This information is invaluable and can change the whole course of future trials. Besides sharing the outcomes, POs should update each other about ongoing CTs, which will give members an opportunity to select trials in which they would like to be involved.

9.2.4 Recommendations for patient organisations

- ✓ Lobby for the CTs that are most wanted by your members.

- ✓ Identify the special contribution of children and parents in CT planning and how and where they can be involved most effectively.

- ✓ Seek opportunities to represent members on committees in charge of developing, reviewing and approving the CT protocol.

- ✓ Define the type of psychological, informational and practical support children and parents need in order to feel in control and empowered.

- ✓ Provide information to members on proposed and ongoing CTs.

- ✓ Act in a counselling role, advising children and parents about participation.

- ✓ Develop a strategy for communication between the researchers, the children, the parents and the PO representatives, adopting an intermediary role between the CT researchers and the patient.

- ✓ Provide emotional support and practical help to participants.

- ✓ Develop a strategy for monitoring and evaluating the trial from the perspective of children and parents, in particular their sense of meaningful involvement and empowerment during their participation in the trial.

- ✓ Provide children with tools and resources to explain their experience to their peers.

- ✓ Take on the role of collecting CT results for distribution to the members.

- ✓ Lobby the European Medicines Agency (EMA) to extend public access to the Clinical Trials Register to include the following information that would be of special interest to parents of sick children and CT participants:
  - the process for joining any CT published on the Clinical Trials Register website;
  - the opinion document from the relevant ethics committee for a particular CT;
  - the research results of each CT.

9.3 Principal investigator and CT staff: role and recommendations

One of the major themes described by the RESPECT project is the need for the participants to be treated as a partner in the CT process; therefore, fulfilment of the families' motivation for participation should be incorporated into the CT protocol. Below are some suggestions of how this can be done. The empowerment model predicts that involvement through *self-determination, accountability, cooperation* and *knowledge* is necessary to increase the feeling of control.

Empowerment can be increased by the children, parents and their patient organisations having access to all parts of the process.

It is necessary to indicate to parents when the clinician is discussing trial-related issues and when they are discussing standard treatment issues (Simon et al., 2004). It is the role and responsibility of the investigator and CT staff to make sure that the difference between research and health care is clearly understood. Creating opportunities, both formal and informal, for patients to influence, design, create, and implement CT procedures makes this distinction much clearer.

9.3.1 Create opportunities for the family to influence the CT protocol

The patient has a unique view of their condition and, in the same way that PROs are developed to give the patient a voice in the CT outcome measures, the involvement of patients at the outset of the project to give their opinions will be of value to the research and increase the chances of the patient group getting the outcomes that matter to them. This could be achieved via a consultation procedure at the CT planning phase.

9.3.2 Create opportunities to include the child's perspective in the outcome measurements

As in the structure of the protocol, the patient representatives should have the possibility to not only have input to the design of the outcome measures but also to be able to suggest methods for data collection. It may be most convenient for the researchers to have questionnaires but, for the child, an opportunity to provide verbal feedback may be preferred. A variety of methods should be considered where children are involved.

9.3.3 Monitor the child's perspective in the CT

How the project is monitored is set down by GCP regulations concerning the conduct of a paediatric CT. However, the child's perspective is not included in this and the necessary structures are not well developed. If there are opportunities to include PRO measures then these should be monitored by an independent body or by the patient representatives. This would give a voice to the child and increase empowerment.

9.3.4 Develop structures that include the patient as research partner

Normally, patients are recruited after the CT protocol has been written and there is no opportunity to change the structure of the trial at the point of patient recruitment. However, if a patient panel composed of similar patients were formed in advance in order to discuss the trial then they would have the opportunity to influence how the trial was structured, which research questions to explore and which outcomes are most important to the patient group.

The paediatric CT should be a team effort between clinician, sponsor, child and others. If children are to become partners in the research, with responsibilities of compliance, then they should also have higher status than that of a patient. This means that they should be included in making decisions about the CT. Some CT organisations give patients information on how the recruitment to the CT is going and how many patients are in the trial, usually in the form of a newsletter. This type of information is important in order to encourage empowerment. There should also be opportunities for the children to pose questions about their participation in the trial.

Note that not all children want this kind of involvement. They may want the doctor to 'carry the burden' for them. It is important to be sensitive to how much the child wants to be involved and informed and to review this over time as the child matures. Staff should be trained in person-centred care, which emphasises the need for active listening, skilled questioning and establishing a shared agenda. Training on how to facilitate the participants' empowerment should be provided for all staff. It is important to let children acquire competencies related to CTs as the trial progresses. Discussing issues related to participating in research with the families gives an opportunity for the researchers to learn from the children themselves.

9.3.5 Helping the child to reach an informed opinion

Children and young people should be involved as much as possible in decisions about their health care. Tools to build children's confidence and skills in making decisions and to improve their understanding about CTs should be made available in all trials. Investigators could for example provide a decision aid as part of the informed consent or assent process in order to help children ask the right questions.

It is not sufficient to describe the study to the child and parents without taking into consideration whether they understood this information or the level of risk involved. It is clear that risk is poorly understood by the majority of people. GCP guidelines refer to defining and monitoring the risk threshold. It is anticipated here that the doctor defines the risk threshold and conveys this information to the child and parent. However, defining the risk is complex and is often hard to communicate. The clinician does not always attempt to ascertain whether or not the patient has fully understood the risks involved.

In order to decrease possible confusion between a trial and normal health care, the CT team should seek ways to make it clear that they belong to a research team and that this is different from the medical team. Investigators should view the informed consent process as a method to increase the potential participants' understanding of the study that continues beyond the start of the trial. It should therefore be seen as a process that is started together with the family. It does not simply involve providing materials created or reviewed by the patient panel. Rather, this process has to take into account that a child will probably need extra time to understand what is involved and that the informed consent process is not completed with a signature on the consent form but continues for the duration of the trial.

9.3.6 Recommendations for the principal investigator and CT staff

- ✓ Provide opportunities for a representative of the patient population to advise on the development of the protocol

- ✓ Include patient representation in the group that decides on the information package for informed consent.

These two activities could be developed into the role of a patient panel that would ensure that the trial is constructed and presented in a way that takes into consideration the child's perspective and the CT information is appropriate to the age group being recruited. The information materials are more likely to fulfil the aim of informing children if they are produced with the help of children themselves.

- ✓ Allow enough time for the family to consider the information contained in the informed consent form prior to consenting or assenting to participation. The time period may vary but at least one week is recommended.

- ✓ Increase transparency by including in the informed consent material a reference to the ethics committee approval and to a publically accessible database where information about the study can be found.

- ✓ Provide a decision aid to help the families and children reach a well-balanced decision.

- ✓ Provide the child and family at each trial visit with the information materials in order to ensure that the information is refreshed and the child has several possibilities to ask questions.

- ✓ Train CT staff in person-centred care.

- ✓ Update children and parents regularly on the progress of the recruitment and the trial itself, thus acknowledging their role as part of the research team.

- ✓ Provide the participants with a short summary of the results of the trial written in non-scientific language. A report on the results of the trial should also be made available to the relevant PO and put on the CT website.

The RESPECT project found that not getting the results of the CT was a major concern expressed in all participant surveys.

- ✓ Provide a written personal health report to the parents and child.

The RESPECT project found that one of the major needs from participation was to get more detailed information about the health of the child. In order to satisfy this need a report could be provided to the participant family. This is in addition to the general report about the CT results.

9.4 Ethics committees: role and recommendations

Ethics committees in Europe work within a common regulatory framework; however, they work independently and there are many national differences. The impact of changes to the paediatric regulatory framework is difficult to evaluate, partly because of the diversity of approaches and partly because, in most Member States, there is no overview of the activities of the ethics committees. This lack of structure makes the implementation of changes difficult and leads to uncertainty about continuity of how applications for paediatric CTs will be treated in different regions. There is also concern among POs, whose opinions are not always formally invited.

In relation to paediatric research, it is the role of ethics committees to guarantee the safety, rights and well-being of the children involved; however, in order to increase empowerment of children and families, a more transparent structure allowing access to patients and their representatives would be desirable.

9.4.1 Criteria to be assessed in relation to paediatric research

It is the role of the ethics committees to guarantee the alignment of researchers and sponsors on the same ethical principles. These principles include:

An approach to patient inclusion
The first guiding principle for approval of paediatric research protocols is that the research should be of direct benefit to the children involved. However, with the expansion of CTs under the new paediatric regulatory framework necessitating the inclusion of more children, a direct benefit cannot be guaranteed. Therefore, this principle needs to be reviewed by ethics committees throughout Europe. They need to consider how to protect the needs of families asked to participate in clinical research even when there is no direct benefit to the child.

Consent and assent of children
The second guiding principle is that children's assent should take account of their maturity. The child's refusal is not always taken seriously if the parents have consented to participation in the study. The application of this principle needs to be standardised to establish how maturity should be measured; some committees consider that the child's assent should be taken into account from the age of six years and that consent should be obtained from the age of 15 years, but such age cut-offs are not harmonised across Europe. Where risk levels are low, a lower age of consent could be considered, thus empowering children at a lower age to take responsibility for their own participation.

In addition to the ethics committees consideration for the child-specific GCP aspects of a paediatric CT, such as minimising risks and discomfort, the clarity and readability of the informed consent information material is considered pivotal; ethics committees assess whether the material is sufficiently child-friendly to ensure that real consent or assent is possible. Children themselves are able to contribute to this evaluation of the information material.

Confidentiality issues
The third guiding principle is that personal information about the child involved in clinical research should be kept to a minimum and not disclosed for purposes other than those for which it was collected, as indicated in the informed consent process. The empowered participant should have some control over this personal information and the ethics committee should ensure that this is included in the protocol and added to the informed consent form.

Paediatric expertise of ethics committees
In order to guarantee that these principles are adhered to and that ethical research is undertaken, ethics committees should involve experts in paediatric research with expertise in the special needs of children. We recognise that to require this level of paediatric expertise on every ethics committee will be difficult; however, criteria for membership should be discussed across Europe. Obtaining the opinions of children themselves should also be considered.

9.4.2 The role of ethics committee networks

Special attention in our discussions has been paid to developing networks among ethics committees. The idea of networking ethics committees was raised and the lack of standardisation and transparency between them was considered to be a barrier to further development. A network of ethics committees within a Member State is essential and a network covering all Member States would be a natural progression from this. Harmonisation of ethical issues in paediatric research would be welcome. The concept of networking has been embraced by some countries and national websites have been established to report on the activities of ethics committees. However, there has been no separate recording or reporting of paediatric CTs and the transparency needed to facilitate empowerment is still lacking.

The role of a European ethics committee network in relation to paediatric research could be, first and foremost, to consolidate and clarify the main ethical and scientific issues. It is necessary to continue to increase awareness of, and to stimulate the debate on, ethical issues arising from paediatric clinical research, in the light of the European paediatric regulatory framework and accompanying ethical recommendations. Secondly, such a network could review procedures to verify conformity between ethics committees and, thirdly, establishing a Europe-wide network would stimulate a more rigorous ethical and scientific approach to the drafting of protocols.

In addition, there is a role to be played in relation to dissemination of knowledge about ethics. There is, for example, a need to share ethical guidelines with families through arranging debates or conferences and training courses at national and local levels.

Of course, practical problems with the establishment of networks need to be taken into consideration, such as the fact that, in most Member States, committee members are not remunerated for their work and a funded network secretariat would need to be established.

9.4.3 *Recommendations for ethics committees*

- ✓ Agree a structure of formal guidelines for paediatric CT protocol assessment and make this available for public scrutiny. These guidelines should be approved at a European level and developed in conjunction with POs, sponsors and industry.

- ✓ Ensure that training and education in the field of ethics of paediatric clinical research are undertaken and that courses are accredited at a national or European level.

- ✓ Develop a central ethics committee to enhance networking among regional ethics committees for collaboration and information exchange. This should particularly be promoted among the new Member States.

- ✓ Include patient representation on ethics committees throughout Europe, facilitating a critical review of the need for the research. This is already done in some countries and should be expanded to all Member States.

- ✓ Recommend that an assessment of informed consent information materials be undertaken in conjunction with representatives of the patient group included in the study.

- ✓ Make publicly available information on the CT applications submitted to ethics committees and decisions on these applications. This will fulfil the need for greater transparency as an element of empowerment.

9.5 Sponsors: role and recommendations

The main role of the sponsor in relation to empowerment is encouraging the inclusion of patients in discussions related to generating new protocols. This can be achieved on the macro and micro levels.

9.5.1 *Macro level: Unmet medical needs*

Although the development of a new medication is most often steered by scientific discovery, there are many stages to the development process. Advisory boards review the science and the market potential for a drug before deciding which CTs should be conducted, but the patient's voice is rarely represented here. This should be seen as an opportunity for the children or their representatives to make their voice heard and express their unmet needs. They should be allowed to have an input into what kind of medications the pharmaceutical industry and the health care system should develop.

9.5.2   Micro level: Patient-reported outcomes

At the micro level, sponsors can encourage discussion concerning patient involvement around the input to the procedures, namely, to the structure of the protocol, the trial design, the outcome measurements, and to a lesser extent to the monitoring procedures.

9.5.3   Recommendations for sponsors

There is a general need for further accountability within the system, giving rise to the following recommendations. It is advisable that the sponsor should develop a policy to oversee that these are incorporated and provided.

- ✓ Work with patient organisations to encourage self-determination by soliciting health care needs, as identified by the children and parents (patient-identified needs) and maintain a list of these needs and priorities. This highlights needs for new clinical research that families with sick children would be most interested in supporting.

- ✓ Make time to involve families and the POs and seek their input, focusing on cooperation and mutual respect in addition to purely scientific results.

- ✓ Provide more time for professional development; sponsors should develop and test tools that will assist the research team in educating potential participants about the need for trials, children's rights within a CT, and to demystify the protocol of specific CTs. Improved knowledge increases the likelihood of willingness to participate in CTs.

- ✓ Create partnership opportunities for effective collaboration on education materials, especially encouraging youth engagement.

9.6   Policy makers: role and recommendations

Understanding patterns of disempowerment in CTs and the underlying medical culture is critical in making informed policy choices that encourage empowerment, as well as in designing interventions. The first step is to make exclusion practices visible by monitoring the child's perspective in CTs.

Efforts to address empowerment may require removing the barriers inherent in the way that CTs are carried out; the way that protocols are developed and the regulations governing these, for example the transparency of the process of ethical review. Additionally, to enable paediatric patients to take advantage of the new opportunities developed, it will be necessary to invest in the capabilities of children and their representatives in ways that they value.

One of the major themes described by the RESPECT project is the need for the participants to have access to information about the CT process and the knowledge to interpret this information. Empowerment comes through knowledge and it should be a wider goal for policy makers to identify ways to facilitate education of the general public on the need for CTs on children. We need to go beyond informed consent and ensure that the patient is fully informed and, where necessary, educated. This can happen at various levels. In society, more emphasis can be placed on the importance of medical research and its benefits. The process of conducting a CT can be included in school education and should be a requirement in all health education. It is recommended that an education programme is developed by patient organisations. In addition, decision aids for CT participation should be provided. At the time of being asked to participate, the parent and child should have access to well-tested decision aids, which can stimulate empowerment by encouraging them to pose the appropriate questions to their doctors and the investigators.

Policy makers have a duty to create an environment for patient involvement in CTs. An important aspect of the development of empowerment for children and parents is that the structure of CT management is overseen from the perspective of the child.

GCP training with certification is a requirement in most European Member States and the EMA has regulatory bodies that can conduct audits to ensure that CT researchers are following the ICH GCP guidelines (European Medicines Agency, 2002); however, these guidelines concern the details of data collection and do not cover monitoring the experience of the patient, which is especially important in the case of children; thus, the possibility of creating an independent GCP monitoring body should be explored. This body could draw upon expertise from CT management and from POs. The possible outcome would be to broaden the definition of GCP to ensure that it includes the patient perspective.

It has fallen upon the ethics committees to judge the comprehensibility of the written information material and consent or assent forms provided to children. Expertise in this area is required and the capacities of the ethics committees are limited here. A role for an advisory group on information material to support the ethics committees should be investigated. A separate body with specialist knowledge of child language comprehension, appropriate presentation formats and differences in age, gender and cultural backgrounds would no doubt be welcomed by ethics committees.

9.6.1 Recommendations for policy makers

- ✓ Establish research to incorporate the child's patient-identified needs (PINs) into clinical research and to explore how these PINs can be expressed by the children and communicated to clinical researchers.

- ✓ Propose supportive legislation to strengthen empowerment through self-determination at a community level by providing resources across traditional geographical boundaries for children participating in CTs.

- ✓ Support training programmes on advocacy in CTs. This will strengthen POs by increasing their knowledge about CTs and improving their effectiveness as partners in the CT process. Training programmes would also assist individual participants to have effective input in CT design.

- ✓ Develop a centralised review process for paediatric CT protocols, which would assist in the standardisation of protocols throughout Europe and increase accessibility for potential participants and their representatives.

- ✓ Investigate the possibilities of establishing an independent European GCP monitoring body leading to the broadening of the definition of GCP to include the patient perspective. This body could draw upon expertise from CT management and from POs.

- ✓ Support the development of a comprehensive European guide addressing paediatric ethical issues in accordance with all the relevant international and European ethical and legal sources. This would assist in the development of standardised ethical committee procedures.

- ✓ Create a European advisory group on informed consent materials, gathering in one body experts from different Member States in the area of language comprehension and presentation formats for different ages, gender and cultural backgrounds. This advisory group should develop guidelines for producing informed consent materials appropriate for the various age groups concerned, with a focus on clarity and comprehensibility. Children themselves should be consulted in this process.

- ✓ Support the establishment of a standardised method of designating risk in CTs, to be used for communicating effectively the level of risk to the potential participant.

- ✓ Initiate a Europe-wide debate concerning the indemnity for damages to the patient participating in a CT. A common European approach needs to be established for describing to the patients and their representatives the level of care that will be available in the event that harm does occur, who will provide it, and who will pay for it.

10 RESPECT demonstration projects

RESPECT conducted two demonstration projects that illustrated and explored the practicality of empowering children through the application of the *self-determination* and *knowledge* elements of the SACK model. The first was a decision aid and the second was an education package.

10.1 Self-determination through use of decision aids

10.1.1 Introduction

Given increased pressure to recruit paediatric patients to CTs, families will in turn be under increasing pressure to make decisions, possibly in the absence of expert advice at the time the decision is made. Help in this area might be covered by decision aids, which are a well-known tool for patients facing decisions about or regarding their health. Moreover, if we focus on randomised CTs, the need for improved support increases. Nevertheless, there is only very limited preliminary research about families or even adult patients making a decision about participation in a CT by using a decision aid.

CTs are run in the public interest, not for the direct benefit of the individual patient, but it is not clear that patients understand the main principles of clinical research when invited to participate. Mainly, they hope for personal benefits regarding their health. Often they understand that there is an altruistic aspect to participating but focus more on the possible personal benefit.

Doctors may believe – and say – that the patient will benefit from the test drug, knowing that the existing drug, if there was one at all, does not work well. Sometimes the only chance to receive a new or experimental treatment is a CT and that is why doctors and patients take this option. Patients are often disappointed to find that they are in the placebo arm or that the test drug did not actually help their condition. This indicates that their decision was not based on a complete understanding of the information they were given or that the information was not complete. (It could be that the benefits were stressed more than the risks, for example.)

10.1.2 Aims

We want patients to participate of their own free will and to be aware of the implications. Being empowered to decide (or not) seems strongly related to how much information the family has. If you are confident that you have received enough information, you feel empowered to make the decision for yourself, either for or against participation. If you do not have enough information, you make a judgement (maybe a gut feeling) about whether you trust the doctor enough to participate.

We need to empower patients to decide about participating in a trial that is not necessarily in their interest (which, because of equipoise, should always be the case). Then the patient is treated more as an equal in the decision. Our literature review showed that some patients want this shared decision-making while others want a paternalistic relationship in which the doctor decides on their behalf, so this has to be taken into account. They may not need the detailed medical background to the trial; it may be rather that decision aids help them to decide whom to trust.

10.1.3 Background

Decision aids are interventions designed to support individuals in making specific and deliberate health- or illness-related choices (Kasper & Lenz, 2005). They prepare people to participate in preference-sensitive decisions (O'Connor et al., 2004). Using decision aids improves patient knowledge, comfort and participation (O'Connor et al., 2004).

Decision aids improve patients' decision making by:
- reducing the number of patients who feel uncertain;
- increasing patients' knowledge;
- creating realistic expectations of problems and outcomes;
- improving the agreement between patients' values and choices;
- reducing decisional conflict and emotions connected to it and
- increasing participation in decision making (O'Connor et al., 2003).

Decisional conflict in situations affecting health
This decision situation is characterised by uncertainty in identifying the best alternative given the risks. Other important characteristics are the scientific uncertainty about benefit or harm and the need to make value judgements about potential benefits vs. potential harm. Furthermore, the anticipated regret over the positive aspects of rejected options might play a role here. It is likely that this specific conflict might increase if decision is to be made on behalf of children.

Research demonstrates that individuals vary in their preferences for accepting treatment or not and that the health condition is not in any case a sufficient predictor for the decision (European Medicines Agency 2002).

Factors aggravating the difficulties families will face in making a decision about participation in a randomised CT are:
- lack of knowledge;
- unrealistic perceptions or expectations;
- unclear personal values;
- social pressure to choose an option;
- lack of support;
- lack of skills or self-confidence and
- lack of other resources (O'Connor, Stacey & Jacobsen, 2011).

A well-designed decision aid targeting knowledge and feelings about medical research in general and the principles of randomised CTs in particular will support families in that tough situation.

Hypothetical decision model

Empowering parents and children to have a say in the design and execution of the trial will motivate their participation and increase the likelihood of achieving outcomes that really matter to patients.

Figure 12: Hypothetical decision model

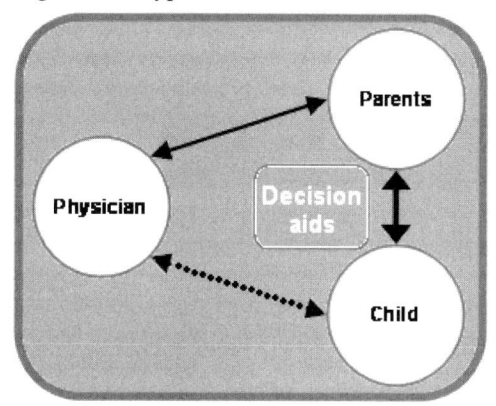

10.1.4 Development

The development process of this generic decision aid supporting families facing a decision about letting their child participate in a randomised CT was conducted following the recommendations given by the Ottawa Health Research Institute (see Figure 13).

Figure 13: Conceptual framework (Ottawa Health Research Institute)

Decision needs
- Decision conflict
- Knowledge & expectations
- Values
- Support & resources
- Decision: type, timing, stage & learning
- Personal / clinical characteristics

Decision support
- Clarity decision and needs
- Provide facts, probabilities
- Clarify values
- Guide/coach/support skills
- Monitor/facilitate progress

Clinical
Decision aids
Coaching

Decision quality
- Informed
- Value based

Actions
- Delay, continuance

Impact
- Value-based health outcomes
- Regret & blame
- Appropriate use & cost of services

Based on their conceptual framework we designed a preliminary version, covering the following topics:
- information about options and possible outcomes,
- presenting probabilities of outcomes (benefit-risk balance),
- values clarification exercises (personal importance of benefits and risks),
- information about others' opinions (examples and case studies) and
- guidance and coaching in decision making and communication.

This first version consisted of two parts: an 18-page brochure and a corresponding workbook of eight pages. It was designed to use them side by side simultaneously, allowing the families first to read a part of the brochure and then collect their ideas and thoughts in the associated part of the workbook.

After making their way through the whole workbook, the family then gathers all thoughts, opinions, fears and hopes connected with the possible participation in the trial. Everything is designed in a visually appealing way, such as a picture of weighing scales to illustrate balancing the risks and benefits. This helps the reader to grasp complex thoughts. For instance, if the family identified a lot more risks than benefits, the scales tip visually towards one side or one decision.

For every particular randomised CT, this generic decision aid should be supplemented by information about the specific conditions, risks, benefits and adverse effects.

10.1.5 Evaluation

According to the recommendations of the Ottawa Health Research Institute, we started with the preliminary version and audited it in a first expert workshop. Then we did a first evaluation with students to test comprehensibility and manageability.

After modifying the brochure and the workbook according to the results of this preliminary evaluation, a second expert workshop was held, to design a first version to be tested with parents considering a health decision for their child. This is still work in progress.

Figure 14: Decision Guide

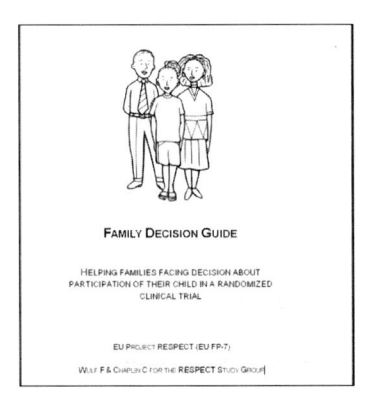

See **Appendix 2** for the complete RESPECT Family Decision Guide and worksheet.

10.1.6 Future issues

It is important for the family to make the best decision regarding the child's health and the physician will be interested to help the patient make a decision that they are comfortable with. However, there is always an element of social (non-peer) pressure that cannot be avoided. Decision tools may help the patient to decide without that pressure.

- How can decision aids be included within the CT process?
- Is it OK to include descriptions of the benefit to the patient from participating (such as that they can get the drug before it is on the market)? If we focus only on the advantages, the family would not be making a balanced decision.
- If we include the opinion of important others (patients with same condition or facing the same decision), would this improve the quality of the decision aid or influence the families in an inappropriate way?
- Should we provide specific versions of the decision aid for children in different age groups as well?

10.2 Knowledge through an education package for schools

10.2.1 Introduction

One part of the RESPECT project is to explore how to empower parents to make an independent decision when asked to consent to their child's participation in a paediatric CT. Although there is a standardised informed consent process that clinicians follow to ensure that parents are given all the necessary information to help them decide, there is always a risk that the parents have not really understood this information; it may be written in technical language or lack an explanation of the basic principles of CTs.

Parents considering whether to consent to the participation of their child in a CT need to be fully informed and educated about the process and principles of a CT (for example, being aware of the concept of equipoise). This enables them to make an adequate and voluntary decision about participation based on what is best for their child as well as considering the benefits of paediatric research from an altruistic perspective.

A person with more knowledge in the area will be more empowered to make his or her own decision. Where awareness of the issues involved in a CT is limited, the person's autonomy to decide about participation might be compromised. He or she may consent based on trust in the clinical staff rather than a truly informed decision and this is likely to increase the probability of withdrawal from the trial if the original (poorly understood) information given is later perceived as misleading. For example, parents often experience the trials as more time-consuming or unpleasant than they had expected, which leads some of them to withdraw prematurely from the trial. This is both time-consuming and costly for the CT and it lowers the parents' and patients' trust in medical research in general, jeopardising the ambition to increase the development of medicines appropriate for children in Europe.

In addition, the fear of adverse events and unpleasant tests for the child to endure are issues that cause parents to decline to consent when approached about participation, leading to recruitment difficulties for the CT staff. The wider altruistic imperative for participation in CTs is harder to appreciate, especially as a certain proportion of participants in CTs are not aware that they are in a trial but rather believe that they are continuing with individual treatment.

Our observations have led us to conclude that parents might benefit from additional education in preparation for the informed consent process.

10.2.2 Identifying possible training needs in order to develop educational material

Information concerning questions and worries from parents regarding children participating in CTs was gathered and evaluated. The purpose was to find out what kind of information a parent might want to know before consenting and what fundamental aspects of a CT seem to be hard to understand.

From the literature review, several articles exploring parents understanding of CTs and their point of view in the informed consent process were compiled as a basis for the education, to find out what parts in the process might be further explained.

Interviews – patients and parents understanding of CTs
To be able to identify what concerns are associated with trial participation and what factors influence the child's willingness to participate or the parents' willingness to have their child participate, two children and three parents were interviewed, all of them with many years of experiences from CTs, either a diabetes trial or a growth hormone trial. The questions in the interviews were collected from earlier interview sessions from an ongoing study developing patient-reported outcome measures for children in growth hormone trials.

From these interviews we learned that, before participation, they felt that the following areas were unclear to them: the informed consent process; the details of the CT process; the benefits their child would have from participation; and what was meant by certain technical terms such as 'standard treatment' and 'randomisation'. The main reasons for agreeing to participation were receiving better treatment, additional medical oversight and access to medical staff. Safety risks were assumed to be minor.

Interviews – how to conduct and educate focus groups
Interviews with people performing focus groups in a medical context were conducted to get an idea of what principles are of importance in educating people in rare situations, such as parents of hospitalised children. A nurse at the department of Cystic Fibrosis at the Östra hospital in Gothenburg and one doctor at the centre for evidence-based dermatology at the University of Nottingham were asked to explain how they conduct focus groups and what educational form they used in their groups.

Video interview – CT participant
A video interview with a paediatric trial participant was conducted to be used as a part of the educational material. This was an idea proposed in the interviews on how to conduct and educate focus groups. The interviewed girl was Swedish, aged 14 years, highly motivated and with several years of trial experience in a growth hormone study. She consented to the film potentially being used as education material. The questions that were asked were the same as those used in the interviews of parent and paediatric patients.

Focus groups - clinicians and nurses
Clinicians and nurses in two focus groups were asked to speak freely from their own experience of the consent process and what parts in the process that might be hard to understand. The purpose was to understand what they felt was missing in the consent process, the parents' lack of knowledge when consenting to their child's participation and to encourage self-criticism. All of them had several years of experience, working in different CTs at the Queen Silvia Children's Hospital in Gothenburg. They welcomed the opportunity to share their knowledge from CTs before giving their view of the initial draft education material.

The first focus group consisted of clinicians and nurses from the department of endocrinology. They were all experienced from running paediatric CTs such as growth hormone and diabetes trials and had extensive experience of recruiting patients; they were completely familiar with the information that is provided in the informed consent process. They felt that their way to inform the parents and patients was adequate and they explained that they encourage them to ask questions in connection to the information. They admitted that sometimes, if they are in a hurry or if the parents ask for more time, they let the parents take the consent form home to read properly. However, both the clinicians and nurses agreed to that in these cases, some of the information might not be considered thoroughly or even read, which means that some of the concepts are not fully appreciated by the parents. This might result in parents consenting with some parts not clearly explained and feeling taken by surprised.

The clinicians and nurses proposed from their own experience what information is not fully understood by parents, which might be of importance in the education material. They stated that one of the greatest factors to empower the patients is to clearly explain the advantages of being in a trial, such as benefiting research in order to produce quality drugs adapted for children in different stages of physiological development and to explain the deficient knowledge about drug interactions that differ in children and adults.

Also, educating parents and patients about adverse events and the adverse event reporting procedures is of importance. Families, they reported, seem to be unaware of why this is conducted and do not understand the importance. Also, the safety of a paediatric participant is a critical aspect to be mentioned in the empowerment process that might not be totally explained in the consent form.

The group confirmed what the literature already stated, what the families in the interviews said, and what the teenage groups later expressed: that the main benefit of participating in a study is seen as the chance to get a new medicine more rapidly by being randomised to the test drug arm of the trial.

The second group consisted of clinicians and nurses at the department of cystic fibrosis. The group was different from the endocrinology group, in that they have a close relationship to their patients throughout their lifetime, which makes it easier to encourage them to participate in trials. They reported a low dropout rate and attributed this to the close relationship between the patient and the medical team. The group stated that the verbal information that is given during the informed consent process is mostly understood by the parents who will ask the questions they need to ask to enable them to understand.

To show the differences in the recruitment-process, the situation of being a patient at the department of oncology was brought as an example of opposite characteristics. A family of a patient, with a newly diagnosed cancer who arrives at the hospital without being familiar to the medical research team, does not have the same ability to consider participation since this adds one more decision to their agenda and there is limited time for the clinicians to be able to inform the parents truly and to establish a sense of trust. This might limit the parent's ability to make that decision, which slows the oncology trial recruitment significantly.

Both these situations are extreme in both ways and therefore, the group stated that it is not clear that any family in this predicament is in a position to be helped by additional education. They stated that the patients who have been in several trials get 'study-fatigue' and are thereby not always able to participate, but not because of fear of adverse drug reactions, which leaves the medical team to persuade them that it is necessary to participate in paediatric trials.

One study nurse reported that healthy children recruited to a trial performing gastrointestinal examinations had no regrets since they felt they were treated with a special status. To elevate the importance of being trial participants might be an empowering tool.

10.2.3 Development of the educational material

Figure 15: Steps of the study

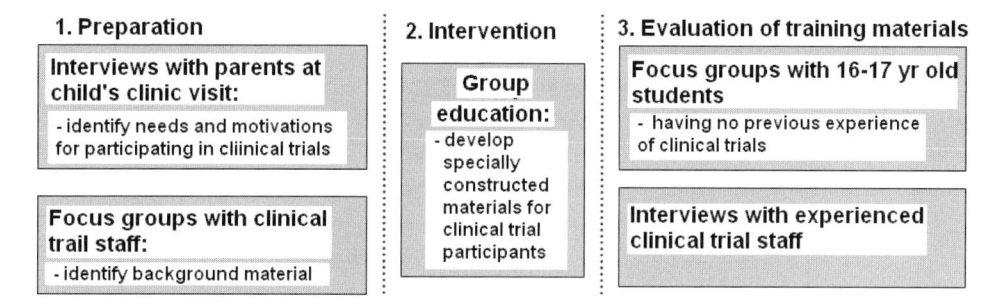

1. Preparation	2. Intervention	3. Evaluation of training materials
Interviews with parents at child's clinic visit: - identify needs and motivations for participating in clinical trials	**Group education:** - develop specially constructed materials for clinical trial participants	**Focus groups with 16-17 yr old students** - having no previous experience of clinical trials
Focus groups with clinical trail staff: - identify background material		**Interviews with experienced clinical trial staff**

Based on the literature survey and the interview and focus group material collected from children, parents and clinical staff, an education package was constructed and piloted with experienced clinical staff to evaluate the content, degree of difficulty and effectiveness. See **Appendix 3a** for the education material.

The educational material was then presented to Swedish secondary school pupils in two groups. They also completed a questionnaire on their attitudes to CTs before and after the presentation of the educational material.

The responses from these two perspectives (CT staff and teenagers) were used to evaluate whether additional education is powerful as an empowering method complementing the standard informed consent procedures, to facilitate the decision process.

10.2.4 Evaluation of the educational material

Evaluation by clinicians
The same educational material that was used in the teenager groups was presented to physicians and nurses from the endocrinology and cystic fibrosis departments. After receiving the oral presentation, the material was openly evaluated without standard questions.

They confirmed that it covered the main issues, though they suggested that trained health educators would be needed to present it. Interestingly, they expressed concern that this kind of education might be discouraging to participation in paediatric CTs.

The material was evaluated as understandable but that some information still might be too technical and the group agreed that education material in addition to the consent might increase the parents' and patients' knowledge about CTs, leading them to give a voluntary consent. Nonetheless, as stated by some of the nurses in the group, the drawbacks were that being aware of all investigations, details and aspects of a CT might lower the ratio of trial participants, since the consenter has the possibility to re-think their decision and weigh their choice against the risks of possible adverse drug reactions or the extra time spent at the hospital.

The clinicians and nurses did not, however, think that empowerment might slow the recruiting process but rather that it would increase the parents' and patients' autonomy to accept or decline trial participation. This might lead to a higher proportion of patients declining participation, but this would be compensated by fewer of the participating patients withdrawing because of insufficient knowledge about the importance of conducting paediatric research.

They also proposed that informed consent, given according to standard regulations, might be enough in the cases where the parents and patients have time to read the form are well informed and have sufficient time to answer.

Piloting the education material with teenager focus groups
Two focus groups were held with 42 teenagers (21 in each group). They were 16-17 year old students who were all studying the natural sciences program. Approximately 50% were boys and 50% girls. In this group a simple questionnaire was used, evaluating adolescents' thoughts about issues in the informed consent process. The teenagers were all free to discuss their thoughts among themselves before they answered the questions by raising an arm.

To establish the teenagers' knowledge about CTs, they all got to answer the question *"Do you know what a clinical trial is?"* One teenager in the first group was able to define some parts of what a trial is, but mixed it up with animal testing in the pre-clinical phase. No one in the second group had ever heard about the concept or the expression *clinical trial* and required a brief explanation of the subject. Their attitude was mostly neutral when given the first questionnaire.

In the second step, the educational material was presented in a 25-minute education session. The teenagers were highly engaged by the material and discussed openly the ethical dilemma surrounding the consenting process. Several of the teenagers expressed a dislike of copious texts and felt that an education session would reduce this stress factor.

After the presentation, the teenagers were asked again to explain the concept of a CT. All 42 reported that they understood the basic principles of a CT. To confirm if the presentation that was used was comprehensible, the groups had to define a CT in their own words. Both groups of participants were able to identify a CT as a study to evaluate the efficacy and safety of a test drug, to be able to develop a drug with good quality and adequate safety.

The discussions continued to examine the teenagers' attitude towards children in CTs. In the first group, all 21 participants had a positive attitude towards paediatric medical research in comparison to the second group, where 16 of 21 agreed with this.

The reasons for encouragement were given in both groups as:
1) the possibility to receive careful observation more frequently, the extra care and to be able to contact the trial clinician 24 hours a day;
2) a chance to be randomised to a candidate-treatment;
3) the significance for children to contribute to other children's medical health.

This factor was actually voted as first priority in the second group. Even those who were not positive to CTs were able to agree with this advantage (Figure 16). Since no one was able to recognise the concept of a CT in the beginning, no-one prioritised media or other resources as a factor affecting attitudes towards CTs. Also, no one had other explanations for why they were positive.

Figure 16: Reasons for positive attitudes to paediatric CTs

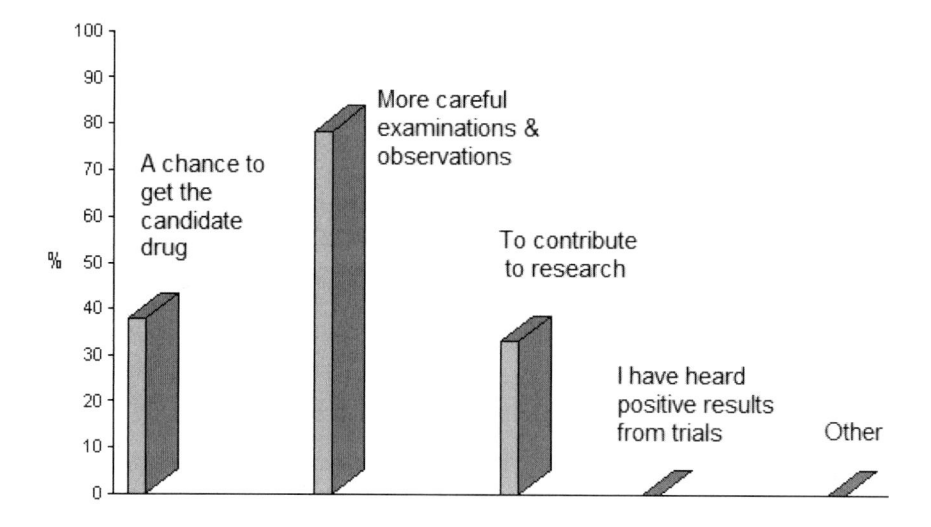

Sixteen per cent had a negative attitude to CTs conducted in children. The reasons for this were discussed and prioritised according to the following: 1) the main-reason was that they did not think that children should be treated as a 'guinea pig' in research. 2) They were not keen on the idea of children being placed at risk of adverse drug reactions (Figure 17).

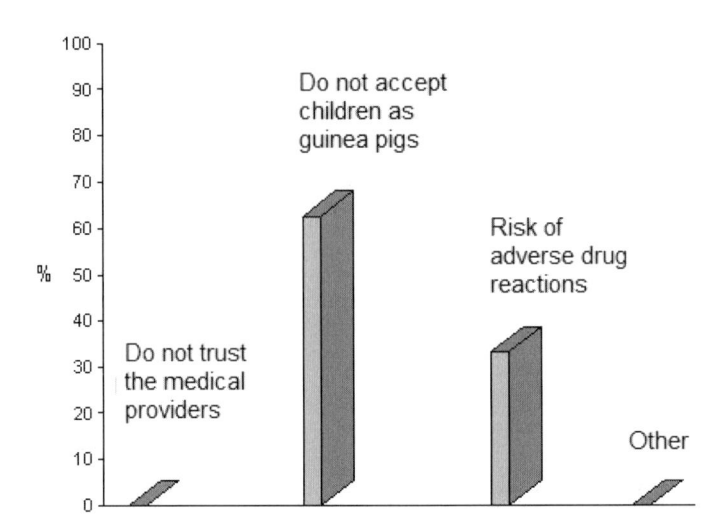

Figure 17: Reasons for negative attitudes to paediatric CTs

The next test was for the teenagers to imagine themselves having a disease, getting a request to participate in a CT of a test drug that in the best case would benefit them or other people with the same conditions. The groups were asked if they would say yes or no to this. The first group included nine teenagers willing to say yes. 1) The main reason was to contribute to the medical research, since there were no guarantees. 2) According to this group, an important motivation to participate was the extra care that a trial provides. 3) They considered hope to receive the candidate important but stated that this was just an extra advantage, since not all get the drug being developed.

All participants agreed that altruism was the most important factor when considering consenting, regardless of whether or not they would say yes. Twelve participants in the first group declined participation with the reasons: 1) having an illness would make them both physiologically and psychologically drained, and being exposed to additional tests with more visits would probably exhaust them and therefore they would be concerned about the illness worsening.

The second group was of another opinion. None of them could decide if they would decline or participate. They all agreed that it depends on 1) the severity of the disease, 2) the availability of adequate drugs and 3) the test drug's proposed efficacy compared to the standard drug. However; they all agreed that the fear of adverse drug reactions and the extra visits were the reasons for not participating if they were hesitant. About half of the group said that they would put their own interests first when participating in a CT, hoping to get the test drug, and half the group stated they would do it for altruistic reasons.

Both groups agreed that educational material in addition to informed consent would make it easier to decide about potential participation. Especially a brief and simple education was desirable in hurried situations, as some of the teenagers expressed their dislike of copious texts being an additional stress factor. Some of their proposals for desired additions to the information they got in the education session are presented below:

- Statistical frequency of severe adverse drug reactions.
- Actual number of paediatric drugs that are authorised after phase III.
- The opportunity to talk with other participants or to see an interview with a participant.

10.2.5 Conclusions

The RESPECT project did not set out to find ways to convince parents to consent to their child's trial participation in a CT; rather, the aim was to investigate the needs and motivation of paediatric patients and their parents who will or have participated in a CT that underlie the informed consent process and possible trial participation in order to empower them in their voluntary choice.

Even though the informed consent process is strictly regulated to enable the consenter to make a voluntary decision, human factors such as the clinician's ability to provide information and the strenuous difficulties involved in taking a decision concerning someone else might lower the learning capability of the parent. We have seen that some aspects of the information in the informed consent process are not easily absorbed by the parents. In some cases, not all of the information has been provided during this process and some aspects of the study come as a surprise to the child and even to the parents.

With this in mind, additional education to the informed consent process as an empowering method was developed and evaluated in pilot focus groups. The conclusions are that some defined groups of parents might need or appreciate additional education about CTs as an empowering tool to be able to make an autonomous decision. This might decrease the frequency of withdrawal, increase compliance and develop a positive attitude toward future trial participation.

This pilot study indicates that education for potential CT participants would make it easier to decide about potential participation in a CT. It is thus an empowering tool. However, substantial research in this area is needed in terms of defining which groups of parents may benefit from training as an empowering tool when considering consent. It is also recommended that specially constructed materials should be presented by a health educator as a valuable addition to CT routines.

11 Best practice examples of empowering children

This chapter gives brief notes and links to projects and organisations that have worked towards empowering families in paediatric CTs. The examples are categorised into the four areas of empowerment - Self-determination, Accountability, Cooperation, and Knowledge.

11.1 Self-determination

MRC CTU
The Medical Research Council's Clinical Trials Unit (MRC CTU) is one of the UK's leading centres for clinical research. On their website, they provide information in accessible language on each trial they run. In addition, they give advice on self-referral to a trial.
http://www.ctu.mrc.ac.uk/

MCRN
In 2006 the UK Medicines for Children Research Network (MCRN), with support from the National Children's Bureau (NCB), set up a pilot Children and Young Person's Advisory Group, to explore how children and young people could be involved and have their say in the design of clinical research. The pilot group, based in Liverpool, was such a success that the group was re-launched with more children and young people. It currently has 15 members aged between 8 and 19 years old. The group has been a great success and one particular accolade of the group is that is has provided invaluable advice to researchers, including the pharmaceutical industry, on various stages of their research design. It has, for example, offered views on patient information leaflets for children; developed guidance for researchers designing patient information leaflets; worked with researchers on the design of interview schedules; offered opinions about various study websites; and helped with the design of leaflets to promote the work of MCRN.
http://www.mcrn.org.uk/

PEAR
PEAR (Public health, Education, Awareness, Research) was a UK National Children's Bureau Research Centre project supporting young people's involvement in public health research. The project ran from 2008-2010, supported by the Wellcome Trust. The PEAR group was made up of 20 young people, aged 13-18.

The project supported young people to contribute to UK public health research and decisions being made about public health issues by:
- Helping young people to learn about public health research and policy (policy is what the government is saying and doing about public health issues)
- Supporting young people to share their views and priorities about public health research and policy
- Supporting young people to explain and publicise research findings to other young people
- Helping young people to explain to other young people what research is saying and how things might affect them.

http://www.ncb.org.uk/pear

Centre of Evidence Based Dermatology: A CTs network eliciting outcome measures
By gathering rich information from patients in CTs, it is possible to use this information when stipulating the significant outcomes to measure in future trials for the same disorder. Some CT groups are already doing this, for example, the Centre of Evidence Based Dermatology:

We spoke with staff at the UK Dermatology Clinical Trials Network. This network is a good example of getting nearer to the patient by identifying patient outcomes that are important to the patient themselves when conducting CTs. They report that the typical CT protocol does not specify recording the outcomes described by the patient in their words. Their classification of what is an adverse event is unclear to clinicians and is not defined as a patient adverse outcome.
http://www.nottingham.ac.uk/scs/divisions/evidencebaseddermatology/

11.2 Accountability

11.2.1 Making requirements on researchers

Asthma UK
In 2009, Asthma UK introduced greater involvement of lay people in their grant round process. They now have a group of lay reviewers and lay members of a Research Review Panel who comment on and score all grant applications.

Asthma UK requires scientists to include a lay description of their research in all funding applications. These 'plain English' lay abstracts play a vital role in helping Asthma UK fund research that is relevant and important to people with asthma. Asthma UK's lay reviewers are there to comment on the relevance of the research to people affected by asthma and, for example, the practicalities of recruiting and involving participants.

Lay reviewers are not expected to comment on the science – this is the role of the peer reviewers and scientific members of the Research Review Panel. Therefore, it is vitally important that a lay abstract passes the *'so what?'* test and communicate why the research is important to people with asthma.

Asthma UK requires that researchers fulfil certain criteria before they will assist them in recruiting participants. The application must show, among other things, the benefit of the research to people living with asthma in the UK, who will conduct the research and how they will communicate with the participants. Once the results of the research are publicly available, they must provide a summary of the outcomes in easy-to-read, jargon-free language, appropriate to the needs of the participants. If the research study is a drug trial, participants should be given clear information about whether or not they are likely to be able to access this drug after the research study has been completed.
http://www.asthma.org.uk/

Parent Involvement in the MCRN Study Assessment Committee
The MCRN Study Assessment Committee meets to consider studies put forward for inclusion within the portfolio of studies that MCRN has adopted and provides support to.

Included on the Committee are five parent/carers all of whom have some experience of either looking after a sick child or being involved in the clinical research process. Their role is:
- to provide a parent/carer perspective, based on personal experience as a parent/carer of a sick child and/or a user of health services;
- to make suggestions, if applicable, on how the study might be improved, particularly in relation to requirements made of children and their parents/carers.

They are sent research applications to review for these issues:
- What is the level of parental involvement in the study design?
- Is the study design ethically sound?
- Does the research address an important and relevant question?
- Is the outcome measure relevant to families, and is it meaningful?
- Are there any concerns from a consumer point of view about the methods used in a study? Are they suitable for children and young people?

The James Lind Alliance
The James Lind Alliance (named after a pioneer of CTs in the 1700s) is a not-for-profit initiative funded by the UK Department of Health and the Medical Research Council. It was established in 2004 to bring patients and clinicians together to agree priorities in treatment uncertainty research. The Alliance's work is based on evidence that a research agenda set in the traditional way - purely by researchers or research funders – can fail to recognise the wishes of those who are ill or those caring for or treating them.

In 2010, the James Lind Alliance published a step-by-step Guidebook in the form of an online resource to enable patients, clinicians or the groups that represent them to ensure that research is grounded in what matters to them jointly. The Guidebook sets out how to:

- establish a Priority Setting Partnership
- involve patients and clinicians
- identify treatment uncertainties
- work with the UK Database of Uncertainties about the Effects of Treatments (UK DUETs)
- prioritise treatment uncertainties
- take priorities to research funders.

Drawn together from five years experience of patient/clinician partnerships in a range of conditions, the Guidebook offers practical advice about and the full protocol for all parts of the priority setting process. It includes templates for questionnaires, terms of reference, draft agendas, and other materials based on case studies of different models of Priority Setting Partnerships. The Guidebook also offers research evidence of why patient and clinician involvement in research priority setting is important, and provides supporting documentation, publications, links and resources.

On the launch of the guidebook, the co-founder of the James Lind Alliance - Sir Iain Chalmers - commented: 'It is surprising how difficult it is to find out how research funders decide what research to fund. What is clear is that patients, carers and ordinary 'jobbing' clinicians are only very rarely involved in these processes. That is probably one of the reasons that the little evidence there is reveals mismatches between the questions that interest researchers and the questions that interest patients and clinicians. The James Lind Alliance Guidebook will help people who want to try to bridge those gaps.'
http://www.jlaguidebook.org/
http://www.lindalliance.org/

11.3 Cooperation

11.3.1 Young patients as research partners

Not Just a Phase
An example of a report advocating cooperation between the patient and researcher is the Not Just a Phase guide, which places the patient as a member of the research team.

Not Just a Phase is a guide to the participation of children and young people in health services and has been developed and published by the Young People's Health Special Interest Group of the Royal College of Paediatrics and Child Health. The guide is designed primarily for paediatricians, senior children's nurses and leaders of organisations which provide general and specialised health services for children and young people. Not Just a Phase practically demonstrates how a culture of participation can be created. The guide points out that it is only through meaningful participation of children and young people that a platform can be created which can influence services and resource allocation. Although the focus of this project was on participation in health care the same process of participation can apply to development of medicines.

This guide had a positive effect on empowerment. Following a presentation of the 'Not Just a Phase' guide to the PDCO by a representative of the Royal College of Paediatrics and Child Health (RCPCH) in January 2011, the PDCO agreed:

- To increase contacts with families representatives
- To support a direct role of children at the EMA and PDCO
- To invite research groups and patients associations to provide proposal on children and parents involvement in CTs
- To identify groups and organisations willing to collaborate in this exercise.

http://www.rcpch.ac.uk/

Listening to Children
Listening to Children is a ten-week training course designed for those who work with children and young people and want to improve their skills of research and consultation. Run by the Centre for Research on Families and Relationships (CRFR), it involves a combination of online

learning and classroom sessions based at the University of Edinburgh. The Listening to Children training is also available as a bespoke option for organisations in a variety of formats.
http://www.crfr.ac.uk/cpd/listeningtochildren/

INVOLVE
INVOLVE was established in 1996 and is part of, and funded by, the UK National Institute for Health Research, to support active public involvement in NHS, public health and social care research. It is one of the few Government-funded programmes of its kind in the world. This national advisory group brings together expertise, insight and experience in the field of public involvement in research, with the aim of advancing it as an essential part of the process by which research is designed, conducted and disseminated.

In 2004, the INVOLVE Support Unit published A Guide to Actively Involving Young People in *Research: For researchers, research commissioners, and managers* by Perpetua Kirby, including input from seventeen young people in two workshops:
http://www.conres.co.uk/pdfs/Involving_Young_People_in_Research_151104_FINAL.pdf
http://www.invo.org.uk/

Participation Works
Participation Works is a partnership of six UK children and young people's agencies that enables organisations to effectively involve children and young people in the development, delivery and evaluation of services that affect their lives.

In 2009 they produced a Guide How to involve children and young people in research:

> 'This guide is about why and how to actively involve young people as researchers within health and social care research. It is about how to **actively involve** them, not as subjects of research and development, but as **partners** in the various stages of research, from commissioning, to evaluation and dissemination. We think it will help professionals to meet article 12 of the UN Convention on the Rights of the Child (ratified by the UK in 1991) which asserts that children and young people should be involved in all decisions affecting their lives.'

http://www.participationworks.org.uk/resources/how-to-involve-children-and-young-people-in-research

NIHR Clinical Research Network Coordinating Centre
The UK Department of Health has a strong commitment to patient and public involvement in many National Health Service (NHS) activities. Of particular interest is the organisation responsible for clinical research, the National Institute for Health Research (NIHR), which invites lay involvement, see Figure 18. These principles have also been adopted by the MCRN for clinical research on children.

The Clinical Research Networks are part of the NIHR and the UK Clinical Research Collaboration. The Networks believe that active patient and public involvement is needed if it is to encourage research that directly benefits and reflects the needs and views of patients and the public. They enable patients and public members to work with researcher professionals and clinicians (e.g. doctors, nurses) and get actively involved in the different stages of research and associated activities. This means research being done with members of the public, not to, about or for them, thus making sure that clinical research is relevant, useful and to the benefit of the public.

Figure 18: The National Institute for Health Research principles for lay involvement in research.

Getting involved in research activities

Many patients and public members work with researcher professionals and clinicians (e.g. doctors, nurses) and get actively involved in the different stages of research and associated activities.

Active involvement in clinical research is very different from being a participant in a study. It means:
- research done with members of the public, not to, about or for them
- getting involved in the research process or activity itself
- making sure that clinical research is relevant, useful and to the benefit of the public.

There are a range of activities that patients and public members may be able to get involved in, with opportunity to choose what interests them. Examples include:
- Helping to identify research that is important and relevant
- Helping to choose important topics for research
- Helping to develop patient information leaflets
- Helping to support a research project or advisory group as a member
- Helping to develop accessible information and research news
- Helping to support and promote good research

Getting actively involved can lead to:
- More relevant research questions being asked resulting in more useful research
- More sensitive approaches to people who take part in studies as 'participants'
- Helping to keep the research on track
- Greater opportunities to share research news with patients and the public.

Patients and the public may benefit from being actively involved:
- By having a say in research
- Through sharing their experience
- By getting research started that is important to them
- By learning more about research activities

---

http://www.crncc.nihr.ac.uk/ppi
http://www.nihr.ac.uk/

Stakeholder Action Group: the DEPICTED study 2010
An example of cooperation was found in the development of a research protocol for an intervention study of diabetes care. The DEPICTED research team (Lowes et al., 2010) initiated a Stakeholder Action Group (SAG) to advise on the formulation of the intervention intended to be more inclusive of the patient's perspective. The SAG advised on the development of the intervention and on a study to evaluate the intervention. The SAG was responsible for the review of evidence provided by the team and for suggesting how the research could be carried out. Members of the SAG were children and young people with type 1 diabetes and their families. Recruitment of members was restricted to people outside of the research team's catchment area to safeguard confidentiality issues and professional relationships. Parents could attend with or without their children. A member of the children's PO was also included. The professional members of the SAG represented all the professional roles that would be involved in the intervention: paediatricians, specialist diabetes nurses, dieticians, psychologists and social workers. The research team included clinical and scientific researchers and administrators.

The SAG met on three occasions over a 10-month period, each meeting being a full day of small group and plenary sessions discussing various aspects of the intervention and research. The SAG small group membership varied in relation to the questions to be considered. So that the lay and professional groups were mixed to consider some questions and separated to discuss others before coming together in the plenary sessions. All stakeholders received reimbursement for their travel expenses, and the lay stakeholders received payment to compensate for time spent. Newsletters were circulated between meetings to update participants on the progress of the research. The stakeholder discussions were audio- recorded and the transcripts analysed.

The SAG meetings were attended by between 13 and 17 lay stakeholders and 10 or 11 professional stakeholders. In addition, there were approximately 14 research team members. The DEPICTED study benefited from the advice provided by the SAG in several key areas, which have been described in the literature (Lowes et al., 2010). In summary, the SAG was evaluated positively with both lay and professional stakeholders reporting value from the joint meetings. The study demonstrated that other research activities could benefit from early involvement of lay stakeholders who had opportunities to contribute to the formation of the research and not just the identification of research topics.

11.3.2 Pharmaceutical companies giving public access to their CT results

Genzyme
Some pharmaceutical companies are committed to transparency and make their results available on their public websites. A good example is Genzyme, whose clinical research program is focused on rare inherited disorders, kidney disease, orthopaedics, cancer, transplant, and immune disease. It also conducts research in cardiovascular disease, neurodegenerative diseases, and other areas of unmet medical need.

Genzyme acts on the belief that access to information is a vital aspect of quality health care and the company has a longstanding commitment to providing health care professionals and patients with the information they need about Genzyme products to make informed medical decisions.

As part of their commitment to transparency throughout the biotechnology and pharmaceutical industries regarding drug-development information, they have posted information about ongoing and completed CTs on their website since 2005 to ensure that physicians and patients can easily obtain all relevant information about the investigational products they are developing.
http://www.genzymeclinicalresearch.com/

11.4 Knowledge

HealthTalkOnline[1]: Parents and children describing their experience of CTs
HealthTalkOnline (part of NSUHR, an international Network to Support Understanding of Health Research) has an area of its website that presents video and textual resources describing the experiences of children and parents of taking part in CTs. Their experiences are put into context by textual description of key issues and background.

Users can choose to watch each individual's story or browse excerpts under the following topic headings:
- Why do we have clinical trials in children and young people?
- Information parents receive when invited to enrol their child
- Involving children in decisions: child assent
- Reasons for wanting your child to take part: child's health
- When the trial ends: feedback of trial results
- Parents messages to health professionals

Interviews with 29 parents were conducted across the country with the aim of gaining a broad range of experiences. Children had taken part in a variety of trials ranging from vaccine trials, drug trials, gene therapy, and screening trials to diet and behaviour management, and a variety of designs including randomised placebo controlled trials, blinded trials, and a Phase 1 trial. The main reason for giving consent was the opportunity to improve their child's health and protect their child. However, parents were also thinking about helping to improve the treatment and care of other children and helping medical research and enhance knowledge.

Sometimes taking part was not an easy decision to make. For example, one parent describes the difficulty of enrolling her child in a placebo controlled drug trial, yet knowing that until the trial is complete no one knows which treatment is best. In addition to receiving personal feedback, receiving the overall outcome of trials was important; as one parent suggested, *"it gives you a sense of being part of a wider community rather than just a number or a box that you tick."* They wanted to know if their child's contribution had made a difference. It was also important for many parents that their children received some feedback too, thus valuing their contribution.

In addition to parents' experiences, interviews with 32 young people, aged 10 to 23 years, were conducted to gain their experiences of being invited to take part in CTs. These interviews can be

---

[1] This information about the HealthTalkOnline project was kindly provided by Louise Locock, Deputy Research Director at the Health Experiences Research Group, University of Oxford.

viewed on the sister website: youthhealthtalk.org. Young people took part in a range of trials including vaccine trials, drug trials, gene therapy trials, and information and psychological trials and research. Young people wanted to take part in trials for a mix of reasons including helping to improve their health, helping other people in the future who may be diagnosed with the same or similar condition, and helping increase knowledge and understanding about conditions. Some young people took part in double-blinded trials that involved a placebo that for a few felt "a bit weird – and a bit worrying", and for a few was "a risky strategy". Despite these initial concerns, young people said the doctors and nurses explained everything about the trial and answered any questions they had and this was very reassuring for young people. In particular, many young people wanted to know about side effects "no matter how horrible they are": openness and honesty was important to young people. On the whole, young people were supportive of CTs in children and young people; they said they would take part in similar trials in the future, yet many found it difficult to describe what a CT is.

The healthtalkonline.org and youthhealthtalk.org websites can be used to help improve understanding about CTs in children and young people, what can be expected when invited to take part in trials, what it means to be randomised or allocated to a treatment group, what is involved and what happens at the end of trials. Watching and listening to other parents' and young people's experiences can help others who may be in similar situations and know that they are not alone.
http://www.healthtalkonline.org/medical_research/clinical_trials_parents
http://www.youthhealthtalk.org/Clinical_trials_in_children_and_young_people/

NHLBI/NIH: 'No More Hand-Me-Down Research'
The NHLBI/NIH (National Heart Lung and blood Institute/National Institute of Health, USA) website is an example of a resource which leads to greater empowerment. Their emphasis is on the need for more paediatric research and a demand that children should no longer have to rely on medicines developed for adults: 'No More Hand-Me-Down Research'. This web site focuses on the **knowledge** element of empowerment providing information about being in a trial. The website also provides information leading to skill development, which is necessary for a **cooperative relationship** such as how to find reliable information and who's who in the research team, which can help to level the balance between the participant and the researcher. There are also videos of children who have participated in CTs describing the positive aspects of participation. It is a good example of information at the right level given in an appropriate format. The website demonstrates that children do understand what they are being asked to do in a CT and the message is that CT procedures should incorporate the child's views and needs to a much larger extent than currently happens.
http://www.nhlbi.nih.gov/childrenandclinicalstudies/index.php
http://www.nhlbi.nih.gov/childrenandclinicalstudies/whatkidssay.php

12 References

Appelbaum, P.S., Roth, L.H., Lidz, C. (1982). The therapeutic misconception: Informed consent in psychiatric research. *International Journal of Law and Psychiatry* 1982;5(3-4):319–29.

Altavilla, A., Giaquinto, C., Ceci, A. (2008). European survey on ethical and legal framework of clinical trials in paediatrics: results and perspectives. *J Int Bioethique* 2008;19(3):17-48, 121–2

Altavilla, A., Giaquinto, C., Giocanti, D., Manfredi, C., Aboulker, J.P., Bartoloni, F., et al. (2009). Activity of ethics committees in Europe on issues related to clinical trials in paediatrics: Results of a survey. *Pharmaceuticals Policy and Law* 2009;11(1,2):79–87

Altavilla, A., Manfredi, C., Baiardi, P., Dehlinger-Kremer, M., Galletti, P., Alemany Pozuelo, A., Chaplin, J. & Ceci, A. (2012). Impact of the new European Paediatric Regulatory framework on ethics committees: overview and perspectives. *Acta Paediatrica*, Jan; 101(1) E27-E32. .

British Medical Association (2001). Consent, rights and choices in health care for children and young people. BMJ Books: London.

Brody, J., Annett, R., Scherer, D., Perryman, M. & Cofrin, K. (2005). Comparisons of Adolescent and Parent Willingness to Participate in Minimal and Above Minimal Risk Pediatric Asthma Research Protocols. *Journal of Adolescent Health*, **37**, 229–235.

Broome, M., Richards, D. & Hall, J. (2001). Children in Research: The Experience of Ill Children and Adolescents. *Journal of Family Nursing*, **7**, 32–49.

Bullinger, M.., Globe, D., Wasserman, J., Young, N.L. & von Mackensen S. (2009). Challenges of patient-reported outcome assessment in hemophilia care — a state of the art review. *Value Health*. 2009 Jul-Aug;12(5):808–20. PubMed PMID: 19490552.

Caldwell. P., Butow, P. & Craig, J. (2003). Parents' attitudes to children's participation in randomized controlled trials. *The Journal of Pediatrics*, **142**, 554–9.

Ceci, A., Giaquinto, C., Aboulker, J.P., Baiardi, P., Bonifazi, F., Della Pasqua, O., Nicolosi, A., Taruscio, D., Sturkenboom, M., & Wong, I. (2009). The Task-force in Europe for Drug Development for the Young (TEDDY) Network of Excellence. *Paediatr Drugs* 11(1):18–21.

CESP (2005). Regulation on new medical products for paediatric patients - Statement from the paediatricians in Europe, 8 June 2005.
http://www.eapaediatrics.eu/index.php?option=com_content&view=article&id=98&Itemid=104 (accessed 5 April 2012).

Chantler, T., Lees, A., Moxon, E., Mant, D., Pollard, A. & Fiztpatrick R. (2007). The Role Familiarity With Science and Medicine Plays in Parents' Decision Making About Enrolling a Child in Vaccine Research. *Qualitative Health Research*, **17**, 311–22.

Chappuy, H., Doz, F., Blanche, S., Gentet, J. & Treluyer, J. (2007). Children's views on their involvement in clinical research. *Pediatric Blood & Cancer*, **50**, 1043–6.

Choonara, I. & Conroy, S. (2002). Unlicensed and off-label drug use in children: implications for safety. *Drug Saf,* 25(1), 1–5.

Clarke, S,A, & Eiser, C, (2004). The measurement of health-related quality of life (QOL) in paediatric clinical trials: a systematic review. *Health Qual Life Outcomes*. 2004; 2: 66. Published online 2004 November 22. doi: 10.1186/1477-7525-2-66

Clarkson, A. & Choonara, I. (2002). Surveillance for fatal suspected adverse drug reactions in the UK. *Archives of Disease in Childhood,* 87(6), 462–66.

Commission of the European Communities. Commission Directive 2005/28/EC of 8 April 2005 laying down principles and detailed guidelines for good clinical practice as regards investigational medicinal products for human use, as well as the requirements for authorisation of the manufacturing or importation of such products. *Official Journal of the European Union* 9.4.2005; L91:13–19

Conroy, S., McIntyre, J., Choonara, I. & Stephenson, T. (2000). Drug trials in children: problems and the way forward. *British Journal of Clinical Pharmacology*, 49, 93–7.

Council of Europe (1997). Convention on Human Rights and Biomedicine. Strasbourg 1997. Entry into force in 1999

Council of Europe (2007). Additional Protocol to the Convention on Human Rights and Biomedicine, concerning Biomedical Research. Strasbourg 2005. Entry into force in 2007

Cressey, D. (2012). Informed consent on trial. *Nature* 482, 16 (02 February 2012) doi:10.1038/482016a. http://www.nature.com/news/informed-consent-on-trial-1.9933 (accessed 10 April 2012).

Crom, D., Tyc, V., Rai, S., Deng, X., Hudson, M., Booth, A., Rodrigues, L., Zhang, L., Mccammon, E. & Kaste, S. (2006). Retention of survivors of acute lymphoblastic leukemia in a longitudinal study of bone mineral density. *Journal of Child Health Care*, **10**, 337–50.

Dolan, L., Sabesan, V., Weinstein, S. & Spratt, K. (2008). Preference Assessment of Recruitment into a Randomized Trial for Adolescent Idiopathic Scoliosis. *The Journal of Bone and Joint Surgery (American)*, **90**, 2594–2605.

Easterbrook, P.J. & Matthews, D.R. (1992). Fate of research studies. *Journal of the Royal Society of Medicine*, 85(2), 71–6.

Easton, K.L., Parsons, B.J., Starr, M, & Brien, J.E. (1998). The incidence of drug-related problems as a cause of hospital admissions in children. *Med J Aust.* 1998 Oct 5;169(7):356–9.

Eiser, C., Davies, H., Jenney, M. & Glaser, A. (2005). Mothers' attitudes to the randomized controlled trial (RCT): the case of acute lymphoblastic leukaemia (ALL) in children. *Child: Care, Health and Development*, 31, 517–23.

Elberse, J.E., Caron-Flinterman, F., & Broerse, J.E.W. (2010). Patient-expert partnerships in research: how to stimulate inclusion of patient perspectives. *Health Expectations*, 14, 225–39.

Erickson, P., Willke, R. & Burke, L. (2009). A concept taxonomy and an instrument hierarchy: Tools for establishing and evaluating the conceptual framework of a patient-reported outcome (pro) instrument as applied to product labeling claims. *Value Health*, 12(8), 1158–67

European Commission Enterprise Directorate General (2002). Better Medicines for Children. Proposed regulatory actions on paediatric medicinal products. Consultation document. Brussels 2002

European Commission Directorate-General for Health and Consumers (2008). Ethical considerations for clinical trials on medicinal products conducted with the paediatric population. Recommendations of the ad hoc group for the development of implementing guidelines for Directive 2001/20/EC relating to good clinical practice in the conduct of clinical trials on medicinal products for human use. http://ec.europa.eu/health/files/eudralex/vol-10/ethical_considerations_en.pdf (accessed 9 Jan 2012).

European Forum for Good Clinical Practice (EFGCP) Ethics Working Party (2010). The Procedure for the Ethical Review of Protocols for Clinical Research Projects in the European Union. Last update April 2010. http://www.efgcp.be/EFGCPReports.asp?L1=5&L2=1 (Accessed 9 Jan 2012.)

European Medicines Agency. (2002) ICH Topic E 6 (R1) Guideline for Good Clinical Practice. http://www.emea.europa.eu/pdfs/human/ich/013595en.pdf (accessed 9 Jan 2012).

European Parliament and the Council of the European Union (2001). Directive 2001/20/EC of the European Parliament and of the Council of 4 April 2001 on the approximation of the laws, regulations and administrative provisions of the Member States relating to the implementation of good clinical practice in the conduct of clinical trials on medicinal products for human use. *Official Journal of the European Union* 1.5.2001; L121:34–44

European Parliament and the Council of the European Union (2006a). Regulation (EC) No 1901/2006 of the European Parliament and of the Council of 12 December 2006 on medicinal products for paediatric use and amending Regulation (EEC) No 1768/92, Directive 2001/20/EC, Directive 2001/83/EC and Regulation (EC) No 726/2004. *Official Journal of the European Union* 27.12.2006; L378:1–19.

European Parliament and the Council of the European Union (2006b). Regulation (EC) No. 1902/2006 of the European Parliament and of the Council of 20 December 2006 amending

Regulation 1901/2006 on medicinal products for paediatric use. *Official Journal of the European Union* 27.12.2006; L378:20–21

EURORDIS (2010). Q&A on off-label use of medicines (4 Nov 2010). http://download.eurordis.org/europlan/3_EURORDIS_Guidance_Documents_for_the_National_Conference/off-label_use_of_medicines_final.pdf (accessed 9 Jan 2012).

Fernandez, C.V., Skedgel, C. & Weijer, C. (2004). Considerations and costs of disclosing study findings to research participants *Canadian Medical Association Journal* 170(9);14171419

Fernandez, C.V., Santor, D., Weijer, C., Strahlendorf, C., Moghrabi, A., Pentz, R., Gao, J. & Kodish, E. (2007). The return of research results to participants: Pilot questionnaire of adolescents and parents of children with cancer. *Pediatric Blood & Cancer*, **48**, 441–6.

Fernandez, C.V., Gao, J., Strahlendorf, C., Moghrabi, A., Pentz, R., Barfield, R., Baker, J., Santor, D., Weijer, C. & Kodish, E. (2009). Providing Research Results to Participants: Attitudes and Needs of Adolescents and Parents of Children With Cancer. *Journal of Clinical Oncology*, **27**, 878–83.

Ford, K., Sankey, J. and Crisp, J. (2007). Development of children's assent documents using a child-centred approach. *Journal of Child Health Care*, **11**, 19–28.

Frosch, D.L. & Kaplan, R.M. (1999). Shared decision making in clinical medicine: past research and future directions. *American Journal of Preventive Medicine*, **17**, 285–94.

Funnell, M.M., Anderson, R.M., Arnold, M.S. et al. (1991). Empowerment: an idea whose time has come in diabetes education. *Diabetes Educ.* 1991;17:37–41

Gibb, D.M., Darbyshire, J.H., Debré, M., Giaquinto, C., Aboulker, J.P., Martinez, M. & Tudor-Williams, G. (1995). Treatment of children with HIV infection. PENTA (Paediatric European Network for Treatment of AIDS). *Lancet*. 1995 Apr 29;345(8957):1115.

Gill, D., Crawley, F.P., LoGiudice, M., Grosek, S., Kurz, R., de Lourdes-Levy, M., et al. (2003). Guidelines for informed consent in biomedical research involving paediatric populations as research participants. *Eur J Pediatr* 2003;162(7-8):455–8

Gómez-Marín, O., Prineas, R. & Sinaiko A. (1991). The sodium-potassium blood pressure trial in children: Design, recruitment, and randomization: The children and adolescent blood pressure program. *Controlled Clinical Trials*, **12**, 408–23.

Hayman, R., Taylor, B., Peart, N., Galland, B. and Sayers, R. (2001). Participation in research: Informed consent, motivation and influence. *Journal of Paediatrics and Child Health*, **37**, 51–54.

Henderson, G.E., Churchill, L.R., Davis, A.M., Easter, M.M., Grady, C., et al. (2007). Clinical Trials and Medical Care: Defining the Therapeutic Misconception. *PLoS Med* 4(11): e324. doi:10.1371/journal.pmed.0040324

Hernandez, R, Cooney, M, Dualé, C et al. (2009). Harmonisation of ethics committees' practice in 10 European countries *J Med Ethics* 2009;35:696–700.

Hoehn, K., Wernovsky, G., Rychik, J., Gaynor, J., Spray, T., Feudtner, C. and Nelson, R. (2005). What factors are important to parents making decisions about neonatal research? *Archives of Disease in Childhood Fetal and Neonatal Edition*, **90**, F267-269.

Huriet, C. (2004). Introduction. In: Ethical Eye: Biomedical research, Council of Europe, 2004;17

ICH E11 (2000). International Conference on Harmonisation of Technical Requirements for Registration of Pharmaceuticals for Human Use (2000). ICH Harmonised Tripartite Guideline - Clinical Investigation of Medicinal Products in the Pediatric Population- E11. Step 4 20 July 2000.
http://www.ich.org/fileadmin/Public_Web_Site/ICH_Products/Guidelines/Efficacy/E11/Step4/E11_Guideline.pdf (accessed 9 Jan 2012).

Janofsky J. & Starfield, B. (1981). Assessment of risk in research on children. *Journal of Pediatrics* **98**, 842-46.

John, J.E. (2007). The child's right to participate in research: myth or misconception? *Br J Nurs* 2007;16(3):157–60

John, T., Hope, T. et al. (2008). Children's consent and paediatric research: is it appropriate for healthy children to be the decision-makers in clinical research? *Archives of Disease in Childhood* 93(5): 379-83.

Jones, P.S. & Meleis, A.I. (1993). Health is empowerment. ANS *Advances in Nursing Science*. 15:1-14

Kasper, J. & Lenz, M. (2005). Kriterien zur Entwicklung und Beurteilung von Decision Aids. *Z ärztl Fortbild Qual Gesundh.wes* 99, 359–65

Kass, NE, Sugarman, J, Faden, R. & Schoch-Spana, M. (1996). Trust, The fragile foundation of contemporary biomedical research. Hastings Cent Rep. 1996 Sep-Oct;26(5):25-9.

Kern, S.E. (2009). Challenges in conducting clinical trials in children: approaches for improving performance. *Expert Rev Clin Pharmacol*. 2009 November 1; 2(6): 609–617. doi:10.1586/ecp.09.40.

Kimland, E., Nydert, P., Odlind, V., Böttiger, Y. and Lindemalm, S. (2012), Paediatric drug use with focus on *off-label* prescriptions at Swedish hospitals – a nationwide study. *Acta Paediatrica*. doi: 10.1111/j.1651-2227.2012.02656.x

Knox, C.A & Burkhart, P.V. (2007). Issues related to children participating in clinical research. *Journal of Pediatric Nursing,* 2007;22:310–8

Kon, A.A. (2006). Assent in Pediatric Research. *Pediatrics* 2006 May 1; 117(5): 1806 -1810. doi: 10.1542/peds.2005–2926.

Leach, A., Hilton, S., Greenwood, B.M., Manneh, E., Dibba, B., Wilkins, A., & Mulholland, E.K. (1999). An evaluation of the informed consent procedure used during a trial of a Haemophilus influenzae type B conjugate vaccine undertaken in The Gambia, West Africa. *Social Science & Medicine,* 1999 Jan;48(2):139–48.

Levi, R., Marsick, R., Drotar, D. & Kodish, E. (2000). Diagnosis, Disclosure, and Informed Consent: Learning From Parents of Children With Cancer. *Journal of Pediatric Hematology/Oncology,* **22**, 3–12.

Lowes, L., Robling, M.R., Bennert, K., Crawley, C., Hambly, H., Hawthorne, K., Gregory, J.W. and the DEPICTED Study Team (2010). Involving lay and professional stakeholders in the development of a research intervention for the DEPICTED study. *Health Expectations,* **14**, 250–60.

Lynch, J. (2010). Consent to Treatment. Radcliffe Publishing; ISBN 9781846192241.

Maslow, A.H. (1943). A Theory of Human Motivation. *Psychological Review* **50** (4):370–96.

McIntyre, J., Conroy, S. et al. (2000). Unlicensed and off label prescribing of drugs in general practice. *Archives of Disease in Childhood* 83(6): 498–501.

Morris, M., Nadkarni, V., Ward, F. & Nelson R. (2004). Exception From Informed Consent for Pediatric Resuscitation Research: Community Consultation for a Trial of Brain Cooling After In-Hospital Cardiac Arrest. *Pediatrics,* **114**, 77–81.

Mulla, H., Tofeig, M., Bullock, F., Samani, N. & Pandya, H.C. (2007). Variations in captopril formulations used to treat children with heart failure: a survey in the United Kingdom. *Archives of Disease in Childhood,* **92**:409–11.

Neubert, A., Wong, I.C., Bonifazi, A., Catapano, M., Felisi, M., Baiardi, P. et al. (2008). Defining off-label and unlicensed use of medicines for children: results of a Delphi survey. *Pharmacol Res* 58(5-6): 316–22.

O'Connor, A.M. & Jacobsen, M.J. (2003). Workbook on Developing and Evaluating Patient Decision Aids. Ottawa Health Research Institute 2003; http://decisionaid.ohri.ca/docs/develop/Develop_DA.pdf (accessed 9 Jan 2012).

O'Connor, A., Stacey, D., Entwistle, V., Llewellyn-Thomas, H., Rovner, D., Holmes-Rovner, M. et al. (2004). Decision aids for people facing health treatment or screening decisions. *Cochrane Database of Systematic Reviews* 2004; 4.

O'Connor, A.M., Stacey, D. & Jacobsen, M.J. (2011). The Ottowa Decision Support Tutorial. Ottowa Hospital Research Institute; https://decisionaid.ohri.ca/ODST/pdfs/ODST.pdf (accessed 9 Jan 2012).

Ondrusek, N., Abramovitch, R., Pencharz, P. & Koren, G. (1998). Empirical examination of the ability of children to consent to clinical research. *Journal of Medical Ethics*, **24**, 158–165.

Pandolfini, C. & Bonati, M . (2005). A literature review on off-label drug use in children. *Eur J Pediatr* 2005;164:552–8

Partridge, A.H., Hackett, N., Blood, E. et al. (2004). Oncology physician and nurse practices and attitudes regarding offering clinical trial results to study participants. *J Natl Cancer Inst* 96:629–32

Partridge, A.H. & Winer, E.P. (2009). Sharing study results with trial participants: Time for action. *Journal of Clinical Oncology* 27:6;838839

Patrick, D. L., Burke, L. B., Powers, J. H., Scott, J. A., Rock, E. P. & Dawisha, S. (2007). Patient-reported outcomes to support medical product labeling claims: FDA perspective. *Value Health, 10 Suppl 2*, S125–37.

Pletsch, P.K. & Stevens, P.E. (2001). Inclusion of Children in Clinical Research: Lessons Learned From Mothers of Diabetic Children. *Clinical Nursing Research*, 10, 140–62.

Prochaska, J. O. & Velicer, W. F. (1997). The transtheoretical model of health behavior change. *American Journal of Health Promotion*, 12; 38–48.

Rappaport J. (1987). Terms of empowerment/exemplars of prevention: toward a theory for community psychology. *Am J Community Psychol*. Apr;15(2):121–48.

Ravens-Sieberer, U., Schmidt, S., Gosch, A., Erhart, M., Petersen, C. & Bullinger, M. (2007). Measuring subjective health in children and adolescents: results of the European KIDSCREEN/DISABKIDS Project. *Psychosoc Med*. 2007 Jul 12;4:Doc08. PubMed PMID: 19742297; PubMed Central PMCID: PMC2736532.

RCN guidance for nurses (2011). Informed consent in health and social care research. 2nd ed. Royal College of Nursing Research Society, London.
http://www.rcn.org.uk/__data/assets/pdf_file/0010/78607/002267.pdf (accessed 9 Jan 2012).

Reitamo, S., Rustin, M., Harper, J., Kalimo, K., Rubins, A., Cambazard, F., Brenninkmeijer, E., Smith, C., Berth-Jones, J., Ruzicka, T., Sharpe, G. & Taieb, A. (2008). A 4-year follow-up study of atopic dermatitis therapy with 0.1% tacrolimus ointment in children and adult patients. *British Journal of Dermatology*, **159**, 942–51.

Rothmier, J.D., Lasley, M.V. & Shapiro, G.G. (2003). Factors Influencing Parental Consent in Pediatric Clinical Research. *Pediatrics*, **111**, 1037–41.

Rotter, J. B. (1980). Interpersonal trust, trustworthiness and gullibility. *American Psychologist*, 35, 1–7.

Saint-Raymond, A. & Seigneuret, N. (2009). The European paediatric initiative: 1 year of experience. *Paediatr Drugs* 2009;11(1):9–10

Sammons, H., Atkinson, M., Choonara, I. & Stephenson, T. (2007). What motivates British parents to consent for research? A questionnaire study. *BMC Pediatrics*, **7**, 12.

Sammons, H. M., Gray, C. et al. (2008). Safety in paediatric clinical trials--a 7-year review. *Acta Paediatrica* 97(4): 474–7.

Samoy, L.J., Zed, P.J., Wilbur, K., Balen, R.M., Abu-Laban, R.B. & Roberts, M. (2006). Drug-related hospitalizations in a tertiary care internal medicine service of a Canadian hospital: a prospective study. *Pharmacotherapy* 26(11): 1578–86.

Sederberg-Olsen, J., Sederberg-Olsen, N., Thomsen, J. & Balle, V. (1998). Problems in recruiting patients to controlled trials on children with secretory otitis media: A demographic comparison of excluded versus included patients. *International Journal of Pediatric Otorhinolaryngology*, 43, 229–233.

Shah, S., Whittle, A., Wilfond, B., Gensle,r G. & Wendler, D. (2004). How do institutional review boards apply the federal risk and benefit standards for pediatric research? *Journal of the American Medical Association* JAMA 2004;**291**:476–82)

Shirkey, H.C. (1968). Therapeutic orphans. *The Journal of Pediatrics* 1968; 72: 119–20

Shirkey, H.C. (1999). Therapeutic orphans. *Pediatrics*. 1999 Sep;104(3 Pt 2):583–4.

Simon, C., Siminoff, L., Kodish, E. & Burant, C. (2004). Comparison of the Informed Consent Process for Randomized Clinical Trials in Pediatric and Adult Oncology. *Journal of Clinical Oncology*, **22**, 2708–17.

Singhal, N., Oberle, K., Burgess, E. & Huber-Okrainec, J. (2002). Parents' perceptions of research with newborns. *Journal of Perinatology*, **22**, 57–63.

Sinha, I.P., Williamson, P.R. & Smyth, R.L. (2009). Outcomes in clinical trials of inhaled corticosteroids for children with asthma are narrowly focussed on short term disease activity. *PLoS One*. 2009 Jul 17;4(7):e6276

Smyth, R. L. (2001) Research with children. *British Medical Journal*, 322, 1377–8.

Snowdon, C., Garcia, J. & Elbourne, D. (1998). Reactions of participants to the results of a randomised controlled trial: exploratory study. *British Medical Journal*, **317**, 21–26.

Snowdon, C., Elbourne, D. & Garcia, J. (2006). "It was a snap decision": Parental and professional perspectives on the speed of decisions about participation in perinatal randomised controlled trials. *Social Science & Medicine*, **62**, 2279–90.

Stafford, R. S. (2008). Regulating off-label drug use--rethinking the role of the FDA. *New England Journal of Medicine, 358*(14), 1427–1429.

Stuijvenberg, M., Suur, M., Vos, S., Tjiang, G., Steyerberg, E., Derksen-Lubsen, G. & Moll, H. (1998). Informed consent, parental awareness, and reasons for participating in a randomised controlled study. *Archives of Disease in Childhood*, **79**, 120–125.

Tait, A., Voepel-Lewis, T. & Malviya, S. (2003). Do they understand? (part II): assent of children participating in clinical anesthesia and surgery research. *Anesthesiology*, **98**, 609–614.

Tait, A., Voepel-Lewis, T. & Malviya, S. (2004). Factors That Influence Parents' Assessments of the Risks and Benefits of Research Involving Their Children. *Pediatrics*, **113**, 727–732.

Tait, A., Voepel-Lewis, T. & Malviya, S. (2007). Presenting Research Information to Children: A Tale of Two Methods. *Anesthesia & Analgesia*, **105**, 358–364.

Tercyak, K., Johnson, S., Kirkpatrick, K. & Silverstein, J. (1998). Offering a randomized trial of intensive therapy for IDDM to adolescents. Reasons for refusal, patient characteristics, and recruiter effects. *Diabetes Care*, **21**, 213–215.

Ufer, M., Kimland, E. & Bergman, U. (2004). Adverse drug reactions and off-label prescribing for paediatric outpatients: a one-year survey of spontaneous reports in Sweden. *Pharmacoepidemiol Drug Safety* **13** (3), 147–52.

Unguru, Y., Sill, A. & Kamani, N. (2010). The Experiences of Children Enrolled in Pediatric Oncology Research: Implications for Assent. *Pediatrics*, **125**, e876–883.

United Nations Committee on the Rights of the Child (2009). Convention on the Rights of the Child, General Comment no.12: The right of the child to be heard. GE.09-43699 (E) 280709. http://www2.ohchr.org/english/bodies/crc/docs/AdvanceVersions/CRC-C-GC-12.doc (accessed 5 April 2012).

US Department of Health and Human Services, (2009). Code of Federal Regulations, title 45: Public Welfare; part 46: Protection of Human Subjects. Revised January 15, 2009. http://www.hhs.gov/ohrp/policy/ohrpregulations.pdf (accessed 11 January 2012).

Varma, S., Jenkins, T. & Wendler, D. (2008). How do children and parents make decisions about pediatric clinical research? *Journal of Pediatric Hematology*, **30**, 823–8.

Wagner, K., Martinez, M. & Joiner, T. (2006). Youths' and their parents' attitudes and experiences about participation in psychopharmacology treatment research. *Journal of Child and Adolescent Psychopharmacology*, **16**, 298–307.

Weijer, C. & Shapiro, S.H. (2000). Clinical equipoise and not the uncertainty principle is the moral underpinning of the randomised controlled trial. *British Medical Journal* 321:23Sept:756–758

Wendler, D., Belsky, L., Thompson, K.M.. & Emanuel, E.J. (2005) Quantifying the federal minimal risk standard: implications for pediatric research without a prospect of direct benefit. *Journal of the American Medical Association* JAMA **294** (7):826–832

Westra, A.E. & de Beaufort, I.D. (2011). The merits of procedure-level risk-benefit assessment. IRB. 2011 Sep-Oct;33(5):7-13. (summary in Chapter 3, of 'The Moral Limits of Medical Research with Children'. PhD thesis by Anna Westra 2011.

Westra, A.E., Wit, J.M., Sukhai, R.N., & de Beaufort, I.D. (2011). How best to Define the Concept of Minimal Risk. *Journal of Pediatrics*, **159 (3)**, 496–500.

Wilson, J.T. (1999). An update on the therapeutic orphan. *Pediatrics*. 1999 Sep;104(3 Pt 2):585–90.

Wulf, F., Krasuska, M. and Bullinger, M. (2012) Determinants of decision-making and patient participation in paediatric clinical trials: A literature review. *Open Journal of Pediatrics*, **2**, 1–17.

Yaffe, S.J. (Editor), Estabrook, R.W., Bouxsein, P., Pitluck, S., Davis, J.R. (2000). Rational Therapeutics for Infants and Children: Workshop Summary, National Academy Press, Washington, DC.

Zupancic, J., Gillie, P., Streiner, D., Watts, J. & Schmidt, B. (1997). Determinants of parental authorization for involvement of newborn infants in clinical trials. *Pediatrics*, **99**, E6.

Appendix 1a:

Children and parents: case study and survey responses

1	OVERVIEW	142
2	CASE STUDIES	142
	2.1 Slovenian parents of children in CTs	142
	2.2 Swedish children and parents in a CT	144
3	SURVEYS	147
	3.1 Italian children and parents in a research study	147
	3.2 German parents of children attending hospital for asthma and eczema	150
	3.3 Slovenian parents of children in study A	151
	3.4 Slovenian parents of children in study B	155
	3.5 Swedish healthy adolescents	156
	3.6 German follow-up study: the 'willingness to participate' construct	160

CONTRIBUTORS:

Ana Fakin
Viktorija Kerin
David Neubauer
John E. Chaplin
Carola Pfeiffer-Mosesson
Catriona Chaplin
Pia-Sophie Wool
Carlo Giaquinto
Adriana Ceci
Falk Wulf
Monika Bullinger
Aliaksandra Mokhar

1 Overview

The RESPECT project is not a quantitative study but rather a 'coordinating action' exploring the issues. As part of this process, we conducted about sixty structured interviews and some small-scale surveys of parents and children in hospital outpatient settings in Slovenia, Sweden, Italy and Germany.

2 Case studies

Various groups of clinical trial participants were interviewed. The majority of participants who participated in clinical trials were families who were being treated for their health care needs at the trial site. In the majority of cases, the participant was asked directly by their health care physician.

2.1 Slovenian parents of children in CTs

Case study interviews were conducted with 30 parents of patients in one CT and 14 parents of patients with a more severe condition participating in another CT in Slovenia.

2.1.1 Parent/child comments:

The research could help me personally
- Wanted to find out a more precise diagnosis. It could lead to improvement of diagnostic procedures.
- Duty towards the child to find out more about the illness. She would do anything to help her son, each study can bring some progress; they still hope that her son's condition will be treatable one day.
- It can give her hope that her daughter will be able to walk better someday. It could lead to finding out if the daughter's condition is improving.
- It is an opportunity to learn something new. Some parents research the disorder on the internet. One mother became interested in the condition because of her daughter. It was interesting to hear another opinion and learn something new.
- She was very interested to see what will come of this.
- She was very interested; she is curious how many children have the same disease as her sons; it would be great if she could receive some information about the results of the study.
- They were happy for the opportunity for an additional medical procedure.
- Might participate if there was something to improve her daughter's health.
- Might participate in future if it involves her child's condition and new approaches.

Duty to participate (altruism)
- It was my duty to participate, to improve cooperation between parents and doctors, and to get doctors to be more open.
- She thought it might help her son, but it was also her duty towards all children who might have a similar condition.
- They would have the procedures done anyway for the diagnostic purposes. She did not even feel like she was participating in a study.
- The study was presented to her daughter, who decided she wanted to participate.
- Perhaps someone will benefit from it – it will only help her personally if they develop a new treatment.
- They did not have any doubts about participating in a study in general but they decided to participate only partially (completing a questionnaire, not the extra medical procedure).
- She is not sure how it could help her or her son.

Painful/unpleasant
- The general anaesthesia and giving blood samples was unpleasant for the child.
- The child was not allowed to eat and drink until after she had the extra medical procedure.
- It was difficult for him watching his child going through it.
- The tests were unpleasant but her daughter handled them well.
- Her son did not say that it was painful but it was probably difficult for him.
- It was unpleasant for her daughter because she had many previous negative experiences with hospitals. She is afraid of the needles and starts crying when she has to go to the doctor.
- One family did not want their daughter to have the additional medical procedure because of the general anaesthesia. The deciding factor was also the fact that this procedure would not have any impact on the daughter's therapy regimen.
- They had doubts regarding the additional medical procedure because they were already planning to have the procedure in the future and did not want her to go through this twice. They decided to only complete the questionnaire.
- Might participate in future research if it does not involve something that would cause harm to her daughter. They would not participate again if it included general anaesthesia.

Inconvenient
- It took them a whole day, because they had to travel far and also wait for the tests.
- They have to wait for a long time in the waiting room.
- Some problems getting permission to spend a whole day with her son in the hospital.

Informed consent / Trust in the child's doctor
- She did not feel pressured to participate. She is always up for anything that could help her child.
- She was not sure what was expected of her and what the study was about.
- He understood only some of what it was about.
- She wishes doctors would give more information in layman's terms, because she is very interested to learn more about her daughter's condition and finds it difficult to understand Latin expressions on the papers.
- They knew they could refuse and they did refuse to participate in a part of it.

- The doctor who was conducting the research was very involved. He asked them politely if they would participate, and he made it clear that it was their decision.
- She hopes that they were serious/responsible people, but it is hard to assess that in such a short time.
- They would not refuse; they decided to do it because it was like any other visit to the doctor.

2.2 Swedish children and parents in a CT

We conducted case studies with paediatric patients and their parents participating in a Swedish CT. The participants had to attend several appointments with a doctor involved in the study, for routine examinations and for taking blood and urine samples.

Parent/child comments:

SV_001

Participant (aged 15) said:
He was not really aware of how much time it would take – would have said no if he had realised. His parents took the decision – he doesn't feel now that he was asked.
He was aware there had been some written information but had not read it himself. He was aware that there was an informed consent form for his parents to sign but not that he had also signed it.

Grandfather was with the child today – he has participated once before but it was the parents who gave informed consent. He had not realised until today that his grandson could have been given a placebo. Grandfather asked if his grandson could have missed out on treatment by participating. "He is in a randomised study but, if he wasn't, could he have got the test drug?"

SV_002

Participant (aged 14) said:
She had read the written description that she had got. Hadn't thought too much about why she was participating. It was just something she had been asked to do by the doctor and her parents had nothing against it. Not sure that it had occurred to them to refuse.

Mother said:
Her daughter might answer differently [if asked again] after she had received the first injection.

SV_003

Participant (aged 12) said:
She did not know about the blood tests and the injections when she agreed to participate. She was not sure what it was all about.

Appendix 1a: Children and parents

Mother said:
They were not sure at first if it was a good idea because of all the tests but when they discussed it with the nurse by phone they saw that this was their only chance to get the possibility of getting the test drug. It was good to have the description on paper so that they could read it and think about it. The mother thought this was the best way and would not have wanted to feel that she was being forced or manipulated into saying yes. It had to be their decision.

It will be interesting to see what the results are. Not sure how she will be informed of the results. Not clear on this.

Conclusion:
They were participating because of the chance to get a benefit from a medicine otherwise not available to them. The child is participating because the parent decides.

SV_004

Participant (aged 10) said:
He was only interested in getting the chocolate drink. He didn't know much about the study, turned to the mother for answers.

> *Was it painful / unpleasant?*
> - I didn't know about the injection

Mother said:
Several reasons for participation –
1) get a chance to try the new drug even if they cannot continue on it;
2) ok to participate if there are no side-effects;
3) good to think that it might lead to helping others in the future.

Nurse said:
They seem motivated to participate due to belief that they get better health care. "That is why I would participate".

Conclusion:
They made a logical decision to participate after being reassured that there were no side effects or disadvantages. They do not express the idea that they get an extra health check by participating. Mother focused on the test drug and its possible benefits.

SV_009

Participant (aged 17) said:
It is hard and boring. I wouldn't like to do another trial after this one. It takes too much time. The diary takes too much time. I don't want to miss school.

RESPECT

SV_101

Participant (aged 16) said:
I would prefer not to do another study after this one. (It takes a lot of time.) I wouldn't do it if there were any personal risk involved.

Father said:
Having the illness in the family is a motivation. I can't see why a healthy person would ever volunteer for a trial.

> *Did you feel you could refuse to participate?*
> - **Participant**: I had no alternative
> - **Father**: We knew that we could say no.

SV_102

Participant (aged 12) said:
I don't mind the visits. I like the nurses but found the injections a bit uncomfortable at first.

Father said:
I had no idea about placebos until after we joined the study. I have total confidence in the medical staff.

SV_103

Participant (aged 11) said:
I wanted to leave the study at first.

Father said:
It's easy to agree to something if you don't know what it actually involves.

SV_104

Participant (aged 11) said:
The injection hurts. [He had just had it.]

Mother said:
I let him decide whether to participate. I would find it hard to make that judgement for him. I would only intervene if the trial involved something that could harm him. Then I would override his judgement and refuse consent. I wouldn't let him be used as a 'guinea pig' in an experiment that could harm him.

Appendix 1a: Children and parents

Conclusion:
They are happy to help other children but are also influenced by the fact that he stands to benefit personally.

SV_105

Participant (aged 13) said:
The injection is painful. The rest is OK and my participation will help others. I am relieved that this was the last visit.

If they said they needed my help with a continuation of this study I would do it, but I would not volunteer for a different study. [He clearly expected to make his own decision if it came up again.]

Mother said: We thought hard about it before agreeing to participate. We read about it in the paper. Being in the study could help him personally and even his children in the future.

We definitely want some report of the results: we want to know which group he was in (placebo / test drug); also what this study found.

Nurse said: We always tell the participants at the end of the trial which arm they were in. We don't give them a report of the findings but in this particular case there is a website with some information about the test drug and the clinical trial

---

3 Surveys

3.1 Italian children and parents in a research study

RESPECT received responses to the online survey from Italians who were undergoing progressive replacement therapy.

These results were interesting because there was a mix of responses from children and parents. Most (8 of 12) had participated in a CT.

Themes that emerged:
- These patients were attending hospital regularly for blood transfusions and thus did not experience the clinical trial as an extra burden when they had to come for appointments anyway.

- It was thus like a continuation of their treatment and they saw a definite benefit for the child. They also noted the potential benefit to other children but this may have been of secondary importance to them.
- They understood that this was a CT and felt it had been clearly explained to them and that it was a worthwhile study.
- They wanted to receive a report on the results after the CT.
- They expressed trust in the clinical staff and most felt appreciated and would participate again if asked.

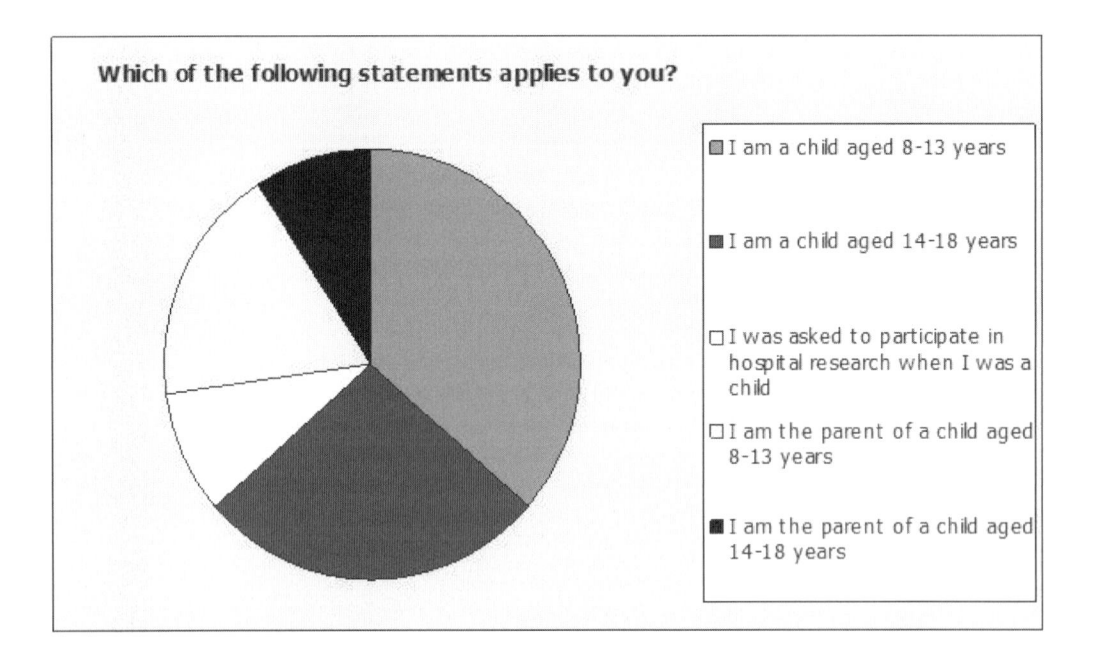

Which of the following statements applies to you?

- I am a child aged 8-13 years
- I am a child aged 14-18 years
- I was asked to participate in hospital research when I was a child
- I am the parent of a child aged 8-13 years
- I am the parent of a child aged 14-18 years

Statement	Agree	Disagree	Not sure
The study could lead to improving other children's health.	8	0	0
The research could help me/my child personally	8	0	0
Research and medicine are interesting to me.	4	0	4
I was interested to see what it was about.	5	1	2
I/we wanted to help the doctors after all the help I/my child has received.	4	2	2
I/we have to come to the hospital anyway for treatment/health checks.	8	0	0

Appendix 1a: Children and parents

Statement	Agree	Disagree	Not sure
I felt that I/we couldn't refuse when others had agreed to participate.	1	5	2
I thought I/my child would get better treatment if I participated.	2	2	4
I thought I/my child would get paid or receive some reward for participating.	1	5	2
They clearly explained the purpose of the research.	7	0	1
They clearly explained what was expected of me/my child.	5	0	2
They clearly explained what they would do with the research results.	5	0	2
I/we like the researcher/doctor/nurse.	8	0	0
I would like to be a researcher/doctor/nurse.	3	4	1
They are serious, responsible people (researcher/doctor/nurse).	8	0	0
They make me/us feel special/valued.	5	1	2
I get/my child gets extra health checks.	4	2	2
It isn't painful or unpleasant.	7	0	1
It isn't difficult.	8	0	0
I/we don't mind the time it takes.	6	1	1
I/we have no problems travelling to the research centre/hospital.	7	1	0
It is better than being at school/at home/at work.	3	5	0
It feels like a competition.	0	7	0
It is fun.	3	2	3
The study is anonymous.	7	1	0
They don't store any personal information.	3	2	3
It is a worthwhile study.	6	0	2
I want to receive a report on the research results at the end of the study.	6	1	0
I/my child would be willing to participate in further research.	5	0	3

Add any comments that may help us understand how you feel
Certainly improved.
In these years of examinations and blood transfusions I felt very much helped by the doctors and all staff and thanks to them I can live happily with my disease.
I think it was helpful for us.

3.2 German parents of children attending hospital for asthma and eczema

The German responses to the online survey gave a different perspective because eight of the nine parents who responded had never been asked to participate in research at a hospital, so they gave an outsider's point of view.

Themes that emerged:
- These respondents were more hesitant at the prospect of participating in a clinical trial.
- It would be a burden to them because they would not otherwise come to the hospital regularly; most indicated that this inconvenience would not be great but they would expect some kind of payment and practical help.
- They did not feel any obligation to the clinical staff and indicated that there would have to be a positive relationship for them to agree to participate.
- They were not totally against the risks involved in a CT and were not particularly interested in having this explained to them, but they were against the child being used as a 'guinea pig' for research. They wanted to know how the results would be used.
- They were unwilling to have their child assigned to a control group and did not want to be tied to one treatment and miss other options because of the trial.

Statement	Agree	Disagree	Not sure
I/my child might be willing to participate in a clinical trial if asked.	4	1	3
I/we would be happy to help other children through participation in a research study.	4	0	4
I/we want to help the doctors after all the help I have/my child has received.	2	5	1
I/we have to come to the hospital anyway for treatment/health checks.	0	8	0
Research and medicine are interesting to me.	8	0	0
It would be interesting to see what the study was about.	4	2	2
I/we would only participate if it was clear what I/my child would have to do.	8	0	0
I/we would only participate if it was clear what the research was about.	8	0	0
I am /my child is not obliged to participate.	8	0	0
I don't want to risk my/my child's health for a new medicine.	1	4	3
I don't want myself/my child to be used as a 'guinea pig' in medical experiments.	8	0	0
I would not want myself/my child to be put in a control group that doesn't get any treatment.	6	0	2

Appendix 1a: Children and parents

Statement	Agree	Disagree	Not sure
I would be worried that I/we might miss out on other new treatment options if I committed myself/my child to a clinical trial of a particular medicine.	5	0	3
I/we would only participate if the research could help me/my child personally.	0	1	7
I/we would only participate if I/we liked the researcher/doctor/nurse.	5	2	1
It would involve too much of my/our time.	0	5	3
It is inconvenient to travel to the testing location.	2	4	2
I/we would only participate if it was clear what they would do with the research results.	6	0	2
I/we would only participate if the study would be anonymous.	2	0	6
I/we would only participate if they removed my/my child's personal information.	3	1	4
I/we would only participate if I/my child would get some payment or other reward.	6	1	1
I/we would only participate if I/my child would get extra treatment in return.	4	2	2
I/we would only participate if I/my child would get practical help (such as with travel arrangements to the research centre / hospital).	5	2	1
I/we would only participate if the risks and benefits of the study were clearly explained.	1	5	2
I/we would only participate if we could receive a report on the research results at the end of the study.	1	5	2

3.3 Slovenian parents of children in study A

The online survey was completed in Slovenia by 27 parents of Slovenian children enrolled at the age of 18 months in a study that involved taking blood samples from the child.

Half of the parents completing the survey gave responses concerning participation in this study, while the other half indicated their opinions on potential participation in a clinical trial.

Themes that emerged (participating in this study):

- This was a long-term study and the parents were aware that they were participating in research and volunteered freely without feeling any pressure. There was no immediate advantage to the child (such as better treatment) and the families would not have been coming to the hospital anyway; they had to make special trips for the study but did not find this a problem.

RESPECT

- They were motivated by interest in worthwhile research that could help all children, including their own, as well as showing a desire to 'pay back' to the medical profession for help already received.
- They indicated respect and trust in the staff but did not feel especially valued for their contribution.
- They wanted to receive the results at the end of the study.
- They would participate in other studies if asked.

Statement	Agree	Disagree	Not sure
The study could lead to improving other children's health.	9	0	1
The research could help me/my child personally.	7	2	1
Research and medicine are interesting to me.	8	1	1
I was interested to see what it was about.	8	2	0
I/we wanted to help the doctors after all the help I/my child has received.	7	0	3
I/we have to come to the hospital anyway for treatment/health checks.	0	10	0
I felt that I/we couldn't refuse when others had agreed to participate.	0	10	0
I thought I/my child would get better treatment by participating.	0	9	1
I thought I/my child would get paid or receive some reward for participating.	1	9	0
They clearly explained the purpose of the research.	10	0	0
They clearly explained what was expected of me/my child.	9	1	0
They clearly explained what they would do with the research results.	8	1	1
I/we like the researcher/doctor/nurse.	7	1	2
I would like to be a researcher/doctor/nurse.	0	5	5
They are serious, responsible people (researcher/doctor/nurse).	7	0	3
They make me/us feel special/valued.	1	5	4
I get/my child gets extra health checks.	1	7	2
It isn't painful or unpleasant.	10	0	0
It isn't difficult.	8	2	0
I/we don't mind the time it takes.	10	0	0
I/we have no problems travelling to the research centre/hospital.	9	1	0

Appendix 1a: Children and parents

Statement	Agree	Disagree	Not sure
It is better than being at school/at home/at work.	2	6	1
It feels like a competition.	0	9	0
It is fun.	7	0	3
The study is anonymous.	5	3	2
They don't store any personal information.	4	2	4
It is a worthwhile study.	6	1	3
I want to receive a report on the research results at the end of the study.	10	0	0
I/my child would be willing to participate in further research.	8	0	1

Themes that emerged (potential participation in clinical trials):

- Altruism, gratitude and an interest in research featured in these responses too.
- The parents would want a lot of information when considering participation. They wanted to see whether it was a worthwhile study and to know exactly what would be expected of the child, as well as the risks and benefits.
- The parents would not expect a direct benefit to their child but, on the other hand, they did not want their child to end up in the control group and thus effectively be a 'guinea pig' in the research.
- They would want a report of the results at the end of the study.

Statement	Agree	Disagree	Not sure
I/my child might be willing to participate in a clinical trial if asked.	10	1	2
I/we would be happy to help other children through participation in a research study.	9	0	3
I/we want to help the doctors after all the help I have/my child has received.	9	0	2
I/we have to come to the hospital anyway for treatment/health checks.	2	9	0
Research and medicine are interesting to me.	8	1	1
It would be interesting to see what the study was about.	8	1	1
I/we would only participate if it was clear what I/my child would have to do.	8	1	1

RESPECT

Statement	Agree	Disagree	Not sure
I/we would only participate if it was clear what the research was about.	9	0	1
I am /my child is not obliged to participate.	8	0	1
I don't want to risk my/my child's health for a new medicine.	0	8	1
I don't want myself/my child to be used as a 'guinea pig' in medical experiments.	8	1	0
I would not want myself/my child to be put in a control group that doesn't get any treatment.	8	1	0
I would be worried that I/we might miss out on other new treatment options if I committed myself/my child to a clinical trial of a particular medicine.	5	3	1
I/we would only participate if the research could help me/my child personally.	2	5	1
I/we would only participate if I/we liked the researcher/doctor/nurse.	0	6	2
It would involve too much of my/our time.	1	3	4
It is inconvenient to travel to the testing location.	2	3	3
I/we would only participate if it was clear what they would do with the research results.	5	2	1
I/we would only participate if the study would be anonymous.	4	3	1
I/we would only participate if they removed my/my child's personal information.	3	4	1
I/we would only participate if I/my child would get some payment or other reward.	0	5	3
I/we would only participate if I/my child would get extra treatment in return.	2	3	3
I/we would only participate if I/my child would get practical help (such as with travel arrangements to the research centre / hospital).	1	3	4
I/we would only participate if the risks and benefits of the study were clearly explained.	6	0	2
I/we would only participate if we could receive a report on the research results at the end of the study.	6	1	1

3.4 Slovenian parents of children in study B

A shorter version of the child-parent questionnaire was filled in manually by 52 Slovenian parents (mostly mothers) of control group adolescents who have been included many times in longitudinal follow-ups in a neonatal outcome study.

The questionnaire was distributed to parents by the adolescents included in the study.

Themes that emerged:
- The parents indicated that participating was of no personal benefit but that they felt a duty to participate for a worthwhile cause. One quarter of the respondents felt that they could not refuse to participate.
- They did not find it painful or difficult and, although it was time-consuming, they were willing to volunteer the time necessary for the research.
- One-third indicated that it was fun to take part in the research and most respondents were interested to see what the research was about.

Statement	Yes	No	Unsure	Missing data
What was your opinion before participation in the study:				
It is a worthwhile study	46	0	2	4
The study can lead to improving people's health	36	5	7	4
I feel it is my duty to participate	39	7	2	4
Research and medicine are interesting to me	44	2	2	4
The research can help me personally	13	21	12	6
Will it involve much of your time?	19	27	1	5
They say I will get paid/something for participation	0	43	4	5
They say I will get better treatment if I participate	7	20	11	5
Participation will take too much of my time	1	47	0	4
It will be difficult	0	48	0	0
It will be painful / unpleasant	0	48	0	0
I feel that I cannot refuse to participate	13	33	1	5
The study is anonymous	44	0	4	4
It will not involve any personal information	34	10	3	5
I might participate in further research	29	7	11	5
It will be like a competition	2	45	1	4
It will be fun	17	22	7	6
It is clear what is expected of me	48	0	1	3
It is clear what the research is about	41	4	4	3
I like the researcher / doctor / nurse	26	0	7	19
I would like to be a researcher / doctor / nurse	2	36	7	7
I am interested to see what it is about	39	4	4	5

3.5 Swedish healthy adolescents

The Swedish version of the healthy child survey was sent by email to healthy adolescents.

The majority (30 of 38) had not even heard of the concept of a clinical trial, so their views were interesting to us to get a snapshot of adolescents' potential reactions to being invited to participate in a trial.

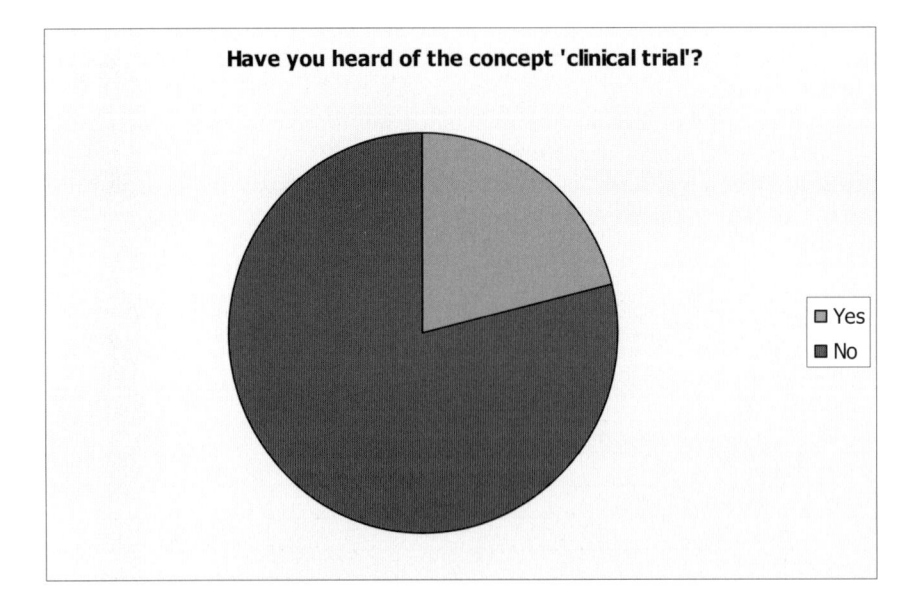

Have you heard of the concept 'clinical trial'?

(Pie chart showing Yes/No responses)

Themes that emerged:

- The response that surprised us most was that they were generally comfortable with the idea of being a 'guinea pig' for medical research.
- They could see the benefits for the progress of medical knowledge, showing an altruistic attitude to societal benefits. (As healthy adolescents, they had no personal need of new medicines, which is often the motivating factor in our other groups studied.)

Appendix 1a: Children and parents

I would participate because ...

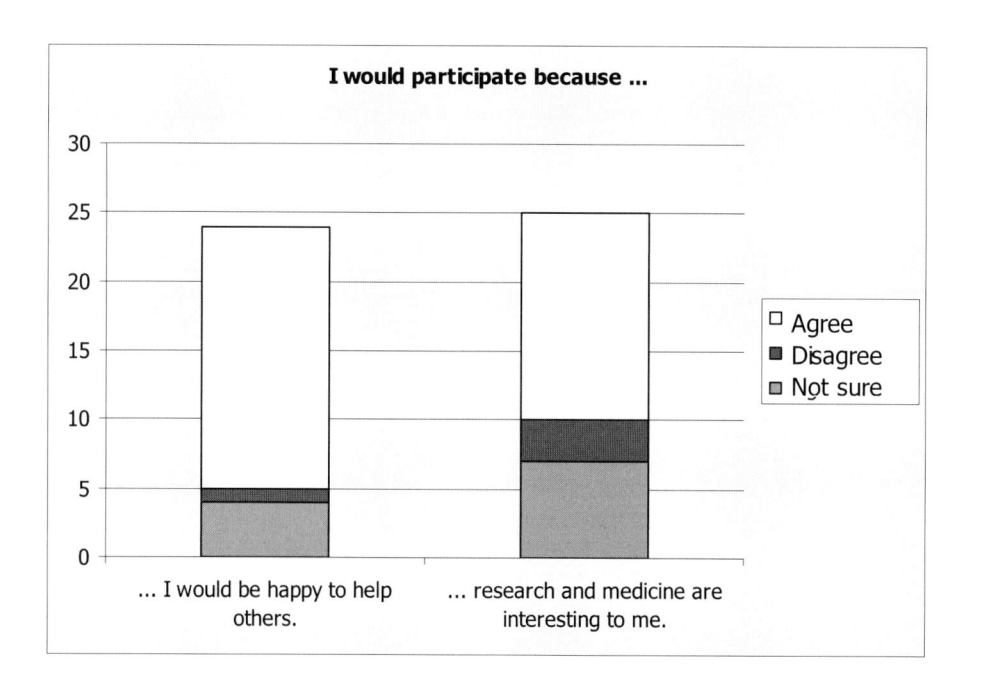

(Bar chart showing two categories with Agree, Disagree, Not sure responses)
- "... I would be happy to help others." — total ~24
- "... research and medicine are interesting to me." — total ~25

Please explain why or add any other comment:
It depends. Preferably nothing I have to put in my body
It depends on the purpose of the test.
It depends on what is being tested, if it is something I could consider being a test subject for, or if it is something I feel uncomfortable about testing.
It is important to keep developing research progress and therefore it is important to participate to see changes and gain more knowldege.
If I were to participate it would be to support people in need and to get a well-developed pharmaceutical industry.
I think that if more people are tested then there can be more results and corrections

I would REFUSE to participate because …

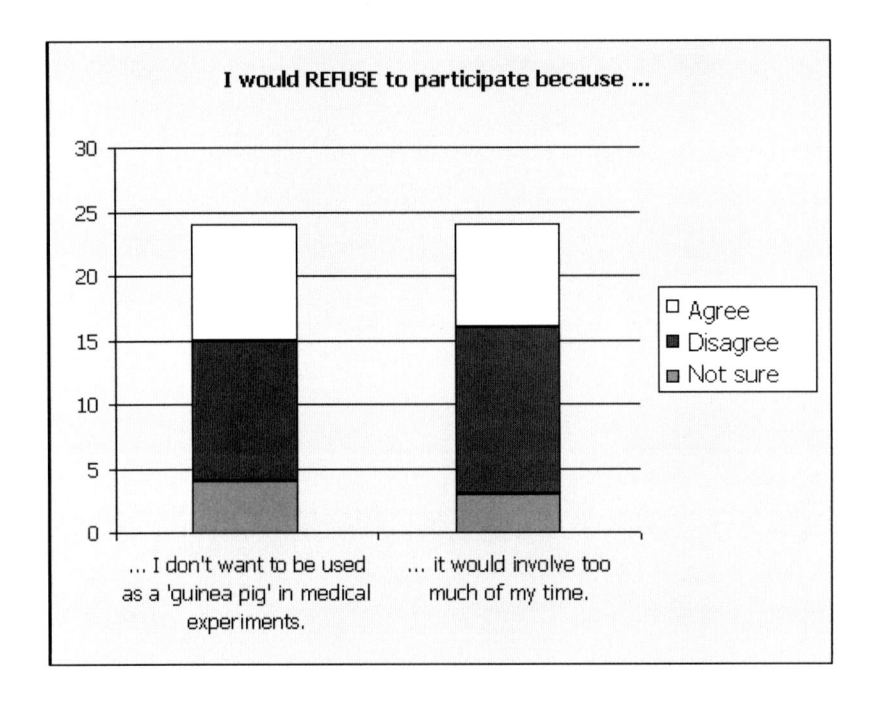

Bar chart showing responses (Agree / Disagree / Not sure) to two statements:
- … I don't want to be used as a 'guinea pig' in medical experiments.
- … it would involve too much of my time.

Please explain why or add any other comment:
I am also afraid of unknown side-effects
I would be happy to participate if it was for a good cause.
I probably wouldn't mind being a 'guinea pig' if the test wasn't something that would make me uncomfortable or frightened or suchlike. If I was asked now, I would not participate because I don't have much spare time, but if my current situation changed and I had the time it requires, I don't think it would be a problem.
Sometimes it feels risky to be the first to try something. It could turn out that the study gave a negative result.
Personally, I wouldn't feel like giving so much of my time. But I see it as a positive thing to be a 'guinea pig'.

Appendix 1a: Children and parents

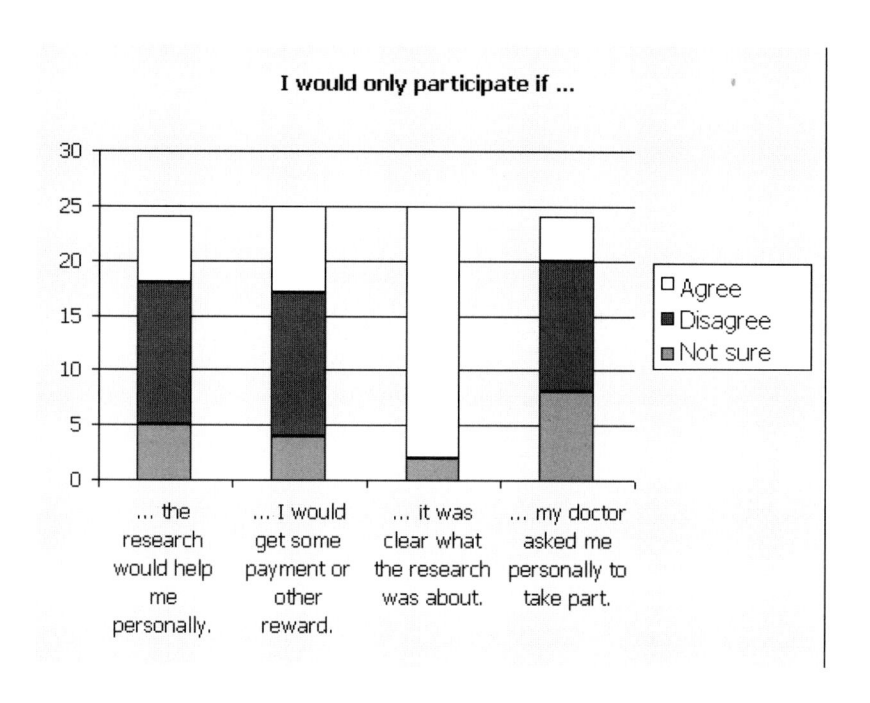

I would only participate if ...

(Bar chart with categories: Agree, Disagree, Not sure)

- ... the research would help me personally.
- ... I would get some payment or other reward.
- ... it was clear what the research was about.
- ... my doctor asked me personally to take part.

Please explain why or add any other comment:
Information is the most important thing. The rest is just a little bonus.
You never know if you will benefit personally from the research in the future; maybe my child would benefit. But I would hopefully be helping others even if I did not benefit personally. A payment is always motivating but it wouldn't have to be much. In many cases a cinema ticket or suchlike would be enough. If it wasn't clear what the research was about, I would probably feel uncomfortable about participating so I would refuse. It depends who poses the question, if I trust that person. But I would probably check with my doctor too.
I would actively look up the clinical trial. I want to know exactly what the substance they are testing is intended to do.
I think it is very important to get a lot of information about the trial, its purpose and the consequences.

3.6 German follow-up study: the 'willingness to participate' construct

3.6.1 Introduction

The decision to participate in a clinical trial or not depends on a series of steps which can be analysed from a motivational psychological standpoint. In health psychology different motivational models have be suggested including the "Transtheoretical Model of action" (Prohaska) which identifies four steps of taking action beginning with lack of intent until carrying out the action, and the Rubicon Model of action theory (Heckhausen).

In psychology, motivation is understood as the totality of subjective motives to engage in the specific behaviour. Readiness to act is traceable back to inner motives and needs or stimuli from outside. In this context action is understood as a goal oriented activity occurring according to specific plans with specific actions expectations.

The construct of "readiness to act" can be defined as the likelihood to perform the action according to a motivation or during an action process. Models of research into action processes in motivational psychology can be distinguishing regarding a more to emotional or more cognitive bass of human behaviour.

Using the more cognitive approach Heckhausen (1989) identified a sequence of motivation and volition phases. According to the "Rubicon Model" the motivation phase starts with the perception of preferences, continues with a reality check to produce expectations of the action process and is results and is concluded by the behaviour itself. Heckhausen (2006) differentiated between the formation of intention, the initiation of intention and activation of intention and action itself. He differentiated four sequences which he called motivation- predecisional, volitional- preactional, volition- actional and motivational- postactional. These relate to phases of weighing decisions, planning of decisions, acting according to the plan and evaluating the decision.

The Hamburg group found this cognitive- motivational model to be useful to identify the construct "willingness to participate" for the RESPECT- project because of the underlying cognitive processes which relate to motives or reasons for or against participation in the clinical trial.

The term willingness to participate has not been defined or operationalised successfully in clinical research; however, several studies have addressed different reasons or motives for or against participation in clinical trials.

For example, Zammar et al. (2010) have identified several variables affecting in the willingness to participate which include motives such as a trust, altruism, reimbursement, personal health benefits, convenience and others. However these are determinants of willingness to participate and they do not contribute to identification of willingness to participate as such. Nevertheless, motives or reasons for or against participating are important aspects of the quantification of willingness to participate.

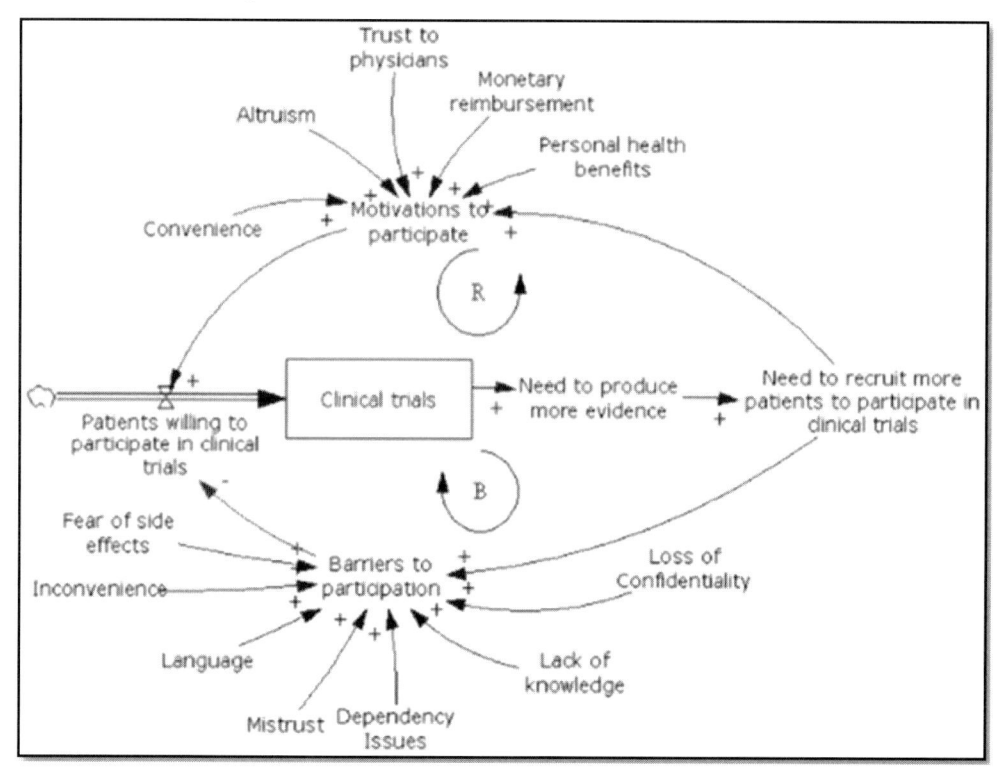

[Figure: Causal loop diagram showing Motivations to participate (Altruism, Trust to physicians, Monetary reimbursement, Personal health benefits, Convenience) feeding into Patients willing to participate in clinical trials (reinforcing loop R), and Barriers to participation (Fear of side effects, Inconvenience, Language, Mistrust, Dependency Issues, Lack of knowledge, Loss of Confidentiality) in balancing loop B, with Clinical trials leading to Need to produce more evidence and Need to recruit more patients to participate in clinical trials.]

Furthermore, Gaul and colleagues identified as important aspects: the personal trust relationship with physician, the efficiency of established treatment regiments, the severity of the diseases and the barriers related to participation (Gaul et al, 2006).

Several studies have underlined these aspects. For example Albrecht et al. (1999) found that interest to participate in the study increases with the degree of personal involvement or concern and with the severity of disease. Rosenbaum et al. (2005) found altruism to be the main reason for participation in clinical research. Finally Llewellyn-Thomas et al. (1991) identified the benefit of receiving more intensive control of the health state as a relevant reason to participate in a clinical trial.

In the RESPECT project, one aspect of the different approaches to understanding participation in clinical trial was a closer investigation into the 'willingness to participate' construct. Using different approaches such as interviews with parents, patients, experts, patient organisations as well as treating physicians and medical staff the construct of the decision to participate or not in a clinical trial was intensively researched and discussed.

3.6.2 Method

The Hamburg group decided to contribute to the construct willingness to participate by using the questionnaire developed within the RESPECT group in its German translation in a convenience sample of medical students, health sciences students and hospital outpatients in the framework of a pilot study. In particular, the empirical question was whether the RESPECT questionnaire contains identifiable underlying dimensions of willingness to participate and whether it is acceptable in terms of psychometric criteria, especially that of reliability. In this evaluation, the majority of the respondents were healthy medical students; that is, patients with serious illnesses were not included in the sample. Sick children and their parents participating in clinical trials should be surveyed after this analysis and subsequent optimisation of the RESPECT questionnaire.

The German version of the questionnaire related to experiences with clinical trials, of which only the questions regarding willingness to participate were given to medical students, health sciences students and patients. Specifically, medical students in their second year of medical training were asked to complete the questionnaire as part of their curriculum in medical psychology, and students of health sciences were asked to do this as part of their curriculum of developmental psychology. In addition, in cooperation with the local hospital in Hamburg, access to outpatients was possible. It was planned to recruit sample of 300 persons to examine psychometrically the questionnaire.

The questionnaire was presented with one of three scenarios: the first scenario in which the participants were instructed that they would participate in pharmaceutical industry sponsored a clinical trial; the second scenario described participation in a university-initiated clinical trial without pharmacy sponsoring and the third version had no specific description of the study sponsor. All samples and versions were used for the psychometric analysis below. In addition, differences between the scenarios were examined.

The aim was to conduct analysis of the 'willingness to participate' part of the questionnaire. Descriptive statistics as well as factor analyses, using principle component analyses with varimax rotation and 'very simple factor structure analyses' were conducted. A calculation of reliability was also included.

3.6.3 Results

In total, 215 questionnaires were returned and analysed in SPSS data mask. An overview of the frequency of patients and healthy respondents shows that 80% were students, 153 of the responders were male, and 62 were female. The mean age was 26 years with a standard deviation of 7.1 years. Descriptive analyses of the questionnaire showed that several items were endorsed more frequently than others were.

In general, the distribution of the items was slightly skewed. The factor analysis was conducted using the Principal Component Methods PCA with a Scree test. This yielded a solution of four factors, which explained 49 percent of the variance. Very Simple Structure analyses also yielded four factors with an acceptable complexity. A varimax rotation of the factors showed that the four factors were equally distributed with a strong first as well as second but very weak fourth factor, which consisted of only three items. Table 1 gives an overview of the results of the factor analyses as well as the loading of items on the factors.

Table 1 Varimax Rotation

Variable	F 1	F 2	F 3	F 4	h³	u²
Possible participation		0,477	0,503		0,56	0,44
Helping others			0,428		0,3	0,7
Gratitude towards doctors			0,405		0,19	0,81
Other appointments at the hospital			0,494		0,25	0,75
Interest in research			0,679		0,55	0,45
Knowledge about the study			0,585		0,38	0,62
Accurate explanation of what is required	0,675	0,367	0,305		0,75	0,25
Precise knowledge of the study	0,687				0,7	0,3
No participation in research		0,611	0,372		0,56	0,44
Threat to health		0,472	0,36		0,37	0,63
Do not be a guinea pig		0,617	0,42		0,57	0,43
No unnecessary medical treatments		0,59			0,46	0,54
Fear of pain		0,558			0,36	0,64
Allocation to the control group		0,603			0,42	0,58
Avoid other treatments		0,444			0,32	0,68
Personal benefits				0,583	0,4	0,6
Doctor knows person		-0,317			0,17	0,83
Claim for time lost		0,491			0,26	0,74
Effort (to get research site)		0,326			0,14	0,86
Knowledge of results	0,652		0,377		0,57	0,43
Anonymity of the study	0,683				0,54	0,46
Personal data anonymity	0,737				0,59	0,41
Expense allowance	0,313			0,571	0,44	0,56
Extra treatment		-0,337		0,531	0,43	0,57
Practical help	0,414				0,26	0,74
Declaration of benefits / risks	0,631				0,59	0,41
Report on the results	0,683				0,51	0,49

A goodness-of-fit test for the factors also showed acceptable proportion of explained variance (see Table 2). The comparison of factor loadings of factor one-two, two-three and three-four showed a clear picture of factor structure of the instrument.

Table 2 Goodness-of-fit test

	F 1	F 2	F 3	F 4
SS loading	3,963	3,476	2,766	1,442
variance	0,147	0,129	0,102	0,053
cumulative variance explained	0,147	0,275	0,378	0,431
Chi-squared test	$\chi^2(351, 220)$ =535,22 $p<0,001$			

As regards items analysis, this was conducted for all 26 items and each factor and showed mean Cronbach's alpha of over .70. Most factors had good item loadings and reliabilities with exception of two items of the first factor. The alpha for factor one was .86. Factor two had a Cronbach's alpha of .72 with two items being suboptimal and in factor three the alpha of 6 items was .74. Factor four consisting of three items had a Cronbach's alpha of .64.

3.6.4 Interpretation of the identified factors

The identified factors were interpreted in terms of factor one (***control***), factor two (***general concerns about participation***), factor three (***general interest in clinical research***) and factor four (***personal benefits of participation***).

The first factor is mainly about a sense of **control** for the trial participants. These respondents are not only interested in basic information about the clinical research, but also in a precise description of the smallest details of the study and its implementation. If the respondents have the impression that they have access to all the information on the use of the data and the results, it will affect their willingness to participate. Apparently, they want to have a say in the study as part of their participation. We also notice that the anonymity of the participants is very important to these respondents; they do not want to be identifiable, thus removing fear of uncontrolled dissemination of the results.

Factor two describes more **general concerns** that lead to participation or non-participation in a clinical trial. The corresponding items concern fears and anxieties of the respondents. Thus, this factor is a good help in planning a clinical trial, indicating that it is important even before the implementation of the study to provide information about possible risks and side effects of the drug to be tested or potential negative consequences from participating in the study. This could be in the form of a brochure or a personal interview. Moreover, this factor also describes the aspect of the time required for participation in a trial, including easy accessibility of the research site. The positive decision to participate in a study also depends upon the patient having a basic general knowledge of clinical research and a certain interest in such projects. One could therefore define the second factor of the general willingness to participate in clinical research, as the patient's interest and the effort involved to participate.

The third factor is a **general interest in clinical research**, with an altruistic attitude being linked to participation. This depends on the person's own experience with clinical research projects, or at least general knowledge about clinical research. The more points of contact there are in this respect, the more likely is a commitment to participate. The prospect of benefit to others is of great importance.

The fourth factor identifies the **personal benefits** to be crucial for a commitment to participate in a clinical trial. The degree of willingness to participate depends greatly on the extent of personal gain the respondent can derive from participation.

Discussion
An almost uniform picture can be found at the first factor. The only distortion here delivers the item "I would participate only if it was explained to me exactly what is required". Although this item loads highly on the first factor, it also influences factors two and three. The item "I would participate only if I would receive practical help (e.g. booking the journey to the research site)", however, has a relatively low item load. The selectivity of the first factor, with the exception of the item "I would participate only if I would receive practical help (e.g. booking the journey to the research site)", is good and the item difficulty is in the satisfactory medium range.

The second factor has, all in all, clear item loading. An exception in this respect, however, is the item "I would refuse because I do not want to put my health at risk." In addition, the item "I would participate only if I knew the researcher / doctor / nurse in person" must be reversed. Finally, the selectivity for the items "I would refuse, because I'm afraid that I would escape through the participation of other treatment options," "I would participate only if I knew the researcher / doctor / nurse personal" and "I would refuse because it would take too much time" is unsatisfactory and therefore needs improvement in future versions of the survey.

The third and fourth factors show - not unexpectedly - low item loading. The reason lies in the variables included here; neither the first nor the second factor could be assigned. The reliability of the first two factors, however, is acceptable, so that further revisions of the questionnaire might focus on these key factors.

3.6.5 Conclusions

This analysis uncovered the largest explanatory factors for the willingness to participate in the survey carried out here. With this factor analysis of the willingness to participate questionnaire, a major step in identifying and assessing the construct was performed. Parents of children with health conditions facing participation in clinical trial may use this and a possible adaptation for children is planned, including suggestions for the improvement of items in terms of wording as well as reducing the number of items. Thus, this work gave empirical insight in to the quantification of the concept of willingness to participate, which is of potential use for research on participation in clinical trials.

Appendix 1b:

Patient organisations: email and online survey responses

1	**OVERVIEW**	167
	1.1 Diseases represented	167
2	**SURVEY RESPONSES**	168
	2.1 Requests from parents for information	168
	2.2 Parents' reasons for consent	168
	2.3 Parents' reasons for refusal	168
	2.4 Good practices	169
	2.5 Role currently	170
	2.6 Future role	170
	2.7 Ideal role	171
	2.8 Additional comments made:	171
3	**CONCLUSIONS**	172

CONTRIBUTORS:

Liuska Sanna
Gaya Ducceschi

1 Overview

RESPECT conducted an email survey of member patient organisations and a larger online survey of patients' organisations (POs) to find out more about their approach to clinical trials (CTs).

The surveys were submitted to 209 patient organisations and we received 33 responses. Eleven of the responses came from the first survey, which was slightly different from the one we made available online.

The type of organisations that replied is quite varied: we go from a strong organisation involved in European projects and funding research to a not-for-profit organisation established by the parents of a sick child whose purpose is to finance the costs of the treatment.

1.1 Diseases represented

Congenital heart diseases (2)
Duchenne muscular dystrophy
Brain tumor
Juvenile chronic arthritis
Rare diseases
Epilepsy (2)
Cystic Fibrosis (2)
Prader-Willi syndrome (3)
Psoriasis
Rheumatism
Stomach and intestinal disorders
Mitochondrial disorders
Adrenoleukodystrophy (ALD) rare, metabolic disorder
Age-related macular degeneration (AMD)
Kidney disease
Asthma
Diabetis
Lupus
Thalassemia
Haemophilia

2 Survey responses

2.1 Requests from parents for information

The respondents were involved to different extents in clinical trials. Most of them were in contact with parents and were consulted to get information and advice about:

- Efficacy and Safety (including side effects)
- If CT were available and if they would recommend them
- How CT proceed
- If they knew other participants
- Goal and eligibility criteria of a CT, how to participate
- If there are medicines specifically tested for children
- If they can try drugs that are not licensed for children

2.2 Parents' reasons for consent

According to the respondents, the main reasons why parents would consent to their child's participation in clinical trials were:

- Make their children benefit from a new effective therapeutic treatment
- Desire for better treatment
- Possibility of an earlier introduction of new drugs
- Despair and Hopelessness – Knowing that there is no cure and that the treatment is the only option/at least gives a better quality of life
- Awareness of the importance to test drugs
- To further research and practice, to develop alternatives

2.3 Parents' reasons for refusal

The POs reported that the main reasons for parents to refuse to let their child participate in clinical trials were:

- Danger
- Fear
- Uncertainty:
- Lack of information and knowledge (of existence, methodology and accountability)
- The feeling that their child will be used as a 'guinea pig';
- Impact of the Media that focus on the negative rather than positive aspects of health systems and gives more space to alternative softer approaches rather than medicines

- Medical risk, side effects, adverse events, concern about long-term effects
- Concern the child would not comply with procedures and behaviour would worsen
- Long journey, limited ability to travel due to illness
- Language problems,
- Ethical reasons
- When procedures are perceived as invasive, and when new tests are foreseen for the trial. No concern if the trial is performed as part of routine checks
- Extra visits
- Extra medicines
- Lack of trust in scientists
- Lack of time if it involves more contact with health services than usual
- Costs
- Unrealistic expectations
- If child is asymptomatic
- Uncertainty to get the tested medication
- Formulation – not child sensitive
- Trial not designed with children in mind
- If it takes a long time to see any results from research done
- Not likely to benefit child directly

2.4 Good practices

With regard to good practices for increasing children's participation, these are those suggested:

- Convince them of the usefulness of the system, of the benefit they could draw and on the safety
- Provide detailed information to parents and stakeholders (also about opportunities abroad)
- Solid contact, strict monitoring of patients, regular feedback
- Transparency and consistency with the home life of the family
- Individual support to children to give them a stronger feeling of the self-determination so that they feel no longer so delivered to the illness
- Provide them with knowledge about clinical research methods through a combination of teaching, testimonies, discussion – individually and/or in groups
- Train the doctors and nurses to face the patients and to listen to the children
- A European focus group could be run with experts and collaboration with patient orgs with children and their parents from diverse disease areas
- Solid legislation framework
- Reach out from physicians to patient associations
- Patient organisations should be more present and improve the information given to parents and children. There must be more cooperation between the different stakeholders

- Key is that the child/parent knows and trusts the person explaining the trial, or introduces the person who will speak to them.

2.5 Role currently

The POs reported playing the following roles in CTs:

- *Providing guidance for trial participants in your brochures (1)*
- *Publishing letters or articles about trial participation in your members magazine or newsletter (10)*
- *Liaising with clinical trial projects (2)*
- *Giving advice and practical help to families in clinical trials (6)*
- *Contributing to health authority guidelines or ethical policy documents (3)*
- *Campaigning/lobbying activities (5)*

- *Other involvement specific to the condition you represent:*
- Support to research projects
- Participate in clinical research projects
- Membership of national and European associations
- Participation to European projects
- Draw attention to ongoing studies in our association magazine and internet media, especially if participants are sought. We report the results of studies. We advise them in advance of conducting the study
- Acting as a liaison between projects and parents, eg mailing out requests from researchers to take part in research to parents
- Bringing together researchers and scientists to discuss with patients' progress on research

2.6 Future role

They reported the following roles desired in the future:

- Same as now (2)
- Continue to fund research projects and start supporting genetic research.
- Lobbying for the people affected and their relatives
- Be involved in the whole CT process, from design to implementation especially in those aspects that are more important in the patients' views
- Inform parents
- More communication about ongoing progress from researchers

- Contribute more actively to the recruitment of participants in trials and help to increase motivation for participation
- Create a platform bringing together patients and the medical research community
- Raise awareness of clinical trials available
- Provide information to parents in close cooperation with doctors
- A role as advocate for Prader-Willi and for research in neurotransmitters
- Greater involvement in discussions about consent issues
- Greater involvement in policy documents or guidelines
- Be involved from the beginning on this issue and how it is presented to individual parents
- To be a resource for parents and for researchers
- Contribute to the development of ethical guidelines and other regulations
- To actively promote trials and research

2.7 Ideal role

The POs should take the supporting role and take the patient's i.e. the child's side in the discussions and support the children to be active.

POs should be involved in the very onset of children trials and in producing the guiding principles/ethics to give guidance.

It should be a requirement that representative POs should be informed when a trial in their disease area is planned and taking place. This would help everyone involved.

2.8 Additional comments made:

- Problems in getting funds to continue the trial, the treatment is not available in our country
- Importance of evaluating the risks against the potential benefit
- Clinical trials are something that are mainly conducted on diseases that are not particularly rare. Research into a rare disease generates less money, which is why we are neglected.
- While I fully understand the reasons why trials involving children are small, I have concerns that the evidence from such small trials is applicable across the wider population of children with the condition. For example, small trials of a new drug /insulin may not detect unexpected adverse events.

3 Conclusions

The low response level may be an indication of low involvement of POs in CTs, as confirmed by findings of the PatientPartner project (PatientPartner: Identifying good practices in patient involvement in clinical trials and research, www.patientpartner-europe.eu).

Apart for the case of one strong PO, most organisations seem to be involved in providing information and advice to parents but had no involvement in ethical committees, in setting up the CT or in the CT itself. Most organisations wished, however, to have a more active role.

We conclude that POs should play a central role for positioning the patients as equal partners in clinical trials (CTs). They must ensure that the ideas, needs and demands of the patients who are about to participate or already participated in CTs are taken into account and addressed. Increased involvement of POs will set the scene for fruitful negotiation between professionals and empowered patients that will lead to more patients participating in more trials.

Appendix 1c:

Paediatricians: survey and interview responses

1	OVERVIEW	174
2	RESPONSES: RECRUITING CHILDREN TO CLINICAL TRIALS	174
3	SUMMARY OF RECOMMENDATIONS FROM PAEDIATRICIANS	190

CONTRIBUTORS:

Monika Bullinger
Falk Wulf
Sylvia von Mackensen
David Neubauer
Catriona Chaplin

1 Overview

This part of the RESPECT project aimed to explore how paediatricians approach the task of recruiting children to clinical trials.

Data collection took place in Nov-Dec 2009. There were four interviews with professors of paediatrics in Sweden, Italy, Germany and the Netherlands. The same questions in the form of a survey were distributed to paediatricians in Slovenia and we received ten responses. These respondents had considerable experience of clinical trials, recruiting on average 85 participants each (ranging from 10 to 300).

2 Responses: recruiting children to clinical trials

Here we report the main questions of interest in the survey. The responses from the interviews have been combined with the survey responses in the results below.

1. What do you think is the best moment for approaching young patients and their families to ask for participation?

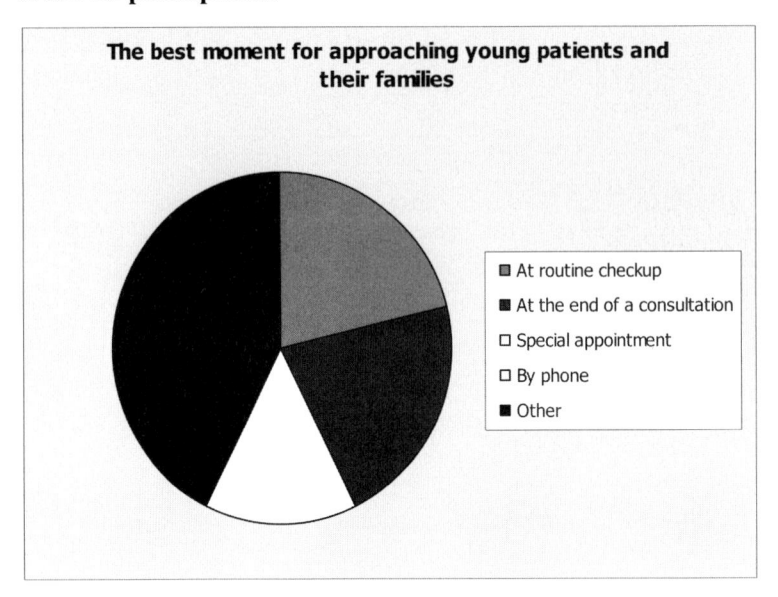

The best moment for approaching young patients and their families
- At routine checkup
- At the end of a consultation
- Special appointment
- By phone
- Other

Comments
- At the time of initial diagnostic workup at the department
- As early as possible
- When they can take time to consider it and have the energy to decide (when they are not at that moment burdened too much with their own health status).
- At the time of the treatment decision

Appendix 1c: Paediatricians

- When necessary to start treatment regardless the study
- After explanation about the condition and possibilities about procedures/treatment.
- After a medical examination or contact with the attending neurologist or physician. In school settings the best time would be at the beginning of the school year in collaboration with the school counselling service.
- After they have received some reassurance their child is being taken care of.
- Should be associated with the end of the consultation, when they know they are going home. A time when they are not stressed and they feel comfortable. A trial is always frightening.
- When they are at the clinic on check-ups and now in advance we would like to talk to them and they reserve time.
- At the check-up, but it is better to arrange a separate appointment to explain the study.
- Not during a medical setting or routine check-up. It should be and extra appointment in which you can focus on the study, but this is not practical.
- With phone follow-up.

2. Is it hard to explain things at their level?

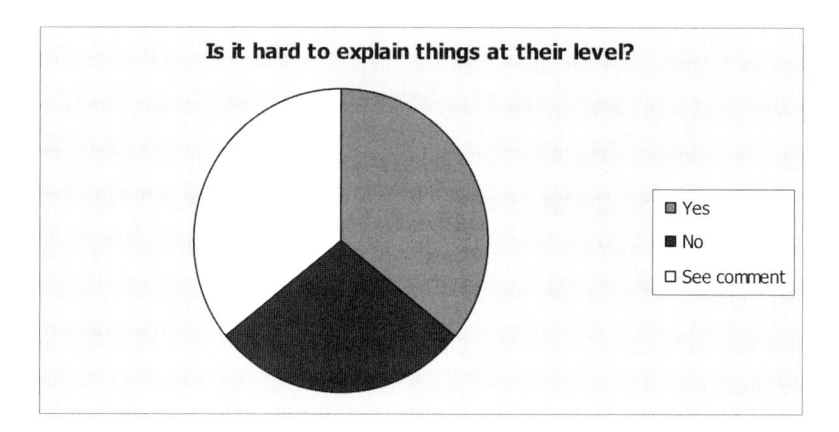

Is it hard to explain things at their level?

- Yes
- No
- See comment

Comments
- Sometimes it is a hard job
- The study purpose is not always clear.
- Yes, it depends on parent's education level.
- It is difficult because children are often not very attentive. The mother/father asks all the questions.
- Yes, I think we have to adjust the way we explain the study to participants according to their age and experience.
- Some aspects of a CT can be a bit harder to explain, but if you are well prepared it is possible to translate it into common language, maybe use some examples for illustration…

- Most of the important information are given at different levels- from practical and theoretical explanation, so that they can have a good picture of the trial.
- As our study deals mostly with adolescents they have are quite capable of understanding the methods and purposes of the study.
- As a paediatrician, I am used to explaining things in a simple way.
- It is the process of explanation similar to any other of medical procedures,

3. What level of knowledge do parents and children show about medical research and RCTs?

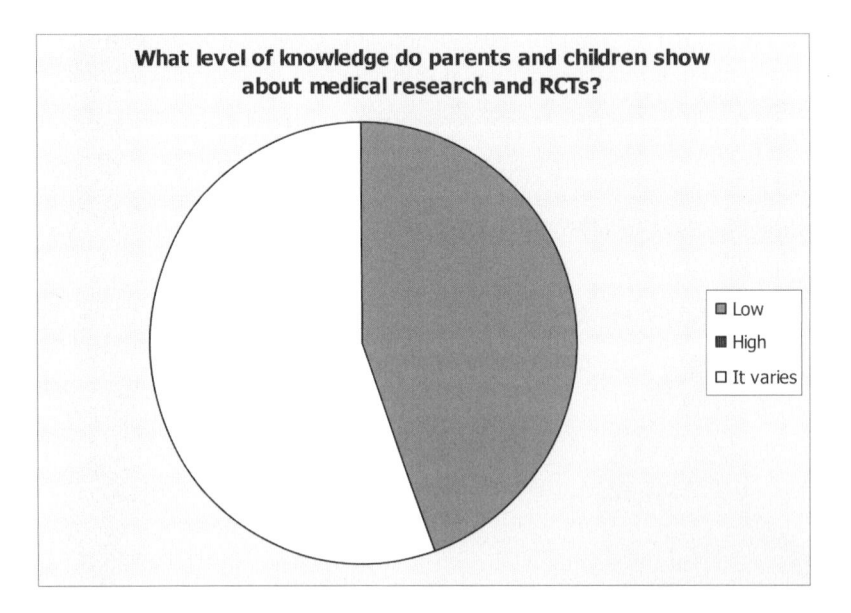

What level of knowledge do parents and children show about medical research and RCTs?

- Low
- High
- It varies

Comments
- Usually they only show basic knowledge about medical research.
- It depends on their education and previous contact with medical staff.
- Level of knowledge differs according to their experience (if they already participated in clinical trials).
- Usually their level is fair.
- Today, parents have a high level of knowledge; children have none.
- It is a bit different for immigrant families and Swedish families due to education differences, but it also varies between families from the same country. It is often difficult for them to understand the concept of randomisation.

Appendix 1c: Paediatricians

4. Do you think the young patients and their parents fully understand what the participant will have to do?

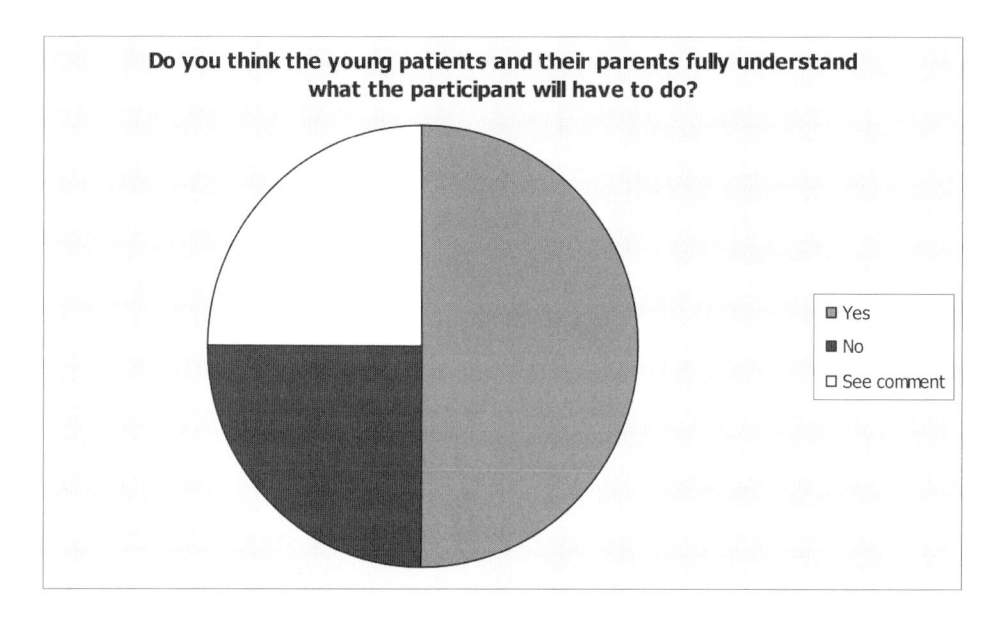

Do you think the young patients and their parents fully understand what the participant will have to do?

- Yes
- No
- See comment

Comments
- They do understand enough, I believe, to have a clear idea of what will happen to their child.
- The majority do.
- Mostly
- In the end
- They understand usually what they will have to do, but not necessarily why is this important for us.
- Many times at the beginning they do not understand fully
- It may not be fully understood by very young patients, but related of their level of understanding. Parents should fully understand the process.
- It is important that they understand what their contribution to the CT will be before they give their consent.
- In terms of psychological methods used, some have different expectations compared to what really happens.
- I am not certain whether they understand everything or not.
- If necessary we have to explain it more times during the study.

RESPECT

5. Are there best ways to inform children and parents about participating in clinical trials?

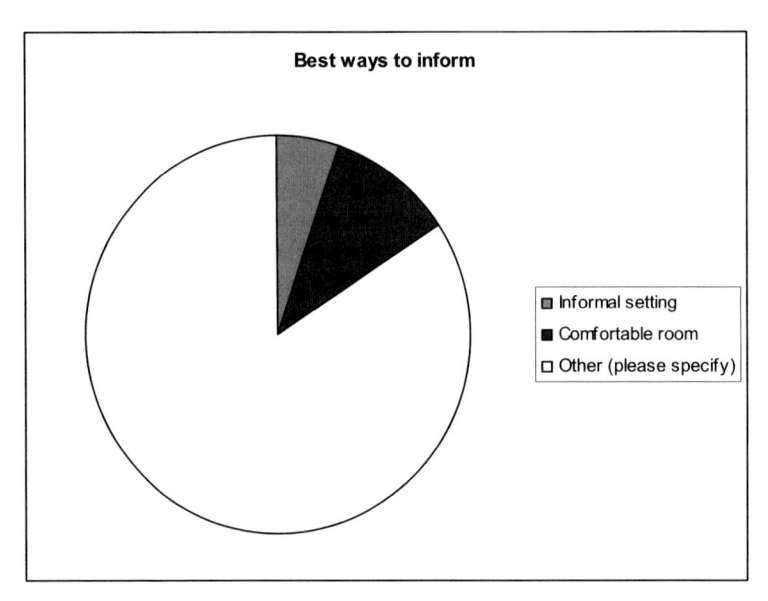

Best ways to inform

- Informal setting
- Comfortable room
- Other (please specify)

Comments
- To explain the whole process quickly but thoroughly.
- If we look at the form of communication, I would prefer verbal – or written information plus verbal explanation.
  As for the informed consent process – I follow the guidelines of APA (American Psychological Association).
- There are basic guidelines legally prescribed by Medical institutions and Ethics Committees, available to any clinical researcher, but subtle instructions how to approach are not always regulated.
- I don't know if there are best ways, since there are many different ways. There are some basic guidelines, but I believe the most important thing is to establish respect, trust and partnership with participants.
- Be honest.
- It has to be appropriate for their age.
- In my opinion it is important to listen to the questions of children and parent and follow them.
- The room should not be sterile – more home-like – and we should be sitting round a table, not behind a desk.

Appendix 1c: Paediatricians

6. From what age onward can children themselves give assent to participate in a clinical trial?

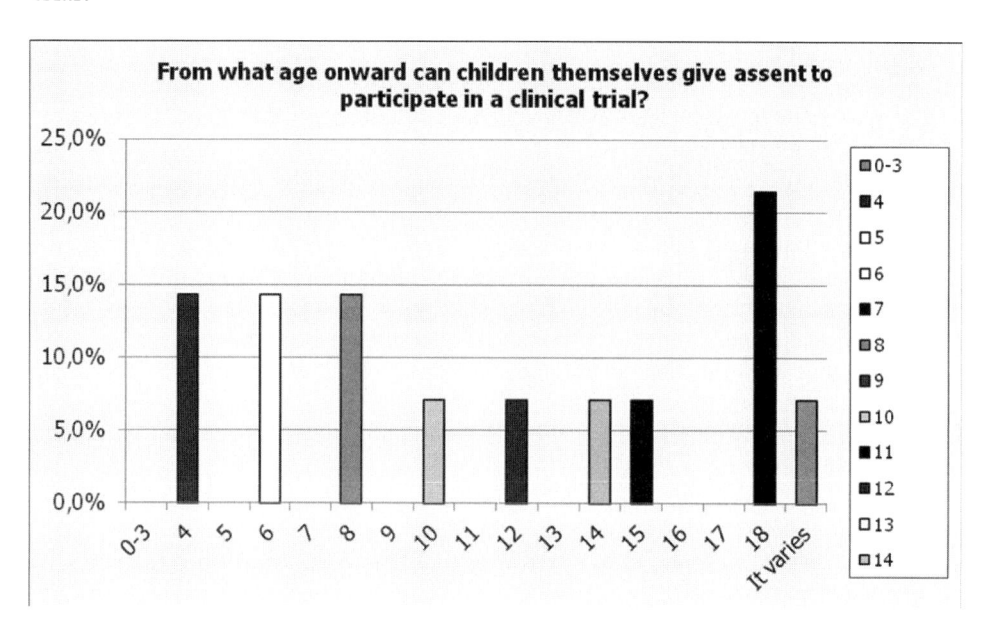

From what age onward can children themselves give assent to participate in a clinical trial?

[Bar chart showing percentages across age categories 0-3, 4, 5, 6, 7, 8, 9, 10, 11, 12, 13, 14, 15, 16, 17, 18, It varies]

Comments
- It depends on the child, his/her medical condition.
- It can be a very young age - since they have their own free will, but of course only their consent is not enough - parent's consent is necessary.
- In our country when they are 18 years old, but I ask also younger adolescents if they agree to the participation.
- Partially form the age of 5-6, fully from the age 10-11.
- It depends on the complexity of the study but, in general, around 8 years old.
- In Sweden, the formal limit is 15 years. We ask at 12 years, or even around 4 years if the child can understand what is going on.
- From 6 years old you can get some assent; from 10-12 years it will be more complete, depending on how mature they are.

7. Can you imagine difficult or special situations when discussing consent/assent?

Distress
- The child can have a devastating disease and bad prognosis and the parents are disappointed about the health care system and doctors and on top of that you try to talk to them about doing a research.
- When a child is severely ill and the type of CT requires talking to the parents at that point.
- When there is a patient who could not participate as a fully conscious person, mentally retarded or dying from chronic illness.
- With the smallest children (under 6 years) when you plan an invasive procedure such as injecting something, especially if they will be able to feel the intervention.
- Parents accept less invasive methods and fewer appointments than adult patients.
- Additional blood tests are often not accepted.
- Problems when the parents and child have different opinions, for example, the child does not want to have blood tests or refuses all of the procedures.

Knowledge gaps
- Randomisation is difficult to explain. When they understand it, some parents have problems accepting that they will be randomised to different treatment arms.
- Double-blind randomisation is even more complicated. They find it hard to accept that the doctor him/herself is not in charge of the treatment decision. It is important to explain the novelty of the new treatment.
- Level of knowledge differs according to their experience (if they already participated in clinical trials).
- It depends on their education and previous contact with medical staff.
- Sometimes parents respond that their child is not a "guinea pig".
- they don't like clinical studies, randomisation or new things.
- It is difficult for a parent since they have to decide on their child's behalf and not for themselves.

Inconvenience
- In situations where parents or patients may feel they would not get the full and appropriate service if they did not participate, although assured otherwise by the staff.
- Parents have time constraints.
- Parents prefer less involvement for themselves, but want to be well informed about child's involvement.

8. Do parents ask for more information than you thought they would need?

Do parents ask for more information than you thought they would need?

- No
- Yes, the results of the study
- Yes, practical details
- Other (please specify)

Risks
- Very rarely they will ask for additional explanations.
- Risks of the medication

Practicalities
- Usually they want more details on the study procedure and practical aspects (number of visits, time, number of days lost).

Results
- Parents are usually interested in the results of the study, especially in the results of their child.
- They rarely ask for the results. I do not give the special individual results routinely but if they ask, I do.

9. How do you explain risks and benefits of participating in clinical trials to children and to parents?

Honesty
- Openly, honestly and allow more times if necessary. I invite them to ask questions.
- I try to be honest and tell them the real information about benefits and their obligations.
- As honestly as possible without scaring them. I draw a comparison with Paracetamol (side-effects).
- Honestly, as I perceive them. That is how I would like somebody to illustrate things if it were my child.
- First I explain benefits and then risks. Risks should be minimal and similar to other routine procedures at the department.

Approaching the child
- A patient briefing with the child and parents together, taking the developmental stage of the child into consideration when explaining.
- With the child, it is very hard to explain the benefit. With older children, it helps to say that the results will benefit the entire patient group.

Appendix 1c: Paediatricians

10. What else could you offer them?

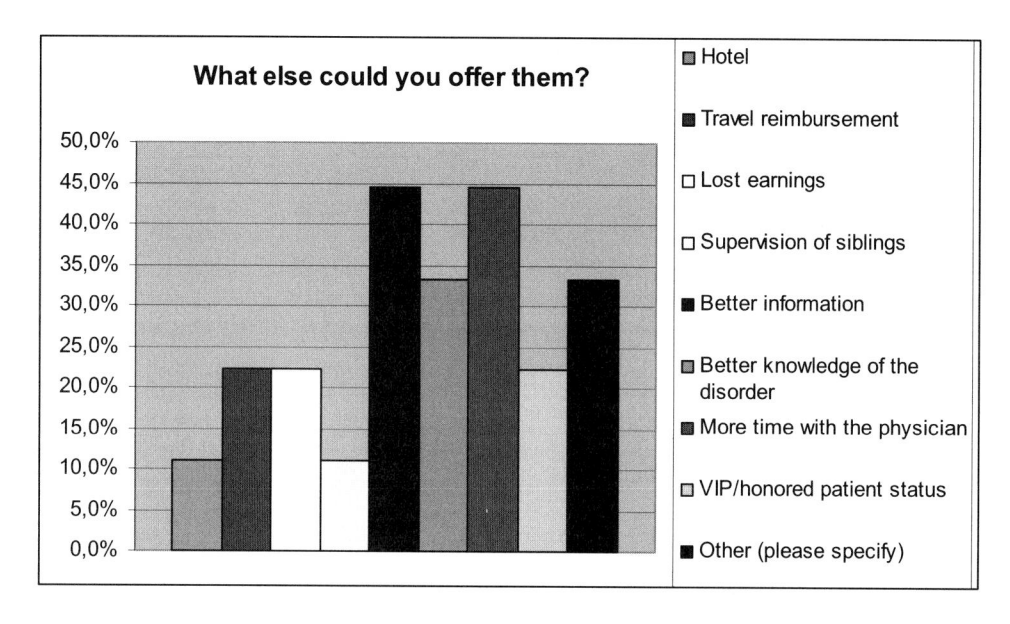

What else could you offer them?

- Hotel
- Travel reimbursement
- Lost earnings
- Supervision of siblings
- Better information
- Better knowledge of the disorder
- More time with the physician
- VIP/honored patient status
- Other (please specify)

Better knowledge
- Better information
- Better knowledge of the disorder
- We offer counselling on learning difficulties and offer information on the cognitive abilities of oneself as incentive.
- We offer other benefits, such as meeting different specialists that are included in the treatment of the child and getting new information. Since the aim of the study is making a psychosocial program for their child and that is a benefit for them in the future.

Extra monitoring, better treatment
- More time with the physician
- Better clinical and/or lab. surveillance during treatment, better drug and /or better efficacy of treatment, *fewer side effects*[1] comparing to standard ones etc.
- I point that out that a CT involves a procedure that is usually not easily available,
- Being a 'VIP patient' is not allowed but they feel this way.

Logistic support
- Travel reimbursement
- Lost earnings
- Hotel
- Supervision of siblings

---

[1] *Shows that this doctor believes the target drug is better*

- Because they usually have to take a day off work it would be nice if we could give them a financial compensation for that day.

Rewards
- Maybe a "fancy" meal (for schoolchildren and adolescents)
- For example to give them a small present after finishing the study, not money.
- VIP/honoured patient status

11. Do you give them a summary of the results?

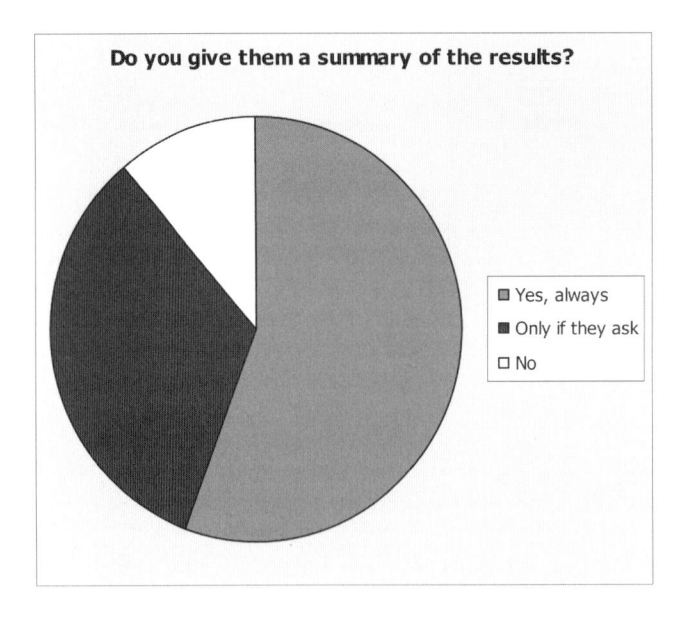

Do you give them a summary of the results?
- Yes, always
- Only if they ask
- No

12. What do you think they would prefer you (or the pharmaceutical company) to offer them?

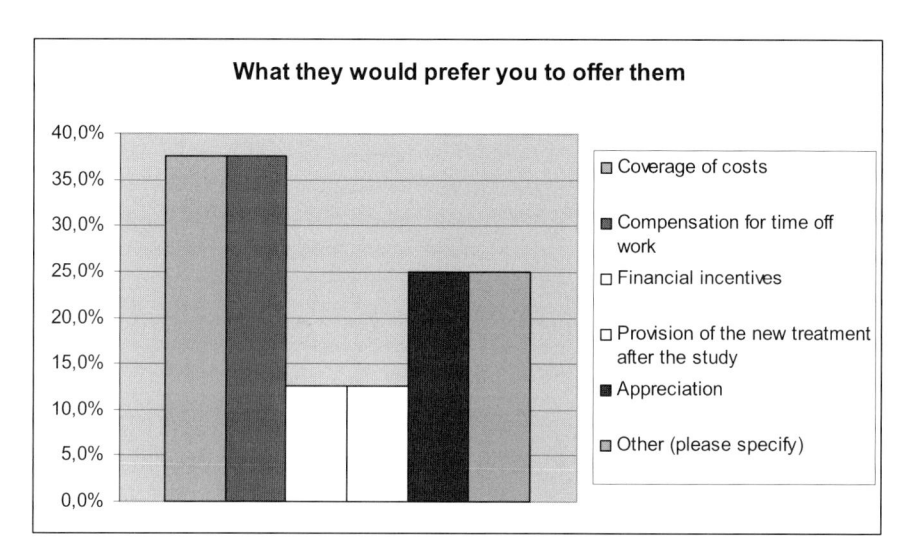

What they would prefer you to offer them

- Coverage of costs
- Compensation for time off work
- Financial incentives
- Provision of the new treatment after the study
- Appreciation
- Other (please specify)

Logistic support
- Coverage of costs
- Compensation for time off work
- Brought to hospital, comfortable room, food & drinks
- Financial incentives

Gratitude /token gestures
- Appreciation
- I think that young participants would prefer other material – non financial kinds or a form of social incentives.
- For a child, a day off the school is usually enough.

Better treatment
- Provision of the new treatment after the study
- Better drug with less side effects and once daily dosing
- If they would start treatment anyway they are usually more interested to participate free.

13. What do you believe are children's / parents' motives or reasons to participate in clinical trials?

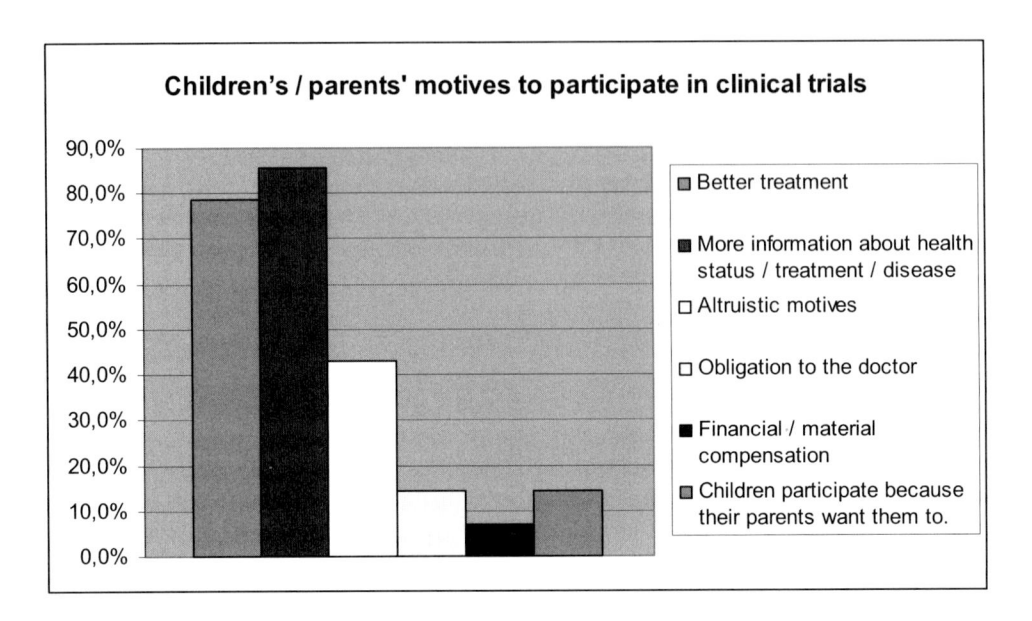

Children's / parents' motives to participate in clinical trials

- Better treatment
- More information about health status / treatment / disease
- Altruistic motives
- Obligation to the doctor
- Financial / material compensation
- Children participate because their parents want them to.

Better treatment / monitoring
- Better treatment
- More information about health status / treatment /
- Additional examinations
- Perhaps new possibilities of treatment.
- Better knowledge of the disease.

Relationship with doctor
- Trust and good relations with the treating doctor
- Obligation to the doctor
- Altruistic motives
- Honoured to be asked

Child's motives
- Children participate because their parents want them to.
- The child has no motivation; participates because the physician asks them to.

Rewards
- Financial / material compensation

Appendix 1c: Paediatricians

14. In your opinion, what are the barriers to participation for children and parents?

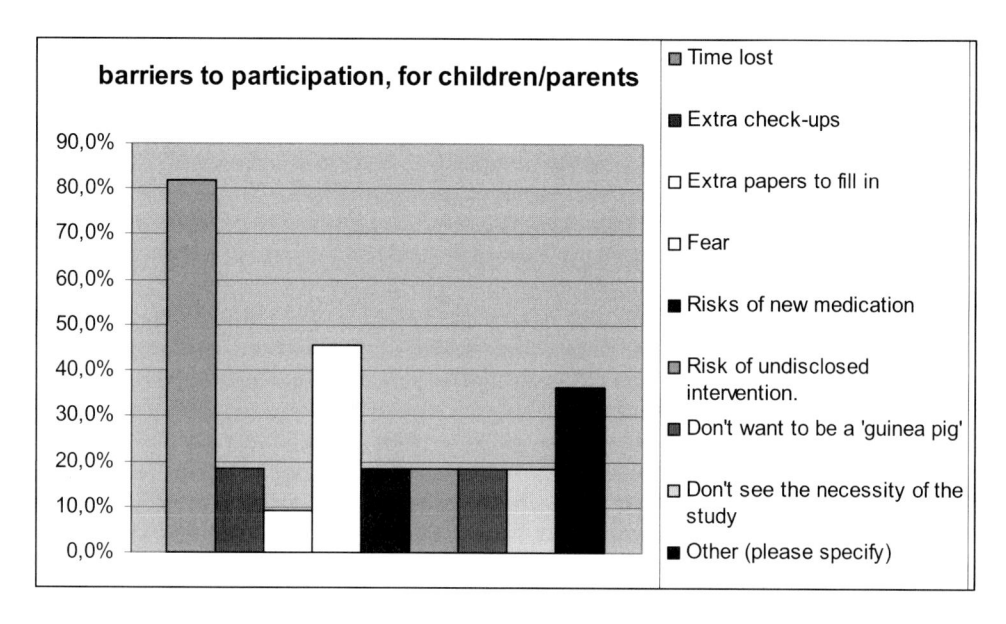

barriers to participation, for children/parents

- Time lost
- Extra check-ups
- Extra papers to fill in
- Fear
- Risks of new medication
- Risk of undisclosed intervention.
- Don't want to be a 'guinea pig'
- Don't see the necessity of the study
- Other (please specify)

Inconvenience
- Extra check-ups
- Extra papers to fill in
- Time constraints
- Difficulties associated in travelling for participants who live further away
- Difficulties at work when parents have to take a day off
- Parents: don't want to invest the time;
- Children: Don't see the necessity of the study

Fear
- Risks of new medication
- Invasive procedures
- Risk of undisclosed intervention
- Worry about the side-effects
- Fear that the child and they could get an infection

Personal disadvantage
- Afraid of their obligations in a longitudinal study
- Overload of clinical trials
- Don't want to be a 'guinea pig'
- Lost hope

15. What are the barriers to participation for clinicians/physicians?

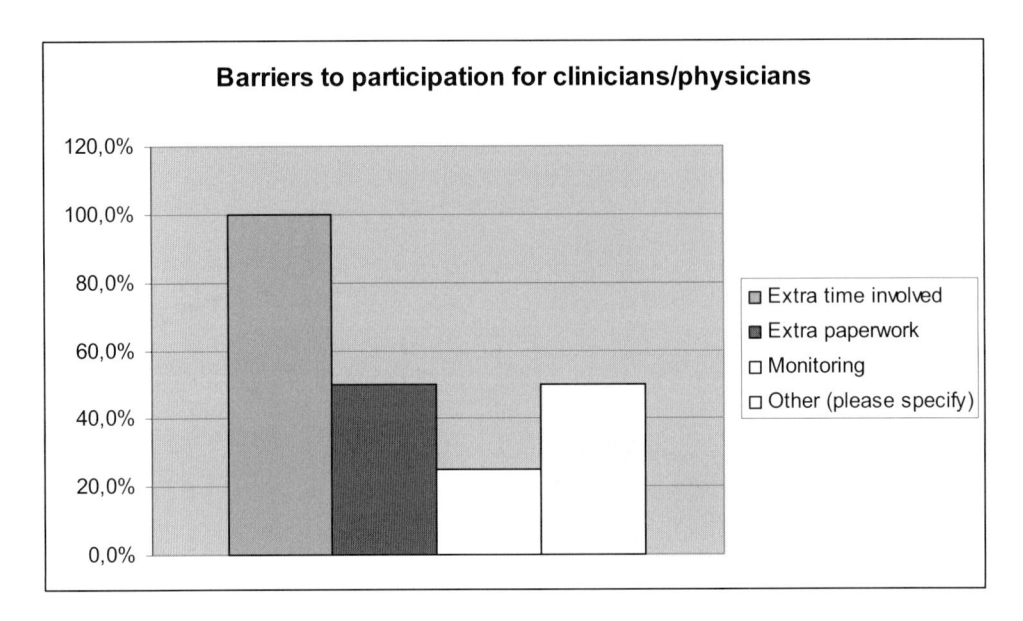

Barriers to participation for clinicians/physicians

- Extra time involved: 100%
- Extra paperwork: 50%
- Monitoring: 25%
- Other (please specify): 50%

Workload
- Extra time involved
- Extra paperwork
- Monitoring
- Lack of medical staff
- High workload on students in schools or at universities
  Difficulty in recruiting participants of control groups that do not come from a clinical population
- Too complicated formal procedures

Appendix 1c: Paediatricians

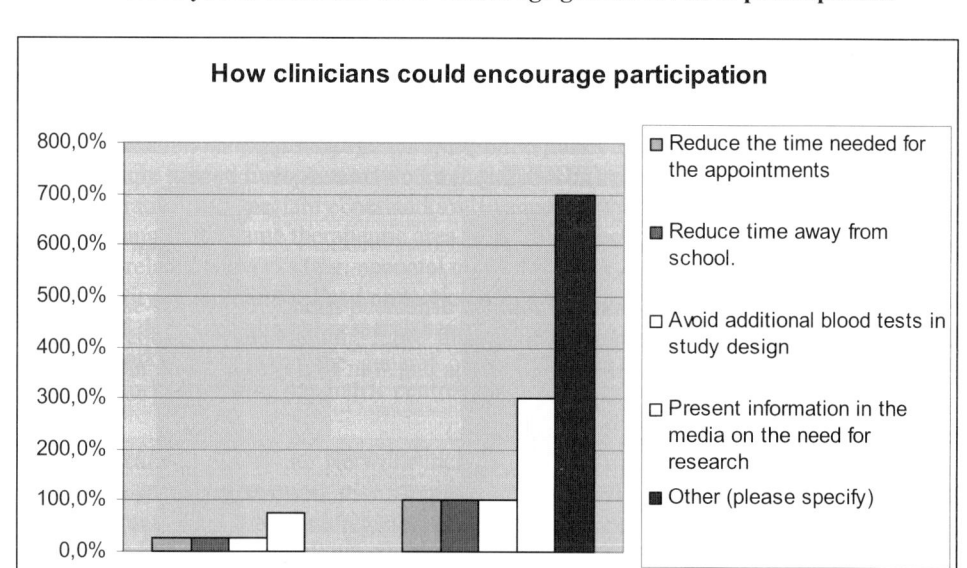

16. What could you as clinicians do to encourage greater levels of participation?

How clinicians could encourage participation

- Reduce the time needed for the appointments
- Reduce time away from school.
- Avoid additional blood tests in study design
- Present information in the media on the need for research
- Other (please specify)

Reduce inconvenience & pain
- Reduce the time needed for the appointments
- Reduce time away from school.
- Avoid additional blood tests in study design
- Try to influence the study design so that additional blood tests could be avoided.
- Some of the above could be improved by better logistical support and the recruitment of a research coordinator (research nurse) who would help facilitate in coordinate efforts in the recruitment process.

More discussion
- Giving more info, taking more time for the conversation.
- Clear explanation
- Encourage them to see the meaning or the benefit for themselves.

Appeal to the public
- A newsletter about ongoing clinical trials, information at patient meetings, flyers & posters.
- Present information in the media on the need for research
- They could be invited in campaigns as "advertising" by posters or radios to facilitate the knowledge about the problem, to let them know where they can come to join the study and to pay for objective expenses when they need to come far to research center.

3   Summary of recommendations from paediatricians

Physicians are in a unique position to inform trial sponsors about the child's unmet medical needs and to influence which trials are conducted.

It is important to ensure that families understand the need for research and are respected for their valuable contribution to CTs. These are the most important points to bear in mind:

- The clinician must gain family's respect and trust;
- randomisation must be clearly explained;
- the clinician must be honest - as one would for one's own child;
- it is important to listen to the family's concerns;
- wherever possible, the clinical staff should strive to reduce distress for the child;
- inconvenience for the family should be kept to a minimum;
- the clinical staff must give and take feedback before, during and after the trial;
- the clinical staff must show appreciation, acknowledging that the child is a 'medical hero'.

Appendix 1d:

CT networks: Survey responses and analysis of the involvement of children within Enpr-EMA

1	**SURVEY**	**192**
	1.1 Introduction	192
	1.2 Definition of CT networks	192
	1.3 Aim of the survey	193
	1.4 Methodology	193
	1.5 Results	194
	1.6 Conclusions	200
2	**ANALYSIS OF THE INVOLVEMENT OF CHILDREN IN CT NETWORKS**	**202**
	2.1 The European network of paediatric research (Enpr-EMA)	202
	2.2 Recognition criteria for self-assessment	202
	2.3 Aim and methodology of this analysis	202
	2.4 Networks evaluated for Enpr-EMA	203
	2.5 Involvement of families or their organisations	204
	2.6 Replies to Criterion 6 from CT networks fulfilling criteria for membership	206
	2.7 Replies to Criterion 6 from CT networks undergoing clarification	214
	2.8 Replies to Criterion 6 from CT networks currently not qualifying for membership	214
	2.9 Conclusions	220

CONTRIBUTORS:

Cristina Manfredi
Adriana Ceci
Catriona Chaplin

1 Survey

1.1 Introduction

The importance of involving children and their representatives early in the development of medicinal products is a well-recognised fact nowadays.

The EU Regulation No. 726/2004/EC [1], for example, lays down the Community procedures for the authorisation and supervision of medicinal products for human and veterinary use and establishes the European Medicines Agency (EMA). Its Articles 78(1) and 78(2), in particular, establish that the EMA must develop interaction with its various stakeholders, particularly representatives of consumers and patients.

Thus, patients and consumers' organisations are involved in EMA activities and they have their representatives in scientific committees and working groups such as the Committee for Orphan Medicinal Products (COMP) and the Paediatric Committee (PDCO). In addition, there is the Patients' and Consumers' Working Party (PCWP) that was created to provide recommendations to the EMA and its human scientific committees on all matters of direct or indirect interest to patients in relation to medicinal products.

However, when it comes to actual clinical research, only 2-3% of all patients actively participate. This is mainly due to a lack of awareness on what exactly CT research is and concerns on ethical issues linked to the trials (e.g. randomisation), but also to lack of feedback of results, inconveniences of the practicalities of the CT, and lack of understanding of the information provided and of the informed consent (http://www.patientpartner-europe.eu).

1.2 Definition of CT networks

The EU Paediatric Regulation [2], with its Recital 3 and Article 44, posed the legal basis for the development of the "European network of existing national and European networks, investigators and centres with specific expertise in the performance of studies in the paediatric population".

The EMA was appointed the responsibility of setting up such a network and the first step taken by the Agency was to draft the implementing strategy where a network was identified as a virtual structure defined by a formal agreement between individuals, organisations or structures sharing and collaborating towards the same objectives, goals and quality standards [3].

A clinical trials (CT) network, in particular, is a network that focused on the development of medicinal products, while paediatric CT networks are those networks with specific expertise in the performance of studies in the paediatric population.

In order to achieve its aim and establish the European Network of Paediatric Networks, the EMA carried out an informal inventory of the existing paediatric clinical trials networks, showing that many different paediatric networks exist or are under construction in the European Community.

According to this inventory, paediatric CT networks can be identified as:
- national networks, generally benefiting from public funding.
- publicly funded European networks (e.g. TEDDY).
- Paediatric 'sub-speciality' networks at European level and beyond, which group centres working in the same therapeutic area (e.g. HIV infection, rheumatology).
- Age-related networks (e.g. neonatal networks).
- Activity or structure-related networks (e.g. community-practitioners networks, hospital-based dedicated clinical-research centres linked by a common structure, pharmacovigilance networks).
- Networks including paediatric centres but not dedicated solely to paediatric research.

1.3 Aim of the survey

Despite the fact that there is wide recognition for the importance of involving patients in the early stages of the planning of clinical research, few studies actually include the active participation of children, parents or their organisation.

In view of the increased number of paediatric clinical trials and the role played by CT networks, RESPECT carried out, in collaboration with TEDDY (Task-force in Europe for Drug Development for the Young), an investigation among paediatric CT networks to better understand how they encourage patients' participation in their clinical research.

1.4 Methodology

A questionnaire was circulated among selected paediatric CT networks.
The survey comprised four open questions that were aimed at understanding how paediatric CT networks encourage patients' participation and involve children or their representatives in their clinical research, and in particular:
- Do families or patient organisation have an input in the design of clinical trials?
- How do paediatric CT networks recruit participants?
- Is there any feedback of results or data collection on patient needs from the families?
- How can the network improve the focus on the child's experience?

The twelve paediatric CT networks contacted for the survey were selected from the inventory carried out by the EMA.

1.5 Results

Answers were collected from eight of the twelve networks contacted.

The survey contained the following questions:
Q1: Does your network allow families or patient organisations any input in the design of clinical trials?
Q2: What is your network's recruitment process?
Q3: Does your network gather and provide feedback from/to families after trial completion?
Q4: Does your network have any examples of best practice in their organisation or suggestions for improved focus on the child's experience of a clinical trial?

A summary of the results of the survey is provided in Table 1.

Table 1: Overview of the survey results

Network no.	Q1: Direct involvement	Q2: Recruitment	Q3: Feedback	Q4: Best practice
1	No	• Network's involved centres • Contact with specialists • Involvement of patients organisation • Ads	Occasionally (only general results)	-
2	No	• Network's involved centres • Ads	Encouraged, but depends on type of trial and sponsor	Templates and picture cards www.finpedmed.com
3	Yes	• Network's involved centres	Newsletters Website	Youth groups
4	Yes	• Individual investigators	General feedback on trial outcome	-
5	No	• Participating centres	No feedback	-
6	No	• Network's Databank • Physicians' direct contact	No feedback	-
7	Yes	• Posters • GP surgeries • Consultant • Access to password protected databases	Encouraged (newsletters, web links, etc.)	MCRN young person's advisory group Topic specific focus groups
8	Depends on study	• Network's involved centres • Contact with specialists • Involvement of patients organisation	Encouraged, but not always attainable	Informative packages for children (videos, picture cards) Recommendations for children and parents

The reported direct involvement of children or their patient organisations in clinical research is achieved through patient organisation representatives in the Executive Committee; alternatively through forums and focus groups, or parents' representatives in the Steering Committee. For others, the participation of patients depends on the type of study and disease.

1.5.1 CT network 1

This network of paediatric clinical investigations centres comprises eight research centres within teaching hospitals and aims to conduct paediatric clinical research in the areas of drug evaluation and pathophysiology (primarily growth and neurosciences) and to contribute to technical innovations

Activities include:
- support to investigators, from design through the conduct of investigator-initiated or industrially sponsored clinical research protocols;
- provide specific training in paediatric clinical research to physicians, pharmacists and nurses;
- conducting research in children.

Below are their answers to the questionnaire.

Q1: Does your network allow families or patient organisations any input in the design of clinical trials?
No real input is collected from patients and their families.

Q2: What is your network's recruitment process?
Feasibility is evaluated with the medical investigator in order to estimate "the number of patients that may participate in the trial.
A team including a paediatrician and a research technician or research nurse is responsible of screening patients.
Recruitment is carried out through the network (hospitalized patients), among specialists and patients organisation (if rare disease). Synopsis and/or short advertisements in hospitals are also used.

Q3: Does your network gather and provide feedback from/to families after trial completion?
Feedback is not always given and usually it concerns general information on results.
Difficult to be accomplished with industry sponsored trials.

1.5.2 CT network 2

This investigators network for paediatric medicines comprises five university hospitals and their paediatric clinics. Its aim is to improve both academic and sponsored paediatric clinical trials for the benefit of children's health and to harmonise and unify research protocol and operations models.

Activities include protocol design, protocol evaluation and development, conduction of clinical research.

Below are their answers to the questionnaire.

Q1: Does your network allow families or patient organisations any input in the design of clinical trials?
This is a coordinating organisation, thus the design of studies is not one of its responsibility. However, the opinion of the network is that input of patient organisations in the design of a clinical trial, or in prioritising proposed clinical trials, is not feasible. Moreover, in our country, patient/family input is systematically included through ethical review process.

Q2: What is your network's recruitment process?
Recruitment is carried out by the investigators, mainly by direct patient contacts from clinics and clinical trial units. In some cases, advertisement in local newspapers is also used.

Q3: Does your network gather and provide feedback from/to families after trial completion?
Feedback to families is always encouraged, however, it depends on type of trial and it is influenced by contract with Sponsor.

Q4: Does your network have any examples of best practice in their organisation or suggestions for improved focus on the child's experience of a clinical trial?
Our network developed a template for providing information on a clinical trial to paediatric patients of all age groups, templates for informed consent in all age groups, and picture cards for use in providing information on a clinical trial for children.

These templates were developed in collaboration with all stakeholders (including families), while the picture cards were developed in collaboration with children of different ages.
The templates have become a national standard and are available in three languages; picture cards have been provided for all network members, and are available for purchase.

1.5.3   CT network 3

This disease-specific European paediatric network was established as a collaboration between paediatric centres in European, South American and Asian countries.

The aims of the network are to address questions about treatment for children with the condition which cannot be answered in adults principally because the natural history of infection differs and the tolerance of drugs may be different; it also aims to collaborate with adult trials networks, and to evaluate primarily safety and tolerability in children to parallel efficacy trials in adults.

Below are their answers to the questionnaire.

Q1: Does your network allow families or patient organisations any input in the design of clinical trials?
There are parents' representatives in the Steering Committee, which has major input in trial design.

Q2: What is your network's recruitment process?
Patients are directly involved in CT by their caring physicians.

Q3: Does your network gather and provide feedback from/to families after trial completion?
Feedback is given through newsletters and website.

Q4: Does your network have any examples of best practice in their organisation or suggestions for improved focus on the child's experience of a clinical trial?
Youth groups who provide feedback on their infectious status, including medical and social care.

1.5.4 CT network 4

This disease-specific European paediatric network includes 18 centres, located in eight different European countries and treating more than 8000 patients. The Network aims to optimise the development and evaluation of new and approved treatments through efficient clinical studies in Europe.

Activities carried out by the Network include advising on optimal study design, identifying the most appropriate target population, improving sample size calculations by using real life data (including data from their own registry) and decreasing the sample size needed by standardisation of outcome parameters.

Below are their answers to the questionnaire.

Q1: Does your network allow families or patient organisations any input in the design of clinical trials?
Protocols are reviewed before being accepted by the Network, including priority rating. This is done by an Executive Committee that includes one Patient Organisation (PO) representative.
A minimum of 2 Patient Organisation representatives are present in the twice-yearly Steering Committee meetings, while the Executive Committee includes one PO representative and meets every two weeks.

Patients have also participated in consensus conferences/workshops on trial design / outcome parameters.

From start-up of the Network, the partnering with patient organisations was seen as the only model possible. Patient representation is asked in every specific Network's activity.

Q2: What is your network's recruitment process?
Recruitment is carried out by individual investigators who consult their internal databases and contact patient / parents.

Studies will soon be listed on the networks website with link to clinicaltrials.gov info and the countries where the study is active.

Q3: Does your network gather and provide feedback from/to families after trial completion?
Individual sites receive a reminder at end of the study to provide information on outcome of research. The Network checks with sponsor to provide such a summary. This general feedback on

RESPECT

trial outcome (in agreement with pharmaceutical companies) is provided to both POs and to the individual participating sites for their use.

1.5.5 CT network 5

This is a non-governmental international disease-specific network including 47 countries and more than 200 centres worldwide. The network's main aim is to foster, facilitate and co-ordinate the development, conduct, analysis, and reporting of multi-centres, international clinical trials and/or outcome standardisation studies in children with these diseases.

Below are their answers to the questionnaire.

Q1: Does your network allow families or patient organisations any input in the design of clinical trials?
No participation from families is foreseen when designing clinical trials.

Q2: What is your network's recruitment process?
Physicians of the network are informed about the possibility to participate in a clinical trial. Participating centres have the responsibility to contact and speak with families for possible enrolment in the trial. Since the Network deals with chronic conditions, this interaction physicians/families is the only and best method to recruit children.

Q3: Does your network gather and provide feedback from/to families after trial completion?
No feedback given.

1.5.6 CT network 6

This national paediatric clinical research network was born in 2005 and members include seven university hospitals.
The aim of the network is to:
- Increase awareness regarding the use of medicines in children;
- Promote GCP in paediatrics nationally;
- Identify unmet needs;
- Monitor off-label use;
- Improve pharmacovigilance reports;
- Organise / facilitate academic research;
- Offer pediatric expertise to ethical committees and health authorities;
- Defend children's right to equal access to medicines;
- Offer established network for pharmaceutical industry pediatric research (in & out patients).

Below are their answers to the questionnaire.

Q1: Does your network allow families or patient organisations any input in the design of clinical trials?
No input from patients or POs.

Q2: What is your network's recruitment process?
Network's databank and physicians' direct contact

Q3: Does your network gather and provide feedback from/to families after trial completion?
No feedback provided.

1.5.7 CT network 7

This national network has been created to improve the co-ordination, speed and quality of randomised controlled trials and other well designed studies of medicines for children and adolescents, including those for prevention, diagnosis and treatment.
The network's main objective is to facilitate the development of medicines that are both safe and effective in the treatment of children. It has a major focus on clinical trials but also includes other study designs relevant to the overall objective.

Below are their answers to the questionnaire.

Q1: Does your network allow families or patient organisations any input in the design of clinical trials?
Yes, the network has a comprehensive patient and public involvement strategy that aims to involve children and families in every stage of the research process, including: priority setting; identifying research ideas; design and delivery of studies; analysis of findings through to the dissemination of research results.

This is achieved through several forums, including:
- A National Young Person's Advisory Group
- Parent/Carer Representatives on all Clinical Studies Groups
- Parent/Carer Representatives on the Study Assessment Committee
- Parent and family involvement in all six Local Research Networks
- Topic Specific Focus Groups
- Engagement of young people in schools.

Q2: What is your network's recruitment process?
This will vary depending on the recruitment strategy identified in the protocol and depends on ethical approval for a particular recruitment approach, for example posters, GP surgeries, consultant etc. Researchers may also have access to password-protected databases that can identify the exact patient population.

Q3: Does your network gather and provide feedback from/to families after trial completion?
As a network, we encourage researchers to feedback the outcomes of the research to families and we have several examples of this.

One particular example is of a qualitative study that investigated how families are recruited to randomised controlled trials (RCTs) of medicines for children. The research team had worked with our young person's advisory group from the beginning of the study, designing patient information leaflets, and interview schedules. They returned to the group to highlight the key findings and worked with the group to produce a child/family-friendly information leaflet to be distributed to participants, the young people also contributed to the dissemination event that was held to highlight the findings to a much wider audience. Our network aims to take forward the recommendations of this study to enhance a child's experience of a clinical trial.

Other examples include feeding back to families during follow up, explaining the outcome of the study. Some researchers produce regular newsletters, web links etc to distribute information to families.

Q4: Does your network have any examples of best practice in their organisation or suggestions for improved focus on the child's experience of a clinical trial?
One example of best practice is to encourage the active involvement of young people and families in the design and delivery of clinical trials (via the young person's advisory group, or topic specific focus groups etc) and to incorporate a feedback mechanism into study design.

1.5.8 CT network 8

This national CT network is a promoter and/or collaborating centre of national and international clinical studies with the ultimate aim of promoting research in the pharmaceutical field.

Activities carried out include design and conduction of CTs, design of CTs in small populations (paediatrics and rare diseases), management of disease registries, pharmacoepidemiological and pharmacoutilisation studies, HTA (pharmacoeconomic studies), and organisation of meetings and workshops targeted to both public bodies and private institutions.

Below are their answers to the questionnaire.

Q1: Does your network allow families or patient organisations any input in the design of clinical trials?
Direct participation of patients and patients organization in the drafting of protocols is not always feasible and depends on the type of study and the type of disease that is being investigated.

Q2: What is your network's recruitment process?
Recruitment is usually carried out by investigators/participating centers by direct patient contacts from clinics and clinical trial units and/or presentations to specialists and/or patients associations.

Q3: Does your network gather and provide feedback from/to families after trial completion?
Feedback is encouraged, but not always attainable.

1.6 Conclusions

Our consultation shows that only three out of the eight paediatric CT networks participating in the survey systematically involve patients and/or patient organisations in their clinical research. Two of the three networks are disease oriented and fall in a very specific *rare diseases* category, while the third is a generic network facilitating the development of medicines that are both safe and effective in the treatment of children.

CT network 8 highlights the fact that the direct participation of patients in the planning stage of clinical research depends on the type of study, and in particular on the investigated disease: if there is a strong patient organisation, it is more likely that their input is sought from the early stages of the research.

Recruitment is usually carried out within the network's members and/or participating centres; if the number of children recruited through the network is not sufficient, specialists and/or POs (in the case of rare diseases) are contacted; only occasionally the clinical trial is publicised through advertisements.

Feedback is systematically given only by one network, while usually it is encouraged, but not always attainable. The amount of information given to families depends on the sponsor, but usually data relate only to the general outcome of the trials, while personal information are typically not given.

Examples of best practice are provided by several networks:
- A national template for providing information on a CT to children of all age groups and templates for informed consent in all age groups. They have also developed picture cards to use when providing information on a clinical trial for children.
- Youth groups that providing feedback on their HIV infectious status and their medical and social care.
- Active involvement of young people and families in the design and delivery of clinical trials via a young person's advisory group, or topic-specific focus groups.

From the results of our survey we conclude that direct involvement of children and patient organisations still is not in the current practice of paediatric CT networks, and it is necessary to increase awareness on the subject.

It might be useful to draft and circulate recommendations targeted to families and children to encourage their aware involvement in clinical trials.

2 Analysis of the involvement of children in CT networks

2.1 The European network of paediatric research (Enpr-EMA)

The European Paediatric Regulation posed the legal basis for the development of the "European network of existing national and European networks, investigators and centres with specific expertise in the performance of studies in the paediatric population". The European Medicines Agency (EMA) was appointed the responsibility to set up such a network and in January 2008, the Agency's Management Board adopted its implementing strategy.

In May 2010, the organisational structure and the recognition criteria requirements to become member of the Network were agreed on by participants from 38 national research networks and clinical trial centres and the European Medicines Agency.

Clinical trial (CT) networks interested in joining the Network were invited to complete a self-assessment form and in January 2011, the EMA published a full listing of applicants for membership of the European network of paediatric research (Enpr-EMA). See: http://www.emea.europa.eu/htms/human/paediatrics/network.htm.

2.2 Recognition criteria for self-assessment

Recognition criteria to become member of the Enpr-EMA have been finalised through a process involving a test pilot phase, public consultation and the outcome of the second workshop organised by EMA with various networks and CT centres.

The following six criteria, with several subcategories (so-called items) that networks should fulfil to be recognised as a member of the Enpr-EMA, were defined:
- Criterion 1: Research experience and ability.
- Criterion 2: Network organisation and processes.
- Criterion 3: Scientific competencies and capacity to provide expert advice.
- Criterion 4: Quality management.
- Criterion 5: Training and educational capacity to build competences.
- Criterion 6: Public involvement.

The self-assessment must be updated annually.

2.3 Aim and methodology of this analysis

This analysis looks specifically at the responses to Criterion 6 to find best practice examples of child, parent or patient organisation involvement.

Within Criterion 6, the minimum requirement was involvement of the public in at least one of the following three component items:

> 6.1 Involvement of patients, parents or their organisations in the protocol design.
> 6.2 Involvement of patients, parents or their organisations in creating the protocol information package.
> 6.3 Involvement of patients, parents or their organisations in the prioritisation of needs for clinical trials in children.

2.4 Networks evaluated for Enpr-EMA

A total of 33 CT networks submitted self-assessment reports to the European Medicines Agency: 18 are now officially members of Enpr-EMA, 1 is currently undergoing clarification and 14 do not qualify for membership (Table 2).

Other networks, such as TEDDY and more recently, GRIP (Global Research in Paediatrics), participate in Enpr-EMA as 'methodological Networks'. These networks do not perform clinical trials directly and do not meet criteria for submitting the self-assessment forms.

Table 2. Networks applying for Enpr-EMA membership

ACRONYM	CLINICAL TRIALS NETWORK NAME
Member Networks	
ECFS-CTN	European Cystic Fibrosis Society - Clinical Trials Network
EPOC	European Paediatric Oncology Off-patent Medicines Consortium
EUNETHYDIS	European Network for Hyperkinetic Disorders
FIMP - MCRN	Italian Paediatric Federation - Medicines for Children Research Network
FINPEDMED	Finnish Investigators Network for Pediatric Medicine
GNN	German Neonatal Network
IBFMSG	International BFM Study Group
ITCC	Innovative Therapies for Children with Cancer
MCRN UK	National Institute for Health Research (NIHR) Medicines for Children Research Network
MCRN NL	Medicines for Children Research Network
MICYRN	Mother Infant Child Youth Research Network
Newcastle CCLG PSG	Newcastle CCLG Pharmacology Studies Group
PENTA	Paediatric European Network for the Treatment of AIDS
PRINTO	Pediatric Rheumatology International Trials Organisation
Scottmcn	Scottish Medicines for Children Network
UKPVG	United Kingdom Paediatric Vaccines Group
CICPed	Paediatric Network of Clinical Investigation Centers
EBMT PD WP	European Group for Blood and Marrow Transplantation

Networks undergoing clarification	
CLG EORTC	Children Leukemia Group
Networks currently not qualifying for membership	
BPDN	Belgian Pediatric Drug Network
EuroNeoNet	EuroNeoNet
ESPGHAN	European Society of Paediatric Gastronenterology Hepatology and Nutrition
Futurenest	Futurenest Clinical Research
IPTA	International Pediatric Transplant Association
IPCRN	Irish Paediatric Clinical Research Network
JSWG PRES	Juvenile Scleroerma Working Group - Paediatric Rheumatology European Society
Neocirculation	Neocirculation
PENTi	Paediatric European Network for the Treatment of Infection
RIPPS	Réseau d'Investigations Pédiatriques des Produits de Santé
BLF	Swedish Pediatric Society
AMIKI	Paediatric Trial Network
NCCHD	National Center for Child Health and Development - Japan
INN	Italian Neonatal Network

2.5 Involvement of families or their organisations

Almost 85% of the applying CT networks involve children, parents or their organisations in at least one of the activities included in Criterion 6 (Public involvement).

In particular, 54.5% include the public in protocol design, 51.5% in the creation of protocol information packages, and 57.6% in the prioritisation of needs for clinical trials in children (Figure 1).

Moreover, 27.3% of these network involve children, parents or their organisations in all three criteria, 24.2% in two of the three criteria, 33.3% in just one criterion and 15.2% do not involve the public at all.

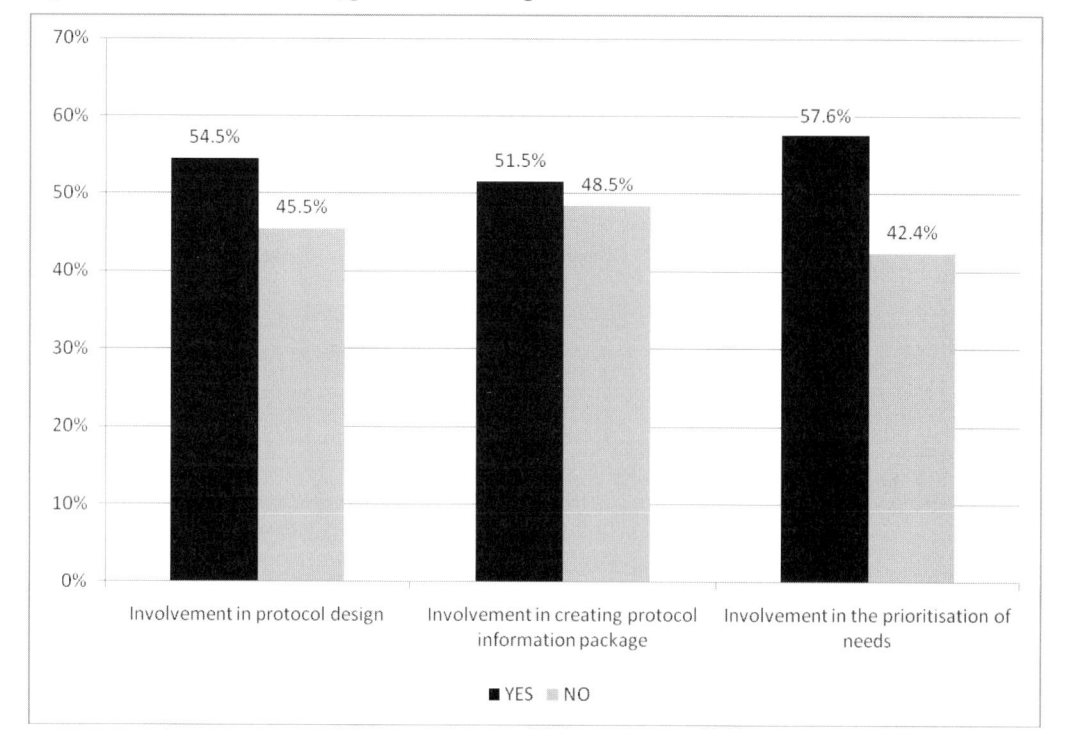

Figure 1: Involvement of children, parents or their organisations

	Involvement in protocol design	Involvement in creating protocol information package	Involvement in the prioritisation of needs
YES	54.5%	51.5%	57.6%
NO	45.5%	48.5%	42.4%

When taking into account the two most represented categories separately, it results that more almost 67% of member Networks involve children, parents or their organisations in protocol design and in the creation of protocol information packages, while 72.2% include them in the prioritisation of needs for clinical trials in children (Figure 2).

Moreover, around 35.7% of networks currently not qualifying for membership at Enpr-EMA declared to involve the public in the protocol design and the creation of protocol information packages, while almost 43% involve them in the prioritisation of needs (Figure 2).

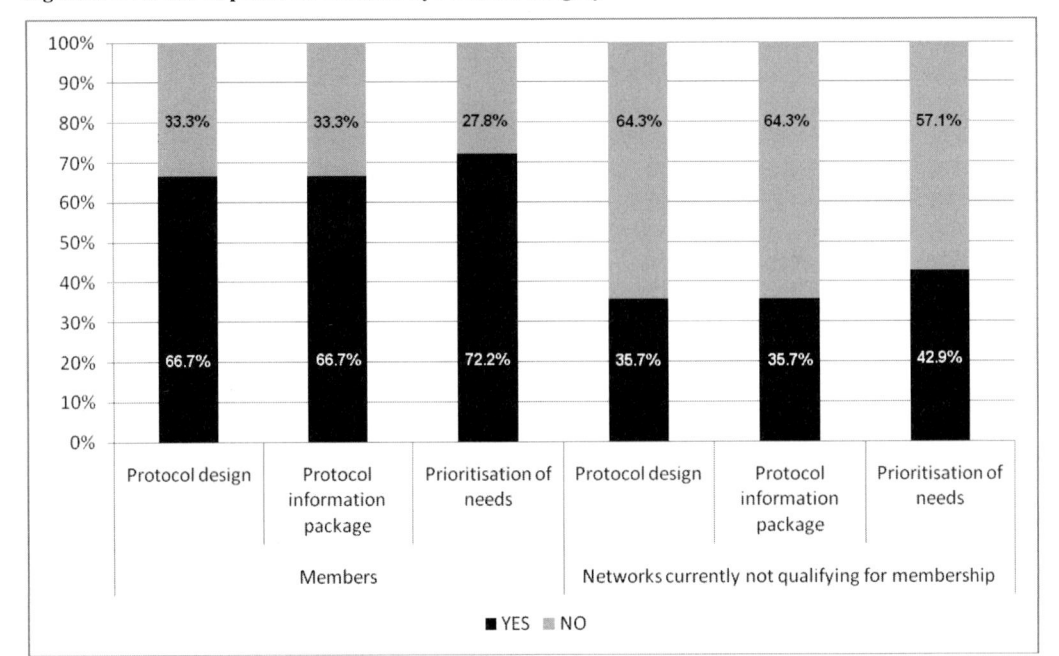

Figure 2: Overview of public involvement by Network category

Bar chart showing YES/NO percentages:

Members:
- Protocol design: YES 66.7%, NO 33.3%
- Protocol information package: YES 66.7%, NO 33.3%
- Prioritisation of needs: YES 72.2%, NO 27.8%

Networks currently not qualifying for membership:
- Protocol design: YES 35.7%, NO 64.3%
- Protocol information package: YES 35.7%, NO 64.3%
- Prioritisation of needs: YES 42.9%, NO 57.1%

2.6 Replies to Criterion 6 from CT networks fulfilling criteria for membership

ECFS-CTN: European Cystic Fibrosis Society - Clinical Trials Network	
The aim of the European Cystic Fibrosis Clinical Trials Network is to intensify clinical research in the area of cystic fibrosis and to bring new medicines to the patients as quickly as possible. Activities: 1. Maintain a network of clinical trial sites according to state-of-the-art quality criteria 2. Keep appropriate structures supporting the network in the acquisition, planning and conduct of clinical trials 3. Attract projects in cooperation with non-profit organizations, academic centres and pharmaceutical or medical-device companies	
6.1 protocol design	No Protocol is designed by pharma company. Protocol acceptance in the CT network is voted in executive committee that includes 1 patient organisation representative.
6.2 protocol information package	Yes Study specific protocol information package is designed by pharma company. General information packages on clinical trials are developed with input from patient organisations.

6.3 prioritisation of needs for clinical trials in children	Yes Taskforce has been created to connect with EMA for prioritization of clinical trials. This taskforce includes patient organization representatives. Two patients representatives attended the consensus conference on outcome parameters. http://www.ecfs.eu/projects/clinical-trials-network/consensus-conference-outcome-parameters for clinical trials (Venice, March 2010)

EPOC: A European paediatric oncology offpatent medicines consortium	
Multinational - aim of conducting and supporting pharmacological studies in paediatric oncology, specifically addressing the EMEA priority lists.	
6.1 protocol design	Yes International Confederation of Childhood Cancer Parent Organisations (ICCCPO). ICCCPO have been a full partner in the development of the project and the protocol.
6.2 protocol information package	Yes ICCCPO have been involved in all discussions regarding the trial design.
6.3 prioritisation of needs for clinical trials in children	Yes ICCCPO have been involved in all discussions regarding the trial design.

EUNETHYDIS: the European Network for Hyperkinetic Disorders	
Eunethydis is primarily concerned with the study of ADHD from a clinical and fundamental research point of view and provides research Guidelines. EUNETHYDIS also supports the development and implementation of clinical research in other areas of child mental health research including paediatric psychopharmacology.	
6.1 protocol design	No
6.2 protocol information package	Yes Several national parent ADHD organizations have been involved in developing patient information packages.
6.3 prioritisation of needs for clinical trials in children	Yes Parental organizations provided information in gaining national support for improved clinical services and lobbying for increased funding for both pharmacological and non-pharmacological clinical trials in ADHD.

FIMP - MCRN (Italian Paediatric Federation- Medicines for Children Research Network)
National, transversal Network, representing community paediatricians/primary care physicians.
It has been created to improve international standards of ethics and scientific quality by means of an agreement between individuals cooperating for the same objectives, goals and quality standards. More than 6000 Italian Family Paediatricians are involved from 20 Italian Regions, covering the entire Italian territory.
The FIMP - MCRN have developed and improved its expertise in Phase 3 and 4 clinical trials: observational and epidemiological studies; long term follow up (LTFU) clinical studies; efficacy studies (DBPC-RCT and/or comparative treatment studies); safety studies (Post-marketing , Pharmacovigilance)
Objectives:
1) To build competences (Training and educational)
2) Infrastructure and organization
3) Quality and ethicality - clinical trials
4) Better communication with families and disease-patients associations
5) Better medicines for children
6) To identify Pediatric Health Care Problems

6.1 protocol design	No
6.2 protocol information package	No
6.3 prioritisation of needs for clinical trials in children	Yes One of the main characteristics of an Italian family paediatrician is a trustful and long-lasting relationship with parents, parent organizations and children which is based on 'family communication'. Families do not contribute to the creation of an institutional list of priorities, but they can certainly give excellent advice and practical suggestions on the priorities for clinical trials in children

FINPEDMED- Finnish Investigators Network for Pediatric Medicines
National network, multispecialty

6.1 protocol design	No
6.2 protocol information package	Yes Involvement of parent representative in work to designing national patient information sheets and informed consents to paediatric trials. Involvement of children in development of picture cards for providing age appropriate trial / clinical care information to children.
6.3 prioritisation of needs for clinical trials in children	No

GNN: German Neonatal Network

National Network foccussed on clinical and genetic influences on the long term development of preterm infants.

6.1 protocol design	Yes Patient organisations were involved in the design of the GNN-study. They are also members of the external advisory committee.
6.2 protocol information package	Yes Patient organisations were involved in the design of the GNN-study. Since the GNN is not developing or marketing medications, we are not able to involve parents organisations in creating package informations.
6.3 prioritisation of needs for clinical trials in children	Yes The need for specific clinical trials is discussed in advisory committee meetings and parents organisations are involved in the priorisation of specific trial proposals.

I-BFM-SG: International BFM Study Group

Network of National Study Groups for the treatment of hematological malignancies

Mission
- To foster the information exchange among the participating groups, including preliminary results.
- To promote research projects in childhood leukemias and related disorders, including non-Hodgkin's lymphomas.
- To activate cooperative projects for biological research.
- To promote prospective randomized clinical trials, using consensus approaches and allowing the participation of other groups.
- To define, detect, register and possibly prevent acute toxicity and late effects

6.1 protocol design	Yes Participation in common sessions at meetings of SIOP with parent groups and (long-term) survivors.
6.2 protocol information package	Yes Indirectly, by involvement of I-BFM partners in the European ENCCA initiative, which aims to foster collaboration with patient/parent groups (ICCPO) on general issues
6.3 prioritisation of needs for clinical trials in children	Yes Through direct and indirect contacts with parent groups and survivors, studies of late effects have a direct impact on design of clinical trials minimizing acute and long-term toxicity. Indirect involvement, as in some studies (e.g. ALL-Rez), parent organizations are able to provide funding. Also, partners of the ENCCA initiative will collect information on concerns and expectations of patients/parents.

ITCC: Innovative Therapies for Children with Cancer	
International Network, Academic European Consortium	
6.1 protocol design	Yes Parents gathering into a Charity asked to review the protocol of academia-sponsored trials.
6.2 protocol information package	Yes Parents gathering into a Charity are asked to review the information package of industry and academia sponsored trials.
6.3 prioritisation of needs for clinical trials in children	Yes The International Confederation of Childhood Cancer Parents Organisations is a partner of ITCC. Parents are partners of the EU project that are submitted, when clinical research activity is part of the proposal

MCRN: National Institute for Health Research (NIHR) Medicines for Children Research Network	
(MCRN Coordinating Centre, University of Liverpool) National network for supporting medicines for children research within England. The NIHR Medicines for Children Research Network supports the development and conduct of randomised controlled trials and other well-designed studies of medicines for children, and is part of the National Institute for Health Research (NIHR) Clinical Research Network which is funded by the Department of Health for England	
6.1 protocol design	Yes The MCRN Coordinating Centre and most of the MCRN Local Research Networks are committed to the involvement of children, parents and families in all aspects of network activity. The MCRN Children and Young Person's group regularly provides input to the design and delivery of MCRN Portfolio studies, and each of the MCRN Clinical Studies Groups has several parent members to ensure that the patient's perspective is considered in the development of new paediatric studies
6.2 protocol information package	Yes The MCRN Children and Young Person's Group have produced a series of guidance documents to support the development of appropriate information leaflets for clinical research involving children. These are available via the MCRN website
6.3 prioritisation of needs for clinical trials in children	Yes The MCRN led a pan-Europe paediatric research prioritisation exercise as part of the ERANET PRIOMEDCHILD project. This included the involvement of parents and carers, and a number of parents presented their perspective on this prioritisation process at the international conference where the findings of the prioritisation exercise were presented and discussed.

MCRN Medicines for Children Research Network [Netherlands]	
National network organisation focused on medicines for children	
6.1 protocol design	Yes via MCRN Patient Participation Platform & CSGs
6.2 protocol information package	Yes via MCRN Patient Participation Platform & CSGs
6.3 prioritisation of needs for clinical trials in children	Yes via MCRN Patient Participation Platform & CSGs

Appendix 1d: CT networks

MICYRN: Mother Infant Child Youth Research Network - Reseau de Recherche en Santé des Enfants et des Mères	
\multicolumn{2}{MICYRN brings together the 17 Canadian academic child/child-maternal health centres and research institutes in a multidisciplinary national initiative committed to removing barriers and building capacity for the conduct of safe and high quality health research.}	
6.1 protocol design	Yes A program modeled after the UK Medicines for Children Research Network "Consumer Engagement Program" is under development. This includes engagement in setting research study direction, protocol development, and identification of meaningful outcome measures.
6.2 protocol information package	No
6.3 prioritisation of needs for clinical trials in children	Yes Patient/disease organizations provide funding to scientifically-competative, peer-reviewed studies (ie. cancer, diabetes, cystic fibrosis, arthritis, immunology, rare diseases, genetics, heart & stroke, etc.). On a national basis, a recent workshop (May 2010) involved patients and families to set research priorities for mental health.

Newcastle CCLG Pharmacology Studies Group	
National. The group previously existed as the Pharmacology Working Group of the UKCCSG (United Kingdom Children's Cancer Study Group) / Working Group of the CCLG (Children's Cancer and Leukaemia Group).	
6.1 protocol design	Yes A member of ICCCPO (International Confederation of Childhood Cancer Parent Organisations) sits on the Data Safety and Ethics Monitoring Committee which independently reviews our studies.
6.2 protocol information package	No
6.3 prioritisation of needs for clinical trials in children	No

PENTA: Paediatric European Network for the Treatment of AIDS.	
Specialty network: paediatric HIV	
6.1 protocol design	Yes Patient advocates are members of the PENTA Steering Committee and are involved in the protocol design. Consultations have been undertaken with children and young people patient groups such as CHIVA youth in the UK about trial issues
6.2 protocol information package	Yes Input on Patient information sheets is received from patient advocates and specialist nursing staff
6.3 prioritisation of needs for clinical trials in children	Yes Patient advocates are formal members of the PENTA Steering Committee which decides which studies to take forward. Questionnaires have been sent to patients about trial priorities

PRINTO : Pediatric Rheumatology International Trials Organisation	
Specialty network: Paediatric Rheumatology PRINTO is a not-for-profit, non-governmental, international research network in more than 50 countries and 396 centres worldwide), with the goal to foster, facilitate and co-ordinate the development, conduct, analysis, and reporting of multi-centre, international clinical trials and/or outcome standardisation studies in children with paediatric rheumatic diseases.	
6.1 protocol design	No
6.2 protocol information package	No
6.3 prioritisation of needs for clinical trials in children	Yes Patients' and parents' organisations have been identified through a specific project funded by the European Union that allowed the creation of a website for families available in more than 50 languages (www.pediatricrheumatology.printo.it). The website provides information on paediatric rheumatic diseases, the list of paediatric rheumatology centres and the list of family help associations. In addition, organisations are invited to attend the annual PRINTO workshop held each year at the PRES scientific meeting.

Scottish Medicines for Children Network	
National Network to support high quality clinical trials in children to increase the safety and efficacy of medicines and/or medical treatments	
6.1 protocol design	Yes Key opinion leaders (professionals, parents and young people) are being consulted as pat of the adopted CHIMES research programme. CHIMES (Child Medical Records for Safer Medicines) is developing pharmacovigilance systems from routinely collated Scottish NHS data.
6.2 protocol information package	Yes All patient information materials and consent forms are commented on by parents and children during their development and this process is being formalised with the development of a children and young persons advisory group to advise on protocol design and patient information sheets.
6.3 prioritisation of needs for clinical trials in children	No

UKPVG: United Kingdom Paediatric Vaccines Group	
Speciality network: paediatric vaccines. UKPVG is an independent network of research institutions that, through collaboration, aims to further education, training and high quality research in the field of paediatric vaccines.	
6.1 protocol design	No
6.2 protocol information package	Yes Individual centres within the network have involved parents or parent groups in studies, especially in design of information sheets
6.3 prioritisation of needs for clinical trials in children	No

CICPed: Paediatric Network of Clinical Investigation Centers	
National French Network dedicated to investigations in children. The CIC are INSERM research structures integrated into teaching hospitals and dedicated to paediatric clinical research. They have both a research team (paediatrician, research nurses and technicians) and facilities specifically adapted to the conduct of trials in children. SPECIFIC OBJECTIVES : -Create interactions between researchers, paediatricians and pharmaceutical industries to conduct clinical research projects under good clinical and laboratory practices.	
6.1 protocol design	Yes Involvement is mainly related to institutional trials Protocol design with Association for rare diseases (Cystic fibrosis, Friedrich) Comments related to informed consent and/or PK sampling (limited to cystic fibrosis)
6.2 protocol information package	No
6.3 prioritisation of needs for clinical trials in children	No

EBMT PD WP – European Group for Blood and Marrow Transplantation; Paediatric Diseases Working Party	
The Paediatric Diseases Working Party was established to support research and education to improve the availability, safety, and efficacy of hematopoietic stem cell transplantation and other cellular therapeutics for children and adolescents. Further aims: • Promote prospective clinical trials • Registration of new drugs, e.g. PIP for Treo • Registration of off patent drugs ("PUMA"), e.g. Etoposide, ATG	
6.1 protocol design	Yes e.g. The Austrian Children Cancer Foundation (Parents organisation). As the EBMT PD WP conducts pan- European trials with different principle investigators, national public stakeholders are involved in the specific study designs.
6.2 protocol information package	No
6.3 prioritisation of needs for clinical trials in children	Yes During the Annual EBMT meeting a specific "Patient and Family Day" covers all issues for paediatric needs in the treatment course of haematopoietic stem cell transplantation.

2.7 Replies to Criterion 6 from CT networks undergoing clarification

	**CLG: Children Leukemia Group of the European Organisation for Research and Treatment of Cancer (EORTC)**
	CLG is an international network working in the field of hematologic malignancies. CLG is also participating in the I-BFM Group. Mission - To improve the cure rates of children and adolescents with leukaemia's and related malignancies (lymphomas, myelodysplastic syndromes, ...) by ameliorating treatment in an evidence-based way (randomised clinical trials).
6.1 protocol design	Yes Ethics committees (national or local) have sometimes representatives from patients
6.2 protocol information package	No
6.3 prioritisation of needs for clinical trials in children	No

2.8 Replies to Criterion 6 from CT networks currently not qualifying for membership

BPDN: Belgian Pediatric Drug Network
Speciality network - Pediatrics.
AIMS:
- To place child health, rights and interest as the primary consideration (Convention on the Rights of the Child)
- Enforce good clinical practice in belgian pediatic research and belgian clinical trials of new drugs
- Propose a network of investigators for clinical trials of existing medicine products for children
    - Establish a network of belgian pediatric units active in clinical research and pediatric clinical trials.
    - Collaborate with other european networks in the field of clinical research and pediatric clinical trials.
- Facilitate exchange of information and promote education on pediatric clinical research and pediatric clinical trials.
- Offer a platform to perform clinical trials in pediatrics in Belgium: protocol proposal, discussion, and organisation
- Offer ethical consideration and advisory board in the field of pediatric research and pediatric clinical trials
- Discuss needs with third parties, in the Best Interest of the Child.
    - Health authorities
    - Patient's organisation
    - Pharmaceutical industry
    - Ethical committees
- Attract attention on the problems related to drug use and clinical tirals in children:
    - Need for children to have access to innovative and old drugs
    - Unlicensed products for children

Appendix1d: CT networks

- o Off label use
- o Lack of pediatric studies
- Extent activities in the field of non pharmaceutical collaborative clinical research

6.1 protocol design	No
6.2 protocol information package	No
6.3 prioritisation of needs for clinical trials in children	No

EuroNeoNet: European Neonatal Network
EuroNeoNet is a platform to promote networking among European neonatologists. The initiative is affiliated to the European Society for Paediatric Research and the European Society for Neonatology (ESPR/ESN).
Its mission is to enhance neonatal networking to help neonatologist to promote a culture for quality of care improvements and patient safety, family-cantered and developmental care and dissemination of evidence-based interventions, e-learning, and to effectively conduct academically-driven clinical trials, case-control, cohort, cluster and nested studies.
EuroNeoNet aims at developing a Network of Excellence of European Neonatal Units, linked by an interactive website.

6.1 protocol design	NA
6.2 protocol information package	NA
6.3 prioritisation of needs for clinical trials in children	No

ESPGHAN: European Society of Paediatric Gastroenterology, Hepatology and Nutrition
The European Society of Paediatric Gastroenterology, Hepatology and Nutrition is an international scientific society based in Europe and founded in 1968.

6.1 protocol design	No
6.2 protocol information package	No
6.3 prioritisation of needs for clinical trials in children	Yes

Futurenest: Futurenest Clinical Research Lc.
Futurenest has been founded in 2009 by paediatricians experienced in paediatric clinical studies. Our mission is to contribute to the development of paediatric clinical studies and research.
We want to take an active role in ensuring that clinical studies in which minors participate are conducted in an efficient way.
Headquarter of the company is in Miskolc, Hungary which is the home of around 20000 children. The paediatric care of over 3000 of them is provided by physicians of our company. We have taken part in epidemiological, phase II and III-IV studies involving both healthy (Vaccines) and unhealthy (infectology, pain relief, etc.) children.

6.1 protocol design	No
6.2 protocol information package	No
6.3 prioritisation of needs for clinical trials in children	No

IPTA: International Pediatric Transplant Association
The International Pediatric Transplant Association (IPTA) is a professional organization of individuals in the field of pediatric transplantation. The purpose of the Association is to advance the science and practice of pediatric transplantation worldwide in order to improve the health of all children who require such treatment. The Association is dedicated to promoting technical and scientific advances in pediatric transplantation and to advocating for the rights of all children who need transplantation.
Goals:
1. Promote the advancement of the science and practice of transplantation in children worldwide
2. Promote research and provide a forum that highlights the most recent advances in clinical and basic sciences related to pediatric transplantation
3. Serve as a unified voice for the special needs of pediatric transplant recipients
4. Develop educational programs for pediatric transplant professionals in underserved regions of the world that enable children to have access to transplantation globally
5. Become the international leader in generating and disseminating information in the field of pediatric transplantation through the publication of our journal, Pediatric Transplantation

6.1 protocol design	No
6.2 protocol information package	No
6.3 prioritisation of needs for clinical trials in children	No

IPCRN: Irish Paediatric Clinical Research Network

The Irish Paediatric Research Network (IPRN), provides advice and support on all aspects of paediatric clinical study design and management. The IPRN is a network of key opinion leaders in paediatric care created to promote high-quality basic and clinical research in children to further our understanding of paediatric illness and develop safe and effective treatment options.

6.1 protocol design	No
6.2 protocol information package	Yes Parent representatives may become involved in the design/review of ageappropriate patient information leaflets, informed consent forms, picture cards etc., via the Irish Platform for Patient's Organisations, Science and Industry (IPPOSI)
6.3 prioritisation of needs for clinical trials in children	Yes The National Children's Research Centre corresponds with the Irish Platform for Patient's Organisations, Science and Industry (IPPOSI)

Juvenile Scleroderma Working Group of the Pediatric Rheumatology European Society

PRES is a European scientific society for healthcare professionals in the field of paediatric rheumatology. Our mission is to:
- Promote knowledge of paediatric rheumatic diseases
- Stimulate research in this field
- Disseminate knowledge through scientific meetings and publications
- Provide guidelines and standards for good clinical practice
- Provide guidelines and standards for the training of doctors and allied health professionals in the practice of paediatric rheumatology

6.1 protocol design	Yes FESCA (European scleroderma patient organisation) for the inceptions cohort project
6.2 protocol information package	Yes Hamburger Elterninitiative Rheumakranker Kinder
6.3 prioritisation of needs for clinical trials in children	No

Neo-circulation
Speciality network in Neonatology

6.1 protocol design	Yes We have two parents from the European Forum for Care of the newborn Infant (EFCNI) in our steering group.
6.2 protocol information package	Yes See above
6.3 prioritisation of needs for clinical trials in children	Yes See above

RESPECT

PENTI: Paediatric European Network for the Treatment of Infection
Emerging speciality network in Paediatric Infectious Diseases - Linked to PENTA and utilising the same clinical trial network as PENTA. The aim of PENTI is to develop in collaboration with PENTA and ESPID a new clinical trial network conducting both academic and pharma led clinical trials and cohort studies in antimicrobials.

6.1 protocol design	Yes via PENTA, MCRN.
6.2 protocol information package	Yes via PENTA, MCRN
6.3 prioritisation of needs for clinical trials in children	Yes via PENTA, MCRN

RIPPS: Réseau d'Investigations Pédiatriques des Produits de Santé - Investigation Network for Paediatric Health Products
The RIPPS is designed to bring existing skills together, to optimize on their operation and their performances. Thus, France can increase its attractivity in relation to other countries (both European and non European) in terms of development of children's health products.

6.1 protocol design	Yes Association for Rett syndrome, Association for Tuberous sclerosis, Fondation Lejeune, Fondation Motrice
6.2 protocol information package	Yes Representatives of patient associations at INSERM
6.3 prioritisation of needs for clinical trials in children	No

BLF: Swedish Paediatric Society
National network with the majority of paediatricians in Sweden. BLF is working to promote the development of paediatrics in Sweden and ensure high quality health care for children and adolescents. One task force is Medicines for Children and patient safety.

6.1 protocol design	No
6.2 protocol information package	No
6.3 prioritisation of needs for clinical trials in children	Yes

Appendix 1d: CT networks

AMIKI: The Paediatric Trial Network
AMIKI is a private and public organisation specialized in clinical studies in Paediatrics, with a past emphasis on Paediatric Endocrinology and Diabetology, but offers clinical trial services in all areas of Paediatrics.
The network combines paediatric experts in clinic (childrens hospital, Univ. of Hamburg), medical practice (Inst. of Paediatric Endocrinology & Diabetology, Frankfurt) with CRO (CTCNnorth) and a publishing Company (Biomedpark), specialized for paediatric diseases.

6.1 protocol design	No
6.2 protocol information package	No
6.3 prioritisation of needs for clinical trials in children	No

NCCHD Japan: National Center for Child Health and Development
National Center (Independent Administrative Agencies) that is allied with major paediatric hospitals in Japan.

6.1 protocol design	Yes In some of the trials including allergy. Will officially have representatives of a patient organization involved starting 2011
6.2 protocol information package	No
6.3 prioritisation of needs for clinical trials in children	No

INN: Italian Neonatal Network
National network for monitoring outcome of preterm newborns and for conducting clinical trials and research.

6.1 protocol design	No
6.2 protocol information package	No
6.3 prioritisation of needs for clinical trials in children	Yes Meeting with associations of patients

2.9 Conclusions

It is sometimes assumed that involving families in making the informed consent material clearer is the closest children, families and/or patient organisations (POs) can get to involvement in the design of clinical trials, but this report shows that much greater involvement is possible and is already practised by these organisations to some extent.

Public involvement is required by European Authorities. The inclusion of children, parents or their organisations in the networks' activities as one of the qualifying criteria for membership in Enpr-EMA is just one of many examples within the European Medicines Agency, which includes PO representatives in their various committees and working groups.

The fact that those networks not qualifying as members of Enpr-EMA are also those that apparently have weaker links with children is a fact that should not be taken lightly, especially if compared with the very different approach employed by Enpr-EMA member networks that on the other hand more systematically involve children and their representatives.

Making children able to have a direct input in the design and execution of the trial, as well as in the prioritisation of needs, will motivate their participation. In addition, a closer cooperation between researchers and children or their representatives as active research partners enriches the understanding of the medical condition and the outcomes.

There are many initiatives aimed at promoting and encouraging the involvement of children and their representatives in clinical research and many examples of how to make these initiatives successful. These networks prove that the involvement of the public does work.

Appendix 1e:

Survey of ethics committees' involvement in paediatric research

1	BACKGROUND	222
2	AIM OF THE STUDY	223
3	METHODOLOGY	223
4	RESULTS	224
5	DISCUSSION	228
6	CONCLUSIONS	229

CONTRIBUTORS:

Annagrazia Altavilla
Adriana Ceci

1 Background

Clinical research develops at an astonishing rate and new drugs and therapeutic options are constantly discovered and applied in clinical practice.

Any type of scientific research on human subjects always has to take into account ethical guidelines and legal rules (Huriet, 2004; European Medicines Agency, 2002; Commission of the European Communities, 2005) and special attention and specific guarantees are required when vulnerable populations, such as children, are involved in clinical research (European Commission Enterprise Directorate General, 2002; Gill et al., 2003; John, 2007; Knox & Burkhart, 2007; ICH harmonised tripartite guideline, 2000).

In Europe, the rights and well-being of children participating in clinical research are currently assured by the provisions of Directive 2001/20/EC (CT-Dir), a reference legislative instrument which entered into force in 2001 and aimed at providing a homogeneous legal and ethical framework for the conduct of clinical trials in the European Economic Area. The Directive includes a specific article, Article 4, aimed at ensuring the protection of minors, taking into account their emotional, physiological and psychological vulnerabilities.

Between 2006 and 2007, the Task-force in Europe for Drug Development for the Young (TEDDY), a Network of Excellence funded by the European Commission under the 6th Framework Programme, carried out a survey to examine the measures enforced by Member States (MS) to implement the CT-Dir and other relevant European norms. Results showed that many differences exist in the protection of minors involved in clinical trials across Europe, mainly due to the Directive implementation process and a lack of coordination among MS (Altavilla, Giaquinto & Ceci, 2008; Altavilla et al., 2009).

In January 2007, the European Paediatric Regulation (European Parliament and the Council of the European Union, 2006a, 2006b) entered into force with the aim of increasing availability of medicines specifically studied in children, stimulating high quality, ethical paediatric research, and making information and data on clinical trials in children and paediatric medicines easily accessible to the public (Saint-Raymond & Seigneuret, 2009). The Regulation is binding in its entirety and directly applicable in all Member States.

In February 2008, the European Commission released the "European Ethical recommendations for clinical trials on medicinal products conducted with the paediatric population" (European Ethical Recommendations) aiming at developing safe and effective medicines for children while ensuring their protection. The document defines rules related to the risk/benefit balance assessment, the information and consent/assent process, and the process of ethical review of paediatric protocols (European Commission's Directorate-General for Health and Consumers, 2011). Individual data protection and insurance issues are also addressed. This non-binding, declaratory instrument provides recommendations on ethical aspects of clinical trials involving children and introduces a new ethical and regulatory context integrating principles contained in various other European/international ethical/legal sources (Council of Europe, 1999, 2007). It constitutes a reference document for Ethics Committees.

Since the approval of clinical trials, including their ethical review, is performed at Member State level by national or local ethics committees (ECs), the correct implementation of the European regulatory framework (especially of the European Ethical Recommendations) is also under their responsibility and it directly influences their activities.

2 Aim of the study

This study was carried out as a collaboration between TEDDY (Task-force in Europe for the Drug Development for the Young) Network of Excellence and RESPECT. The survey was addressed to ECs with the objective of pointing out proposals to facilitate the integration of ethics committees interested in paediatric research across Europe, and to determine a road map to enhance the role of ECs in promoting the development of medicine tailored for children.

In particular, this investigation aimed at:
- identifying ECs operating in Europe;
- identifying the ECs that are entitled to review paediatric protocols, according to their national legislation;
- evaluating how paediatric expertise is guaranteed in ECs;
- assessing their awareness of the new European paediatric regulatory framework;
- monitoring and assessing the impact of the new paediatric regulatory framework on the activities of ECs;
- identifying future initiatives aimed at increasing EC involvement in paediatric research.

3 Methodology

An inventory was carried out to identify ethics committees operating in Europe. The results of the first TEDDY survey (Altavilla, Giaquinto & Ceci, 2008; Altavilla et al., 2009) indicated the approximate number of ECs and the website addresses where their contact details are available. Other sources were TEDDY and RESPECT partners, MS medicines agencies and personal communication. When details were not available or easily accessible through the Internet, Paediatric Committee (PDCO) members were contacted for support. The inventory was planned and carried out between April and June 2009 and is continuously updated.

The survey was performed entirely online. ECs received an electronic invitation letter with a link to the questionnaire, which presented first a filter question to establish whether the committee was responsible for reviewing paediatric clinical trial protocols. Only ECs entitled to assess paediatric studies were presented with the remaining questions.

A total of 12 questions, whose replies were either mandatory or optional, were presented. The survey was divided into two main sections:
1. ethics committees and paediatric research under the new regulatory framework in Europe, focusing on the EC's awareness and knowledge of the current regulatory framework in paediatrics and its impact on their activities,
2. interest and involvement of ethics committees in paediatric research, focusing on the EC's interest in being involved in activities related to paediatric research.

The preliminary version of the questionnaire was discussed and shared with members of the PDCO. Two electronic mailings of the invitation were sent and subsequently ECs were contacted directly.

The results below are expressed as frequencies and percentages. Analyses were performed on the whole sample and on subgroups stratified into old EU Member States - the EU-15 (Austria, Belgium, Denmark, Finland, France, Germany, Ireland, Italy, Luxembourg, Portugal, Spain, Sweden, The Netherlands, UK) - and new Member States (Cyprus, Czech Republic, Estonia, Latvia, Malta, Poland, Slovakia). Norway and Iceland, are associated to the European Research Programmes and have been included in the EU-15 group because of their clinical research, legal and ethical framework.

4 Results

One thousand seven ECs in 29 European countries were identified (Table 1) and contact details were collected for more than 830 ECs in 28 countries. Replies were gathered from a total of 154 ECs (18.2%) operating in 22 countries; with a response rate below 10%, in 4 countries (Spain, Finland, Germany, UK) but exceeding 30% in 12 countries.

Table 1: Ethics Committees existing in Europe

COUNTRY	No. of ECs	Inhabitants (millions)	No. ECs / 1.000.000 inh.
Bulgaria	103	7.6	13.55
Iceland	3	0.3	10.00
Finland	25	5.3	4.72
Italy	270	60	4.50
Belgium	38	10.7	3.55
Austria	27	8.3	3.25
Spain	143	45.8	3.12
Ireland	13	4.5	2.89
Slovakia	13	5.4	2.41
UK	143	61.7	2.32
Latvia	5	2.3	2.17
Luxembourg	1	0.5	2.00
Malta	1	0.5	2.00

The Netherlands	32	16.4	1.95
Denmark	9	5.5	1.64
Estonia	2	1.3	1.54
Norway	7	4.7	1.49
Poland	54	38.1	1.42
Cyprus	1	0.8	1.25
Czech Republic	9	10.5	0.86
Sweden	7	9.2	0.76
Germany	54	82	0.66
France	40	64.3	0.62
Lithuania	2	3.3	0.61
Slovenia	1	2	0.50
Hungary	1	10	0.10
Portugal	1	10.6	0.09
Greece	1	11.2	0.09
Romania	1	21.5	0.05
TOTAL	**1007**	**504.3**	**2.00**

Source: TEDDY inventory; EU website (http://europa.eu/about-eu/member-countries/index_en.htm)

One hundred thirty-nine committees reported that they are entitled to review paediatric clinical trial protocols, 73 (52.5%) of which also answered the optional questions.

Almost 59% of 73 responding ECs include paediatric experts as full members, usually a paediatrician, while 28.8% take advice from an external expert case by case (Figure 1).

Figure 1: Paediatric expertise in ECs

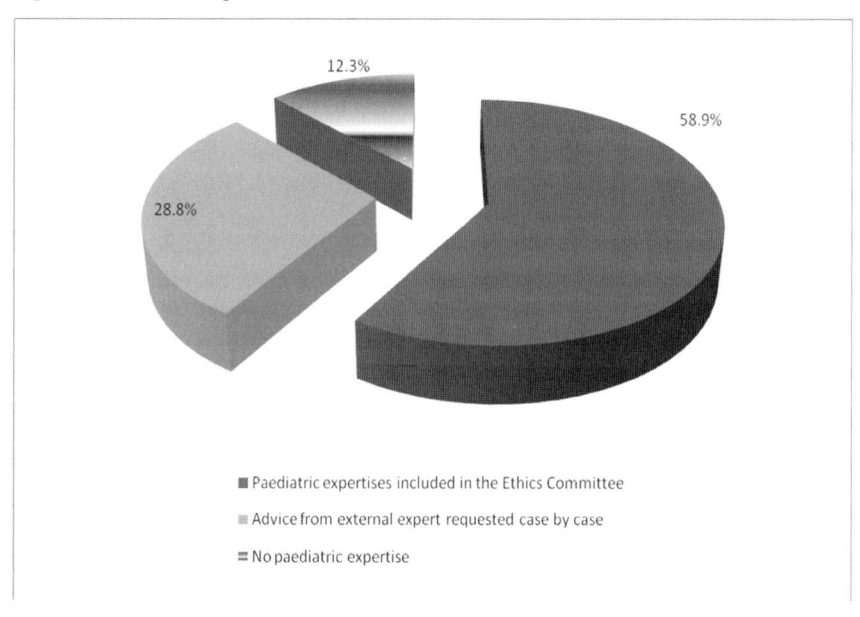

Only 14.4% out of 139 ECs indicated that they had formally discussed and/or analysed the European Paediatric Regulation, and only about 13% reported having formally discussed and/or implemented the European Ethical Recommendations (Figure 2). Analyses were usually carried out through dedicated sessions or training initiatives.

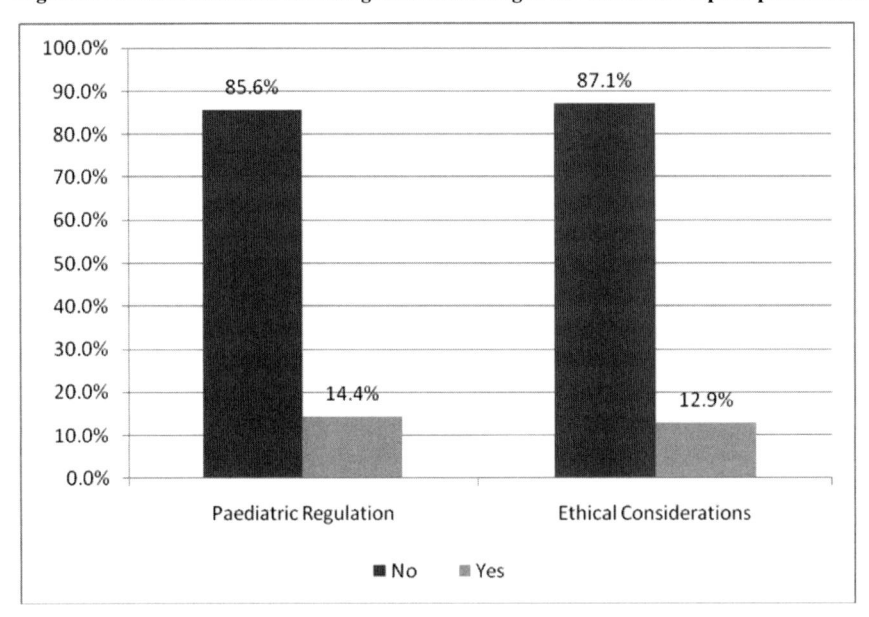

Figure 2: Ethics Committees knowledge/understanding of the current European paediatric framework

	Paediatric Regulation	Ethical Considerations
No	85.6%	87.1%
Yes	14.4%	12.9%

When asked about the influences of the new regulatory framework, 35.6% of the 73 responding ECs reported "no impact" on their work from the Paediatric Regulation, about 29% indicated "low impact", 26% "sufficient" and around 10% "high impact". The trend was confirmed when considering the influence of the European Ethical Recommendations: only 6.8% acknowledged "high impact", 11.8% "sufficient", 26% "low" and 44% "none". Figure 3 details the major types of influences recognised by ECs. Other effects were: increased attention to paediatric protocols; increased facility to carry out paediatric trials; and the necessity to specify ethical requirements.

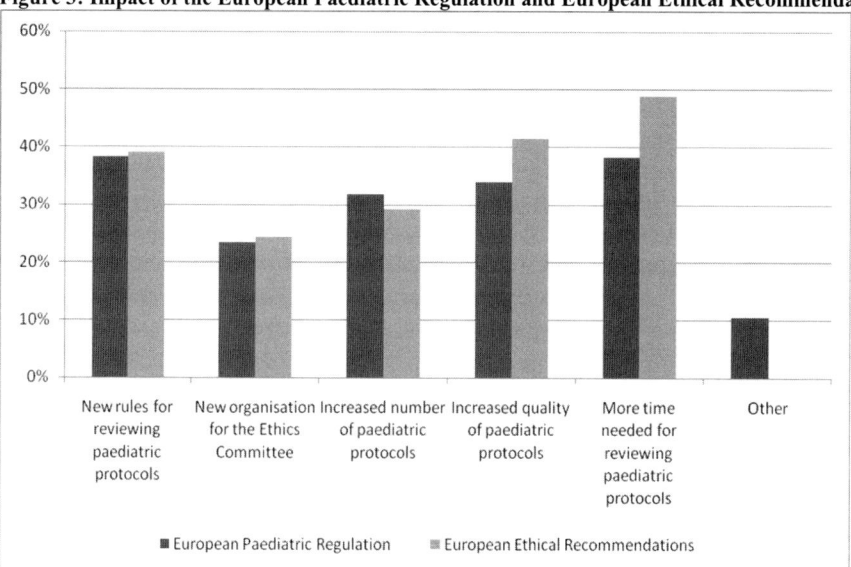

Figure 3: Impact of the European Paediatric Regulation and European Ethical Recommendations

Figure 4 summarises the opinions of ECs on the major issues to be dealt with under the framework; about half of our sample identified the increased need for additional expertise to evaluate paediatric protocols (52.1%) and for measures to minimize pain, distress and fear of children (46.6%). Complexity in evaluating inclusion/exclusion criteria, risk/benefit balance and consent/assent procedures were also highlighted as main concerns. Issues related to compensation for parents and children, insurance, provisions for protection of personal data, and administrative burdens were declared to be unchanged.

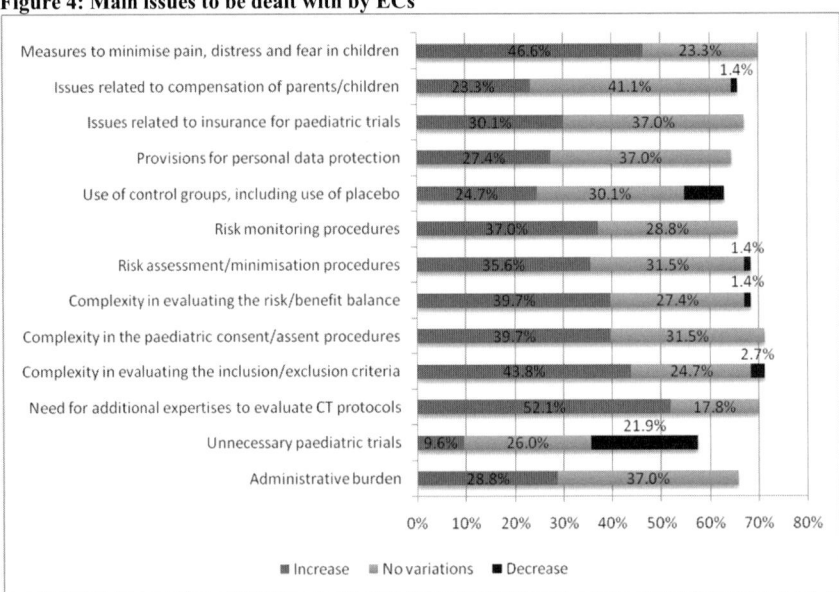

Figure 4: Main issues to be dealt with by ECs

Issue	Increase	No variations	Decrease
Measures to minimise pain, distress and fear in children	46.6%	23.3%	1.4%
Issues related to compensation of parents/children	23.3%	41.1%	
Issues related to insurance for paediatric trials	30.1%	37.0%	
Provisions for personal data protection	27.4%	37.0%	
Use of control groups, including use of placebo	24.7%	30.1%	
Risk monitoring procedures	37.0%	28.8%	1.4%
Risk assessment/minimisation procedures	35.6%	31.5%	1.4%
Complexity in evaluating the risk/benefit balance	39.7%	27.4%	
Complexity in the paediatric consent/assent procedures	39.7%	31.5%	2.7%
Complexity in evaluating the inclusion/exclusion criteria	43.8%	24.7%	
Need for additional expertises to evaluate CT protocols	52.1%	17.8%	
Unnecessary paediatric trials	9.6%	26.0%	21.9%
Administrative burden	28.8%	37.0%	

Only 30% percent of the 73 respondents indicated that they had participated in initiatives in the field of paediatric research and those who did usually took part in conferences (68%) and training activities (32%). Moreover, 74% declared an interest in being involved in European initiatives related to paediatric research, preferring means such as training at national and local level and networking among ECs (59% and 56%, respectively). Debates and conferences (at the national level) and educational initiatives supported by European institutions were less preferred (54% and 50%, respectively). Seventy-three percent of those ethics committees interested in networking belong to the EU-15 (Belgium, France, Germany, Ireland, Italy, Luxembourg, Portugal, Spain, Sweden, The Netherlands), while 27% are established in new Member States (Cyprus, Czech Republic, Estonia, Latvia, Malta, Poland).

5 Discussion

The CT-Dir introduced a number of measures to harmonize the ethical review of clinical trials and facilitate clinical research. It required MS to establish ethics committees legally, including obligations and specifications, formal procedures and timelines, composition and competencies. Specific provisions were also adopted for reviewing clinical trial protocols including children. However, due to the nature and legal force of a Directive, MS had some flexibility in implementing its provisions in their national legislation. Thus, ethical review procedures and the amount and quality of publicly available information vary significantly among European countries (European Forum for Good Clinical Practice (EFGCP) Ethics Working Party, 2010).

Our results show that the number, competence and composition of ECs vary greatly across Europe. For example, Italy has the largest number of ECs, while countries like Malta, Cyprus or Hungary have only one EC (Table 1). Nevertheless, if we relate the number of ECs to the population, Bulgaria has the highest number of ECs per million inhabitants (13.55) and Romania the lowest (0.05). These differences could reflect the diverse legal and social backgrounds and the different organisation and funding of healthcare systems across the EU. An inventory of ECs operating in Europe, updated on a regular basis, is an important tool to facilitate the exchange of adequate and reliable information on their activities and procedures.

Moreover, our results demonstrate that a gap exists between the current regulatory framework and ethics committees' awareness, knowledge and understanding of the major issues related to paediatric clinical research; a very limited number of ECs had discussed and analysed the most important European legal instruments devoted to paediatric research. That could explain the lower rate of ECs answering the optional questions related to more specific issues.

Additionally, the majority of ECs operating in EU-15 Member States declared a low impact of the Paediatric Regulation (39%) and the European Ethical Recommendations (50%). On the other hand, 33% of ECs in new EU MS declared "high impact" of the Paediatric Regulation and are mainly divided between "high" and "sufficient" impact of the European Ethical Recommendations, suggesting that the latter has been identified as a more effective tool for influencing the activities of ECs. These data suggest that ECs in the new EU MS are more actively involved in efforts for integration and harmonization towards EU research and health norms and systems than EU-15 ethics committees (Glasa, 2002).

Overall, ECs recognized, as possible effects of the new European paediatric regulatory framework, the increase in the number of medicines tailored for children, an increase in well-designed paediatric trials and more multicentre paediatric clinical studies. Nevertheless, it has been stressed that there is still a lack of knowledge regarding the risks and burdens that are acceptable for children in different age groups.

Finally, even if the increased involvement of children in clinical research has been recognised as an effect of the Paediatric Regulation, it has also been underlined that it is difficult to adapt information to parents and children in accordance with the new requirements.

6 Conclusions

This survey demonstrated that there is a lack of knowledge of the European paediatric regulatory framework among ethics committees, and that their awareness of ethical issues related to paediatric research is limited, reflecting their low level of involvement in paediatric research, especially in terms of training, education and other similar activities.

Given that ECs are one of the most important actors in guaranteeing the safety, rights and well-being of children involved in clinical research, it is of primary importance to increase their competence and their involvement in paediatric research, and to promote the implementation of the European Ethical Recommendations at the local level.

In this context, training and education in the field of ethics of paediatric clinical research should be an important objective.

Networking may be a fundamental tool to enhance collaboration and experiences and information exchange. It should be particularly important to promote these initiatives in the new Member States, where the number of clinical trials is increasing.

One possible relevant result of networking could be the development of a comprehensive guide practically addressing paediatric ethical issues in accordance with all the relevant international and European ethical and legal sources. This guide, chaired at the EMA level, should address all those specific ethical issues related to paediatrics: information/authorisation-assent process, paediatric expertise of ethics committees in charge of reviewing paediatric protocols (including training and education of the members of the ECs), use of placebo, compensation for damage, as well as other specific aspects to be considered in reviewing paediatric protocols.

Appendix 2:

RESPECT Family Decision Guide and worksheet

CONTRIBUTORS:

Falk Wulf
Monika Bullinger
Catriona Chaplin

RESPECT

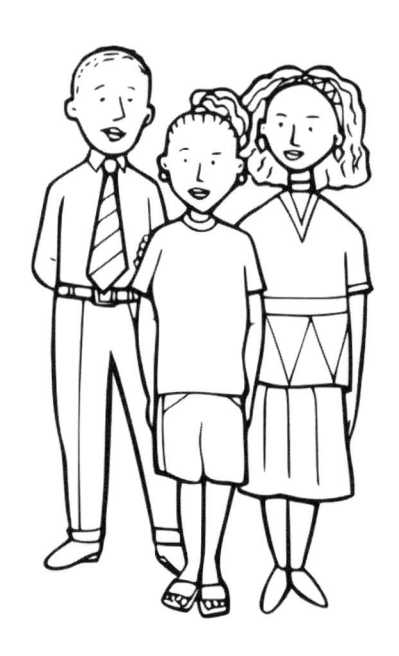

FAMILY DECISION GUIDE – DRAFT

HELPING FAMILIES FACING DECISION ABOUT PARTICIPATION OF THEIR CHILD IN A RANDOMIZED CLINICAL TRIAL

EU PROJECT RESPECT (EU FP-7)

WULF F & CHAPLIN C FOR THE RESPECT STUDY GROUP

Family Decision Guide

Before you start

Some introductory words

You and your family are in a tough situation. You and maybe your child are considering the child's participation in a randomized clinical trial. This decision is not an easy one!

There are some situations you and your child might face:
- maybe your child has an acute and severe health condition and you are trying to find the best possible treatments for your child
- maybe your child suffered from a disease in the past and was cured by effective medications; now you feel like "giving back" and contributing to the medical progress
- maybe you are convinced of the need for medical research and you like the idea that participation in a clinical trial might help other children or
- maybe it is a mixture of all of the above or something not mentioned here.

Whichever it is, before enrolling your child in a randomized clinical trial, there are some specific points to discuss so that, at the end of this process, you and your child should be clear and feel certain about the decision you made.

To assist you and your child in this decision-making process we designed a brochure which you are reading right now and an accompanying worksheet which you will find attached to this brochure.

Appendix 2: Family Decision Guide & worksheet

Family Decision Guide

The process of deciding about participation in a trial

You may have received this brochure after initial disclosure of a diagnosis. In this consultation your doctor may also have asked you if you or your child would consider participating in a clinical trial.

Participating in clinical trials and medical research is something you probably never thought about before. But, for many people suffering from diseases, it is fruitful to take part in this process of medical research. The following figure denotes one example how the conversation with your doctor can take place.

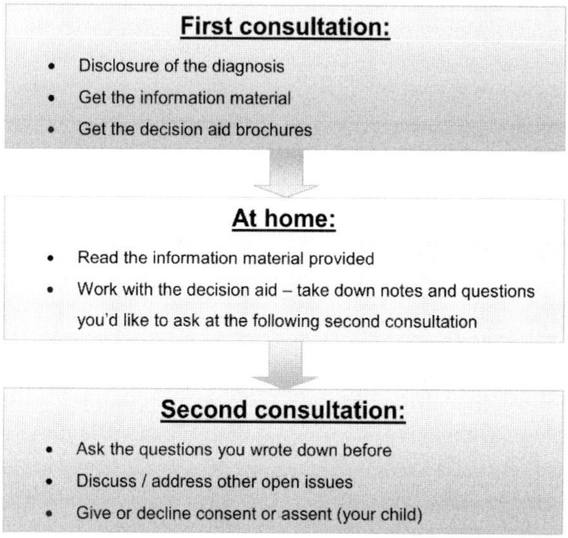

First consultation:
- Disclosure of the diagnosis
- Get the information material
- Get the decision aid brochures

At home:
- Read the information material provided
- Work with the decision aid – take down notes and questions you'd like to ask at the following second consultation

Second consultation:
- Ask the questions you wrote down before
- Discuss / address other open issues
- Give or decline consent or assent (your child)

Figure 1: Conversations with your doctor

RESPECT

Family Decision Guide

Symbols used in this brochure

Table 1: Symbols

(i)	This symbol indicates important information to understand.
(pencil)	Whenever you see this symbol to the right of the text, grab a pen and take some notes in the boxes in that section of the worksheet.
(cloud)	This cloud symbol represents thinking. Whenever you see this you should analyze your thoughts, feelings and concerns thoroughly.
(warning)	This is a warning sign. If you see this you should read carefully.
(?)	This yellow question mark indicates a decision. If this is printed to the right of the text you should make a decision.

OK, now it's time to start the decision making process – please move on to the next section and turn the page.

Appendix 2: Family Decision Guide & worksheet

Family Decision Guide

Clarify the situation

Medical research in general

The aims of medical research are:

- to improve the understanding of the causes and development of medical conditions;
- to prevent illnesses and reduce the number of people who become ill;
- to find new ways to treat diseases and to develop new treatments and medicines;
- to improve the quality of life for people living with medical conditions.

Why is medical research important?

Without it, there would be no new medicines or tests, improved treatments, or better ways of providing healthcare. Some treatments developed over the last few decades have led to improved rates of survival for major health problems.

What do you think about medical research?

Now it's time to have a look at the worksheet that comes with this brochure. What is your opinion about medical research in general? Please make a mark in the worksheet and make some notes of questions you would like to discuss.

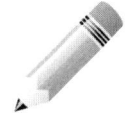

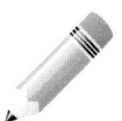

Worksheet page 1

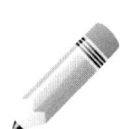

Regulations and conditions of the trial

It is important to distinguish the different stakeholders in the process of conducting a trial. For example, a pharmaceutical company is most likely to have different reasons for funding a trial than a university doing medical research. Have a look at the worksheet again and write down what you know about the goals and the people who are conducting the trial.

Worksheet page 1

Clarify the decision & Things you should know

To be aware of the complexity of the situation you and your family are in, it is important to think about the following questions. Please try to answer all the questions and make notes in the boxes below.

Worksheet page 2 & 3

Family Decision Guide

Get the facts

Key points to remember

- It is extremely rare for participation to be unsafe.
- There is sufficient legal and ethical regulation to assure your child's safety and health.
- Before, during and after the clinical trial, there is extensive monitoring of your child's health. If any problems occur, your child will get immediate help.
- You can withdraw your consent to participation at any time without any negative consequences for your child!
- If you or your family's members have a question or feel unsure, don't hesitate to ask the staff immediately!

Appendix 2: Family Decision Guide & worksheet

Family Decision Guide

Clinical trial groups and placebo

If a new drug is developed, its safety and effectiveness have to be tested in a clinical trial, in which the researchers give the new drug to some volunteer participants. For the study to be as correct and fair as possible, other volunteers are given the standard treatment, which will be compared with the new drug. The standard treatment is always the therapy used normally, the treatment you would receive if you weren't participating in a trial. If there is no standard treatment, a placebo (a drug containing only inactive substances) is used instead. Depending on the design of the study your child might be treated with the standard treatment - or placebo if there is no existing treatment - or the new drug. (In some cases, your child is given each of these during different time phases.)

In the picture below, the measuring scales between the experimental and the control group symbolise clinical equipoise. Clinical equipoise means that the researchers who will conduct the study do not know the comparative effectiveness of each experimental or control group at the time of beginning the research. This is what they want to find out.

Experimental group	Control group	
New drug	Placebo group: Inactive drug / no drug	Standard care group: Similar to standard care prescribed

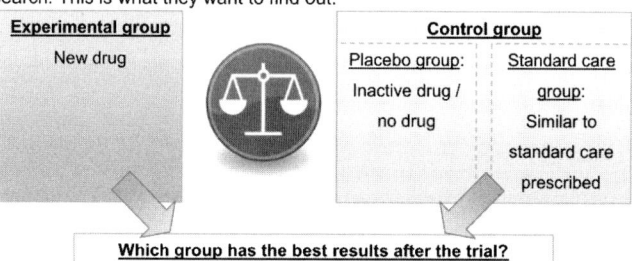

Which group has the best results after the trial?

Figure 2: Trial groups

Good to know:

It is essential to be aware that your child might not get the new treatment during the trial, because he or she may be placed in the control group receiving the standard (existing) treatment. The use of a placebo (a non-active substance) is only allowed in studies where no standard treatment exists, so that in no case will your child receive a placebo when there is a treatment currently available or the standard treatment is no better than the placebo.

Further reading:
http://en.wikipedia.org/wiki/Placebo

Family Decision Guide

Randomisation

After enrolment your child is assigned to one of the groups at random (for example, decided by chance).

It is not possible to choose one group or to say „we will only participate if my child is placed in the group receiving the new drug"

The participants won't know to which group they are assigned to, and even the researchers, doctors and nurses themselves won't know. This is what we call "double-blinded".

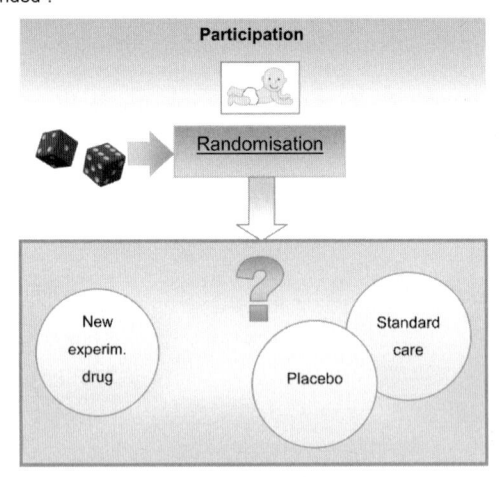

Figure 3: Randomisation

Good to know:

Why is this randomised process so important?
Randomisation is used to reduce bias in the study. For instance, if a study is not randomised, physicians might unconsciously assign participants with a higher chance of recovery to the experimental group, thus making the new therapy seem more effective than it really is. Conversely, participants with a lower chance of recovery might pick the experimental treatment, leading it to look less effective than it really is.

Appendix 2: Family Decision Guide & worksheet

Family Decision Guide

Compare the benefits and risks

What is usually involved?

Participation	Decline
• You get specific information about procedures used in the clinical trial • A series of blood tests and other medical screening procedures • Extra check-ups in the hospital / clinic	• Your child will get standard medical care / treatment. This is safe.

Personal story:

Lorem ipsum dolor sit amet, consectetur adipiscing elit. Cras id neque augue, sed porttitor neque. Pellentesque vitae tellus non risus posuere tincidunt nec non elit. Aliquam pretium eros nec orci dictum eget placerat lacus consequat. Maecenas mauris diam, rhoncus sit amet rutrum quis, vestibulum ac metus. Aenean condimentum interdum imperdiet. Phasellus adipiscing diam non dolor sollicitudin dignissim. Aliquam venenatis tincidunt nunc ornare pharetra. Cras sed tincidunt tortor. In magna diam, euismod at sagittis ac, vulputate ut turpis. Donec sed sodales velit. Cum sociis natoque penatibus et magnis dis parturient montes, nascetur ridiculus mus. Nunc at orci a turpis vestibulum tempor at eget lacus. Integer a magna dolor. Morbi diam tellus, semper a tempus a, pharetra quis mauris. Integer arcu neque, cursus a faucibus id, fermentum non nunc.

Family Decision Guide

What are the benefits?

Participation	Decline
• Complete health screening for your child • *Your child might receive a treatment* • Your child will support important medical research and might help other children with the same condition in the future	• Avoiding burden of participation • Your child is not exposed to new and unknown risks

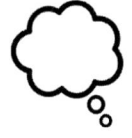

> *Personal story:*
>
> *Lorem ipsum dolor sit amet, consectetur adipiscing elit. Cras id neque augue, sed porttitor neque. Pellentesque vitae tellus non risus posuere tincidunt nec non elit. Aliquam pretium eros nec orci dictum eget placerat lacus consequat. Maecenas mauris diam, rhoncus sit amet rutrum quis, vestibulum ac metus. Aenean condimentum interdum imperdiet. Phasellus adipiscing diam non dolor sollicitudin dignissim. Aliquam venenatis tincidunt nunc ornare pharetra. Cras sed tincidunt tortor. In magna diam, euismod at sagittis ac, vulputate ut turpis. Donec sed sodales velit. Cum sociis natoque penatibus et magnis dis parturient montes, nascetur ridiculus mus. Nunc at orci a turpis vestibulum tempor at eget lacus. Integer a magna dolor. Morbi diam tellus, semper a tempus a, pharetra quis mauris. Integer arcu neque, cursus a faucibus id, fermentum non nunc.*

Appendix 2: Family Decision Guide & worksheet

Family Decision Guide

What are the risks and side effects?

Participation	Decline
• Your child may suffer from minor side effects • Your child may suffer from rare long-term effects • Specific information about risks and side effects of participating in this RCT	• Your child may suffer side-effects of the standard therapy • Your child may suffer from short and long-term effects if untreated.

Personal story:

Lorem ipsum dolor sit amet, consectetur adipiscing elit. Cras id neque augue, sed porttitor neque. Pellentesque vitae tellus non risus posuere tincidunt nec non elit. Aliquam pretium eros nec orci dictum eget placerat lacus consequat. Maecenas mauris diam, rhoncus sit amet rutrum quis, vestibulum ac metus. Aenean condimentum interdum imperdiet. Phasellus adipiscing diam non dolor sollicitudin dignissim. Aliquam venenatis tincidunt nunc ornare pharetra. Cras sed tincidunt tortor. In magna diam, euismod at sagittis ac, vulputate ut turpis. Donec sed sodales velit. Cum sociis natoque penatibus et magnis dis parturient montes, nascetur ridiculus mus. Nunc at orci a turpis vestibulum tempor at eget lacus. Integer a magna dolor. Morbi diam tellus, semper a tempus a, pharetra quis mauris. Integer arcu neque, cursus a faucibus id, fermentum non nunc.

RESPECT

Family Decision Guide

Explore your decision

Now, after reading all this information about trial design, benefits and risks connected to participation in a trial, it's time to list your personal view of the options, benefits and risks. Look at the worksheet section "Compare the benefits and risks".

First you will find a symbolic scale with the heading "If you say 'YES' to participation in the trial": Please list there the risks and benefits which may occur if you or your child participate in the trial. If there is something very important to you, use bigger letters or underline your writing. Do this again at the scale headed "If you say 'NO' and decline participation in the trial".
This is intended to help you visualize the risks and benefits according to participation or declining and how much they matter to you personally.

After that, please look at the whole page and try to identify which risks and benefits matter most to you and if your list of the risks and benefits can give you an idea of whether you prefer to participate or decline.
Have you identified an option (agree to participation / decline participation) which you would prefer? If not, please take some more time to think or discuss it with somebody from the research team or someone else who can help you with your decision.
If you have identified an option you prefer, please make a circle around it and mark at the respective heading the word "YES" or "NO".

Worksheet page 4

Family Decision Guide

Your feelings

In this section it's all about your feelings, views and attitudes. There is a list of statements you may agree or disagree with. Please grab the pen again and mark an X on the line between "agree" and "disagree".
After doing so, you may see that your feelings tend more towards participation or towards declining.

Worksheet page 5

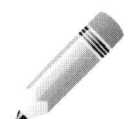

Support

Are there other persons involved? Please go to the worksheet, section "Support" and list persons who are involved in this decision. Then note which option each person prefers and if the person needs support to decide or can be helpful by giving support to you. You can also note here if you feel the person is pressurizing you to choose one option.
Then you should indicate what role you prefer to have in this decision-making process.

Worksheet page 6

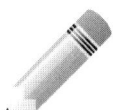

Information needs

Identify your decision-making needs

At this point in the decision-making process, you have gathered information and done a lot of thinking and discussing about your opinions, attitudes and feelings. Now it's time for a short review: let's see if something is still unclear or uncertain. Please go to the worksheet again and read the questions in the section "Information needs – Identify your decision making needs" and tick the corresponding "Yes" or "No" box for each question.
If you still have some marks in the "No" boxes, you should go back to a preceding section and try to solve your information needs.
Remember: you can at any time discuss your thoughts and questions with other people.

Worksheet page 7

Next steps based on your needs

Please reflect, based on your needs, what will be your next steps to get to an informed and definite decision.

Family Decision Guide

Your decision

Worksheet page 8

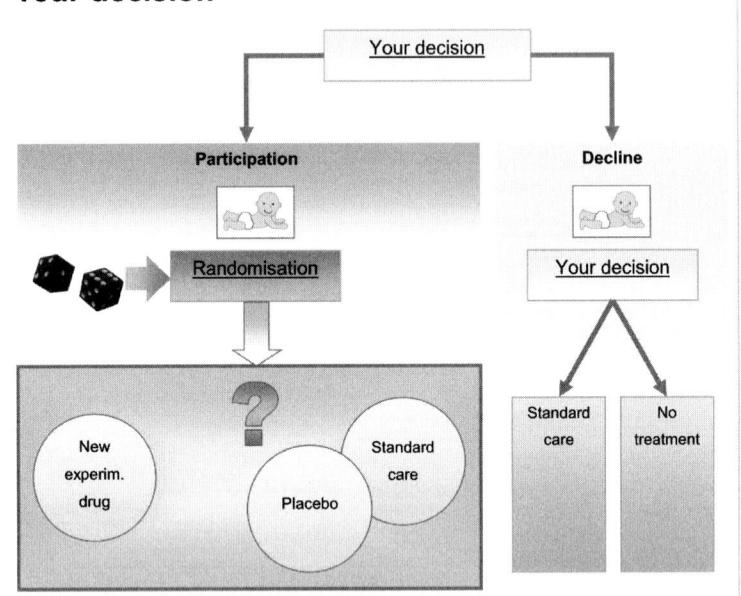

Figure 4: Your decision

Where are you leaning now?
Finally, it's time to make a final decision. Consider everything that you have worked out so far and mark an X on the line in the section "Your decision – Where are you leaning now?" in the worksheet.
Remember: you / your child can withdraw or decline at any time without negative consequences!

How sure you are about your decision?
Please estimate your certainty about this decision and make a corresponding mark in the final section of the worksheet.

Family Decision Guide

Summary

Now you have done a lot of work exploring your thoughts, attitudes, fears and needs. We hope that this little tool has helped you in this difficult process.
You had a look at the different options and identified the one you prefer. Then you reflected about your feelings about randomised clinical trials.
After that you looked at which of the involved persons needs support or can give you support.

That's it – thank you very much for using this tool!

RESPECT

Appendix 2: Family Decision Guide & worksheet

FAMILY DECISION GUIDE
WORKSHEET

Clarify the situation

What do you think about medical research?

Like	Don't like
←	→

How can my child or our family benefit from medical research?

Brochure page 5

Regulations and conditions of the trial

You should know:

Unsure? → Ask

Who conducts the trial? ☐

What is the goal of the trial? ☐

How safety will be monitored ☐

Will insurance or a grant cover the costs? ☐

Brochure page 5

RESPECT

Family Decision Guide - Worksheet

Clarify the decision

What decision do you face?

Why do you need to make this decision?

When do you need to make a choice?

What is your personal feeling towards participation?

Brochure page 5

Family Decision Guide - Worksheet

Things you should know

Unsure? → Ask

| Is this trial / study important? Am I doing a good thing? | ☐ |

| What is the amount of time and commitment involved? | ☐ |

| Does participation include painful interventions? | ☐ |

| What are the possible side effects? | ☐ |

| What are the possible long term effects? | ☐ |

| What will be the chance of getting the desired treatment? | ☐ |

| Does participation include a better health monitoring? | ☐ |

| Will I get answers to my questions? | ☐ |

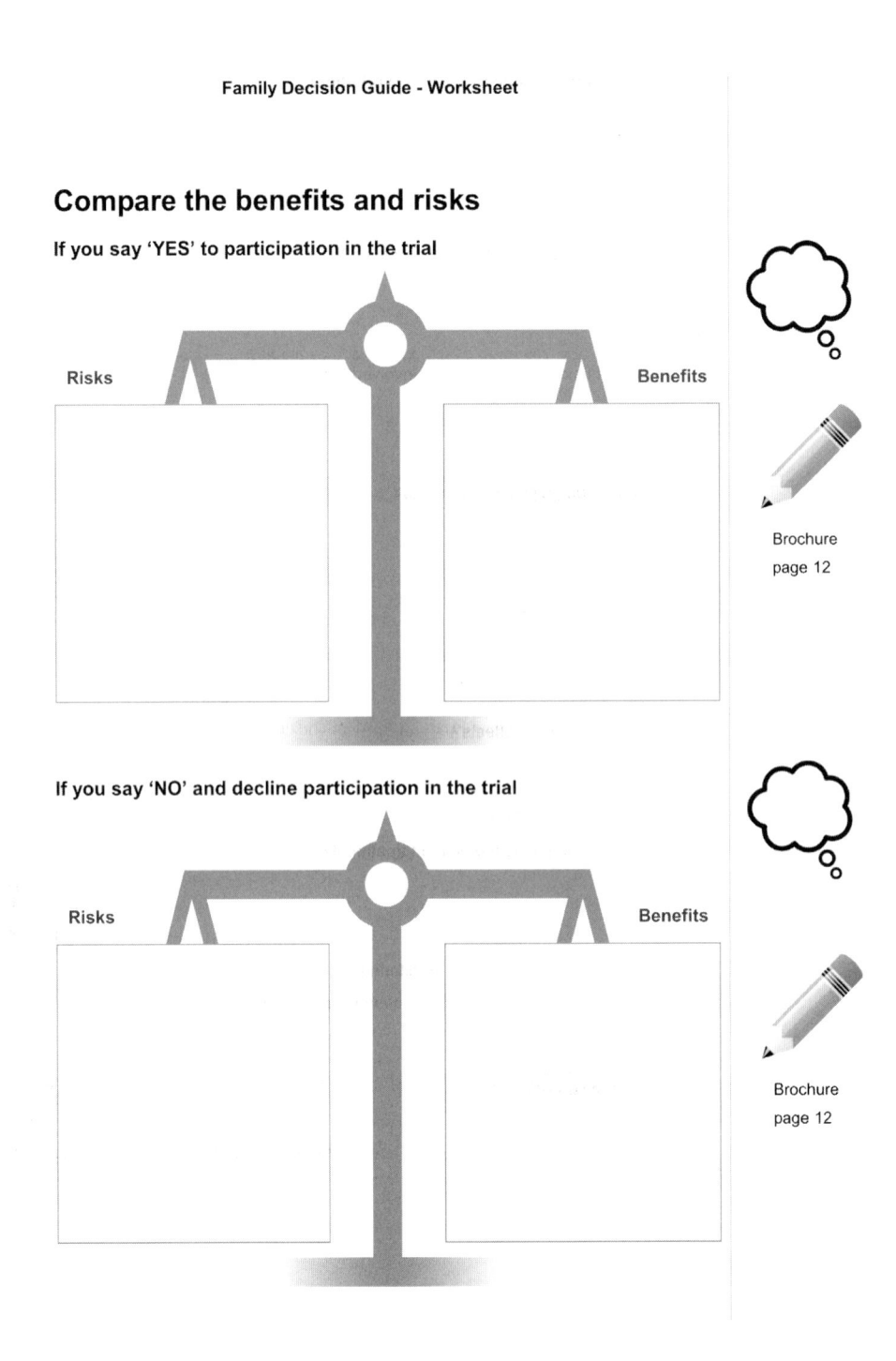

Family Decision Guide - Worksheet

Compare the benefits and risks

If you say 'YES' to participation in the trial

Risks | Benefits

Brochure page 12

If you say 'NO' and decline participation in the trial

Risks | Benefits

Brochure page 12

Family Decision Guide - Worksheet

Your feelings

Participation	Decline

The study could lead to improving other children's health.
agree _____ disagree

I am not worried about my child being in an experiment.
agree _____ disagree

I think my child would get better care through participation.
agree _____ disagree

I trust the research staff.
agree _____ disagree

I expect financial compensation or reimbursement.
agree _____ disagree

Medical research is not done only for economic reasons.
agree _____ disagree

The research could help my child personally.
agree _____ disagree

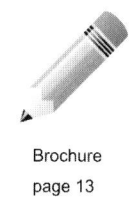

Brochure page 13

RESPECT

Family Decision Guide - Worksheet

Support

Other persons involved

Person involved	Option preferred	Need or give support
Child		☐ Need ☐ Give
		☐ Need ☐ Give
		☐ Need ☐ Give

Brochure page 13

Your desired role

☐ I'd like to decide by myself / after hearing the views of: _____

☐ I'd like to share the decision with: _____

☐ I'd like somebody else to decide. Name: _____

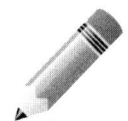

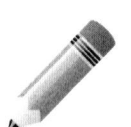

Brochure page 13

Appendix 2: Family Decision Guide & worksheet

Family Decision Guide - Worksheet

Information needs

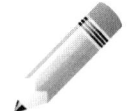

Identify your decision making needs

		Yes	No
Knowledge	Do you know which options are available?	☐	☐
	Do you know both the risks and benefits of every option?	☐	☐
Values	Are you clear about which risks and benefits matter most to you?	☐	☐
Support	Do you have enough support from others to make a choice?	☐	☐
	Are you choosing without pressure from others?	☐	☐
Certainty	Do you feel sure about the best choice?	☐	☐

Brochure page 13

Next steps based on your needs

Knowledge	Find out more about the facts, benefits, risks and options.
	List your questions:
Values	Review the "Compare options" and "Your feelings" sections
	Discuss with others what matters most to you.
	Find other people who have made the decision.
Support	Try to find neutral support.

Brochure page 13

RESPECT

Family Decision Guide - Worksheet

Your decision

Where are you leaning now?

Now that you've thought about the facts and your feelings, you may have a general idea of where you stand on this decision. Show which way you are leaning right now.

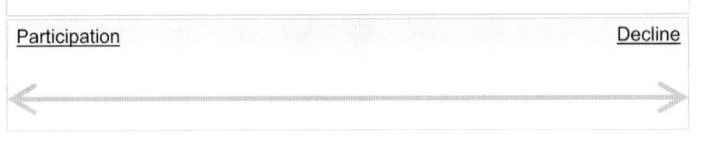

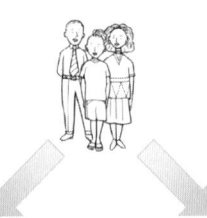

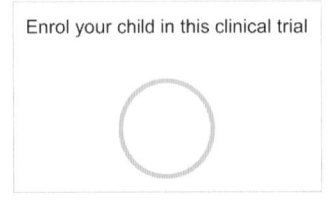

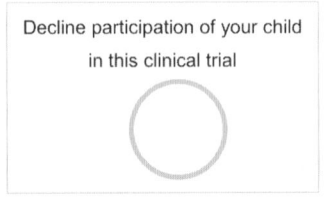

Participation   Decline

Brochure page 14

Enrol your child in this clinical trial	Decline participation of your child in this clinical trial
◯	◯

Brochure page 14

How sure you are about your decision?

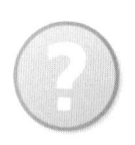

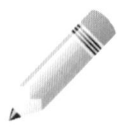

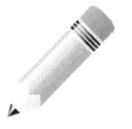

Sure   Not sure

Brochure page 14

Appendix 3a:

Pilot education package for parents

CONTRIBUTORS:

Andrea Sandberg
John E. Chaplin

RESPECT

Appendix 3a: Pilot education package for parents

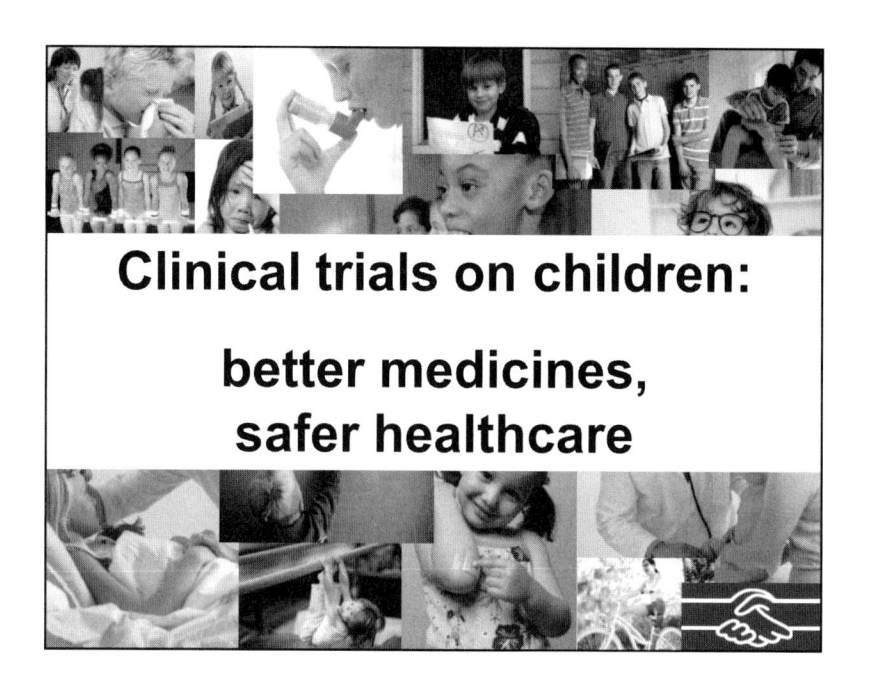

Clinical trials on children:

better medicines, safer healthcare

More than half of the medicines given to children are not approved for children

Doctors use medicines intended for adults and experiment with lower doses or different ways to administer the drug.

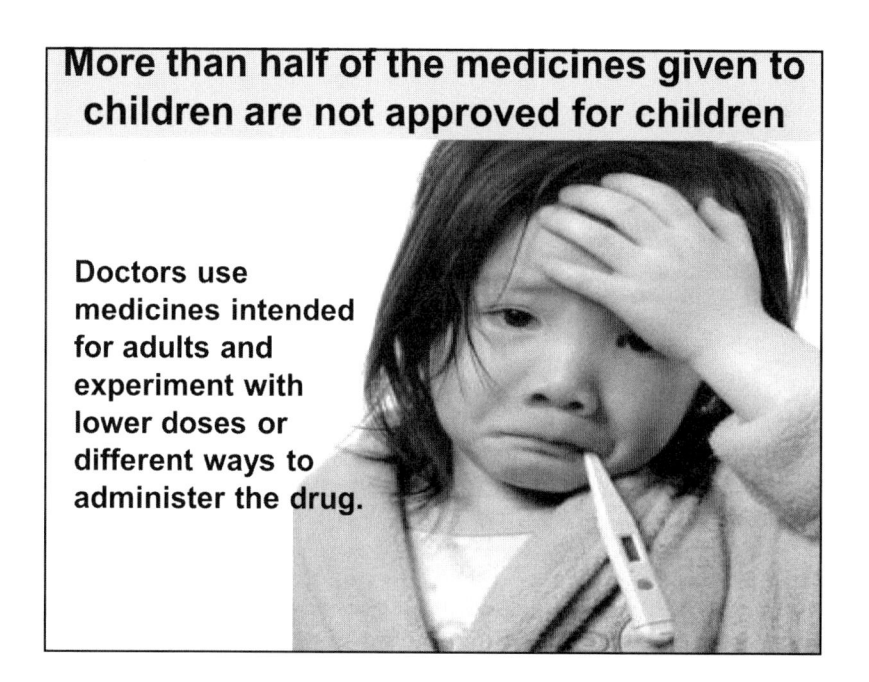

Proportion of non-approved medicines in different age categories

approx 90%   approx 50%   approx 1%

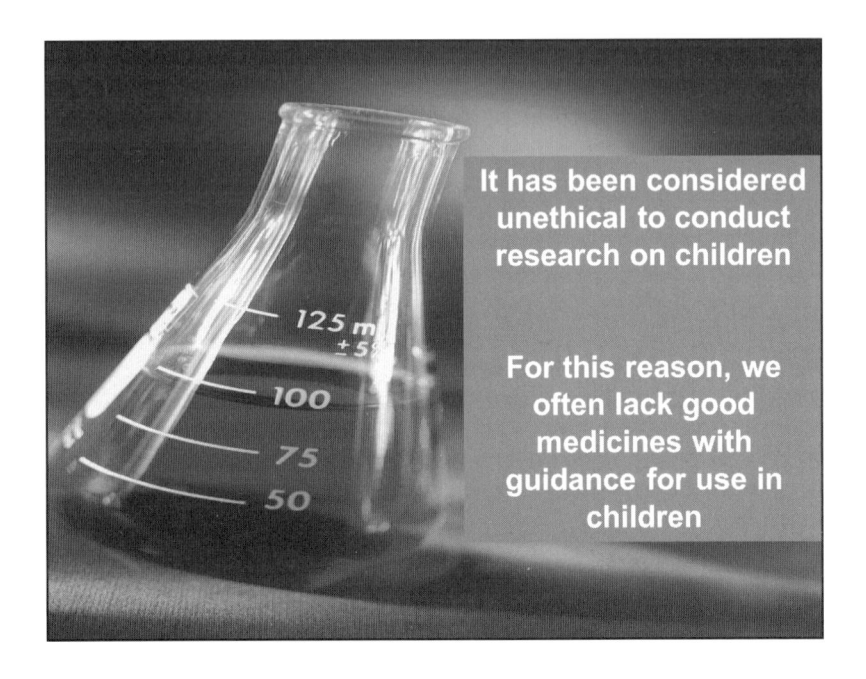

It has been considered unethical to conduct research on children

For this reason, we often lack good medicines with guidance for use in children

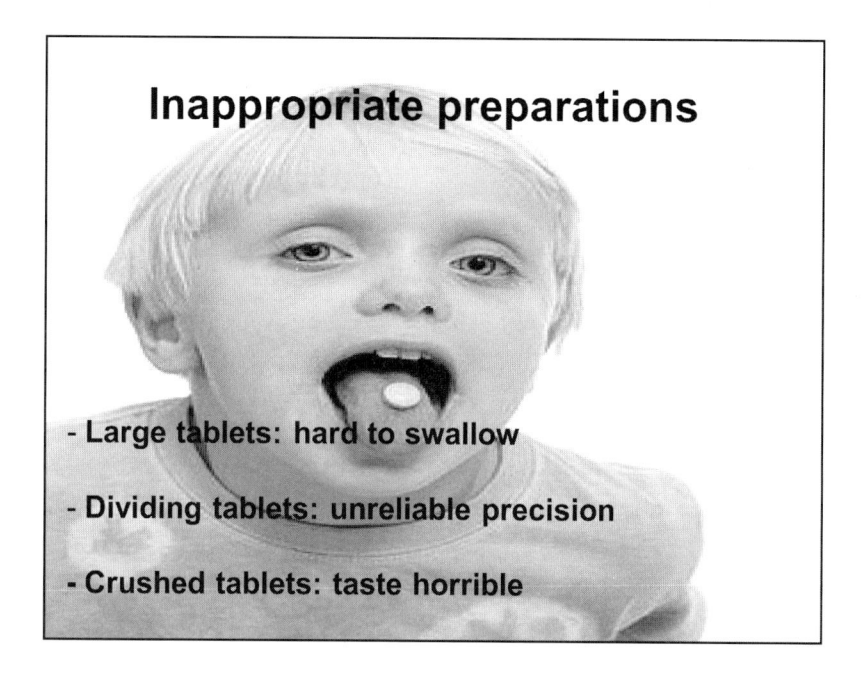

Appendix 3a: Pilot education package for parents

Inappropriate preparations

- Large tablets: hard to swallow
- Dividing tablets: unreliable precision
- Crushed tablets: taste horrible

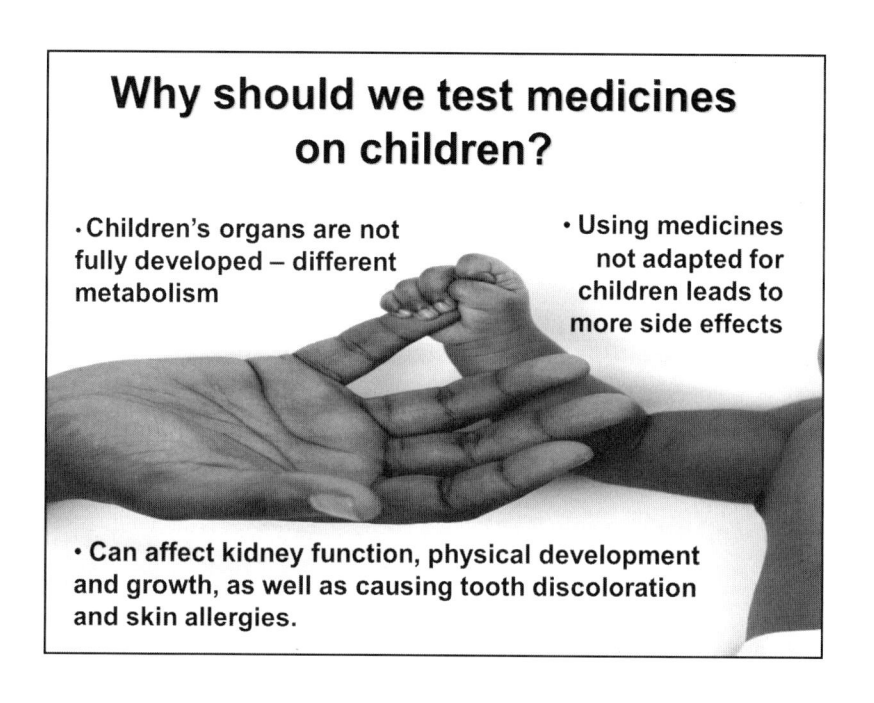

Why should we test medicines on children?

- Children's organs are not fully developed – different metabolism
- Using medicines not adapted for children leads to more side effects
- Can affect kidney function, physical development and growth, as well as causing tooth discoloration and skin allergies.

2007 – the European Paediatric Regulation

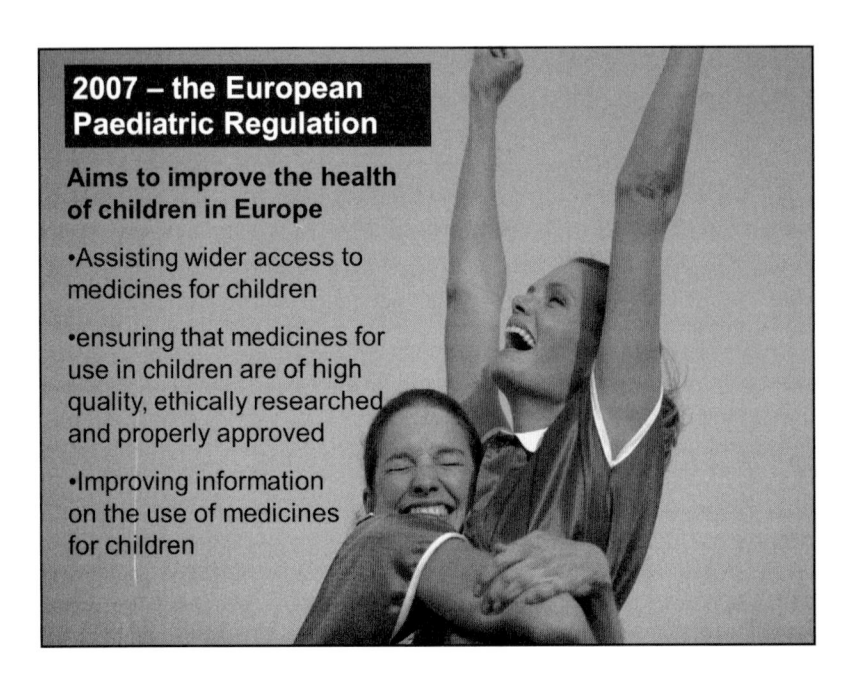

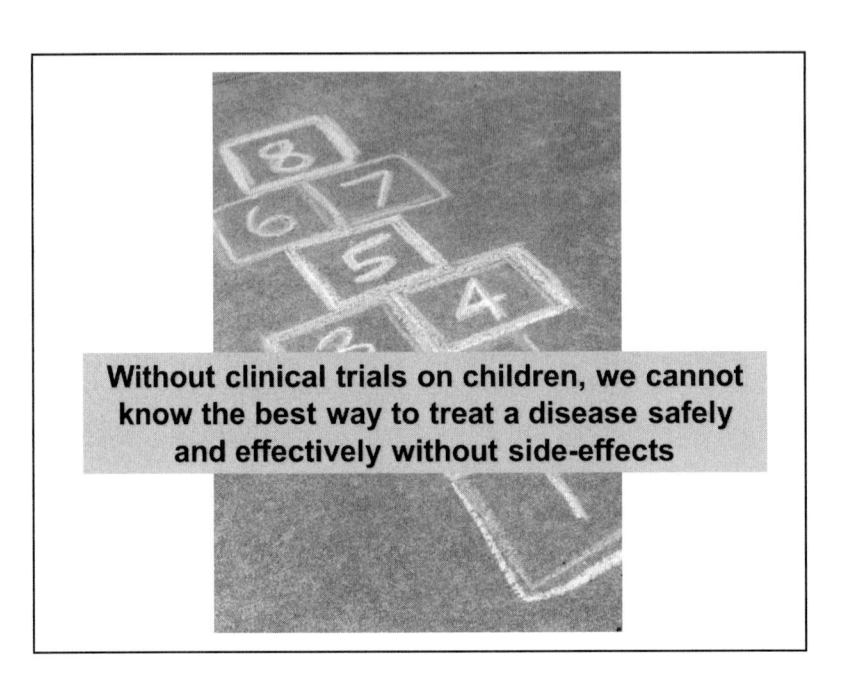

Aims to improve the health of children in Europe

- Assisting wider access to medicines for children

- ensuring that medicines for use in children are of high quality, ethically researched and properly approved

- Improving information on the use of medicines for children

Without clinical trials on children, we cannot know the best way to treat a disease safely and effectively without side-effects

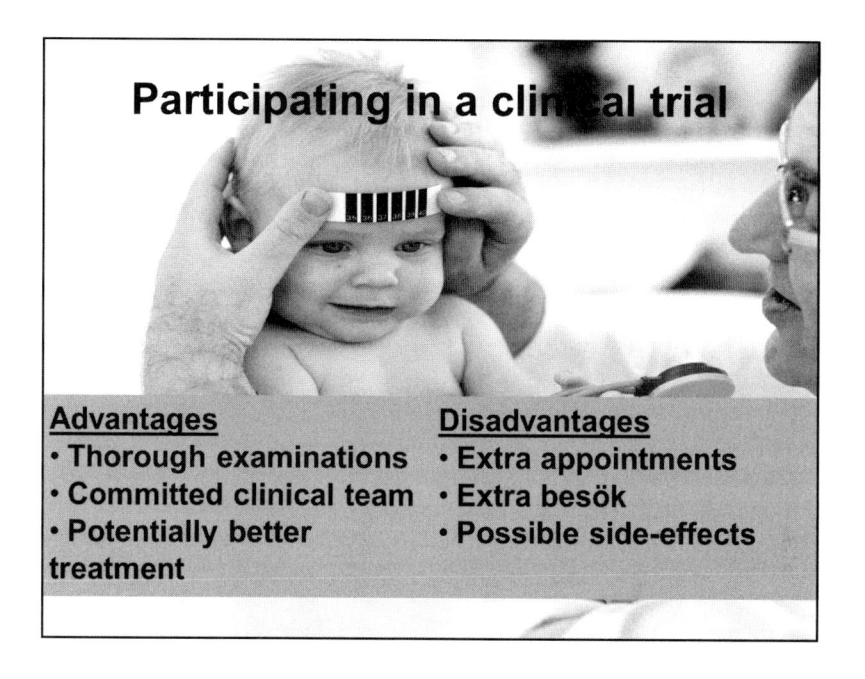

Appendix 3a: Pilot education package for parents

Participating in a clinical trial

Advantages
- Thorough examinations
- Committed clinical team
- Potentially better treatment

Disadvantages
- Extra appointments
- Extra besök
- Possible side-effects

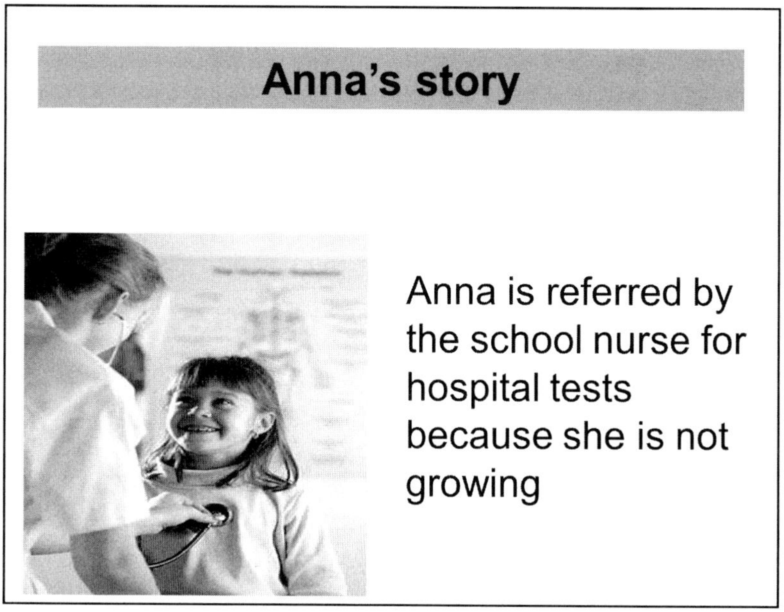

Anna's story

Anna is referred by the school nurse for hospital tests because she is not growing

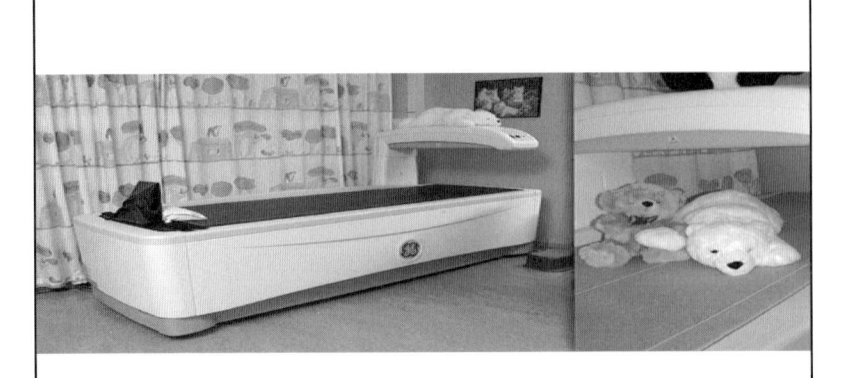

She has a number of tests at the hospital clinic. The results show that she has growth hormone deficiency.

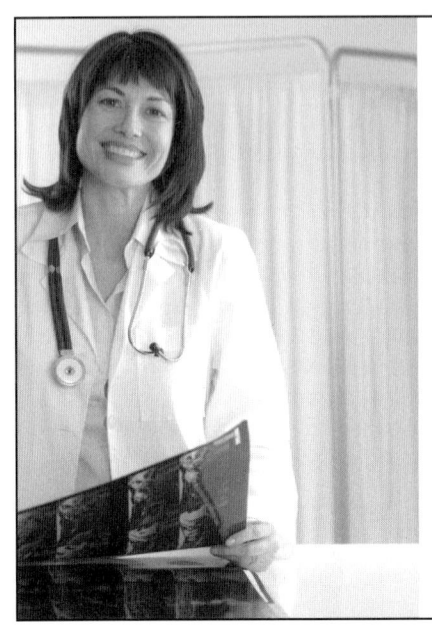

Anna returns to the hospital to find out how she will be treated:

- **medicine under development in a clinical trial?**

- **standard medicine?**

Appendix 3a: Pilot education package for parents

Why do we run clinical trials?

Clinical trials make sure that medicines are of high quality and as safe as possible.

They tell us, for example:
- how safe a medicine is
- what side effects it gives
- how effective it is as a treatment

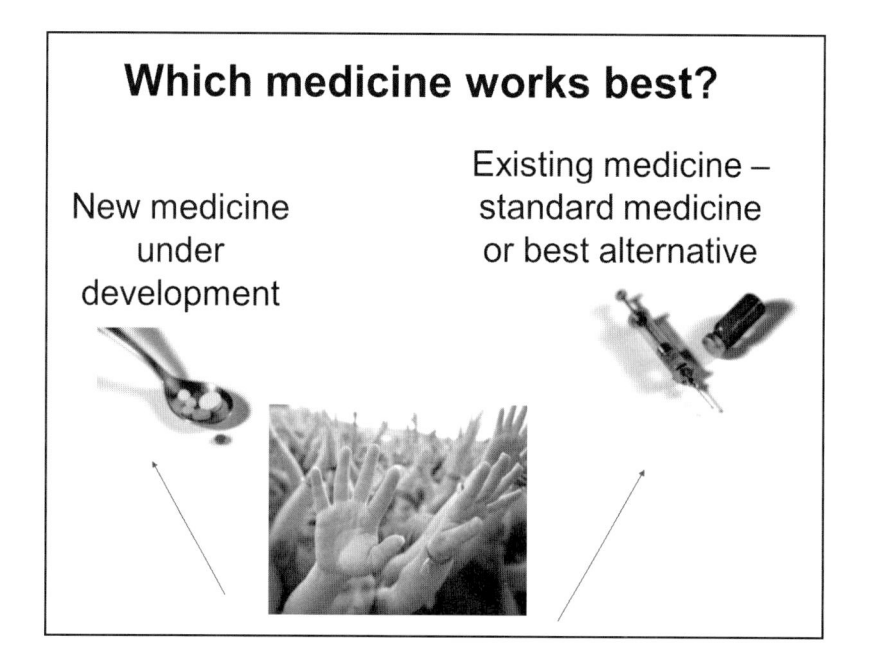

Which medicine works best?

New medicine under development

Existing medicine – standard medicine or best alternative

RESPECT

A trial follows a strict plan – a 'protocol'

The protocol contains information about:

- all the study procedures, how they will be conducted
- which patients will be in the study
- which medical conditions they must have and which ones they must not have.
- laws and regulations to be followed

Informed consent

The clinical staff explain:

- what the medicine is for
- study design
- purpose of the trial
- methods, tests and visits
- risks and benefits
- use of placebo (if applicable)
- freedom to refuse to participate
- rules, laws, insurance

Appendix 3a: Pilot education package for parents

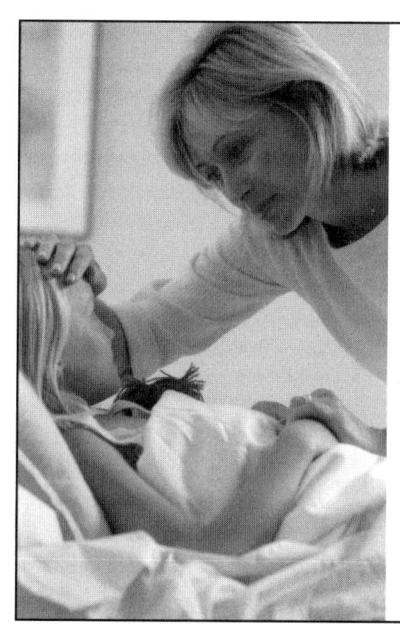

Anna and her family agree to participate – what happens now?

- Anna fulfils the criteria for the trial

- She will have clinic appointments throughout the study. Doctors and nurses will monitor her closely and keep detailed records of her progress.

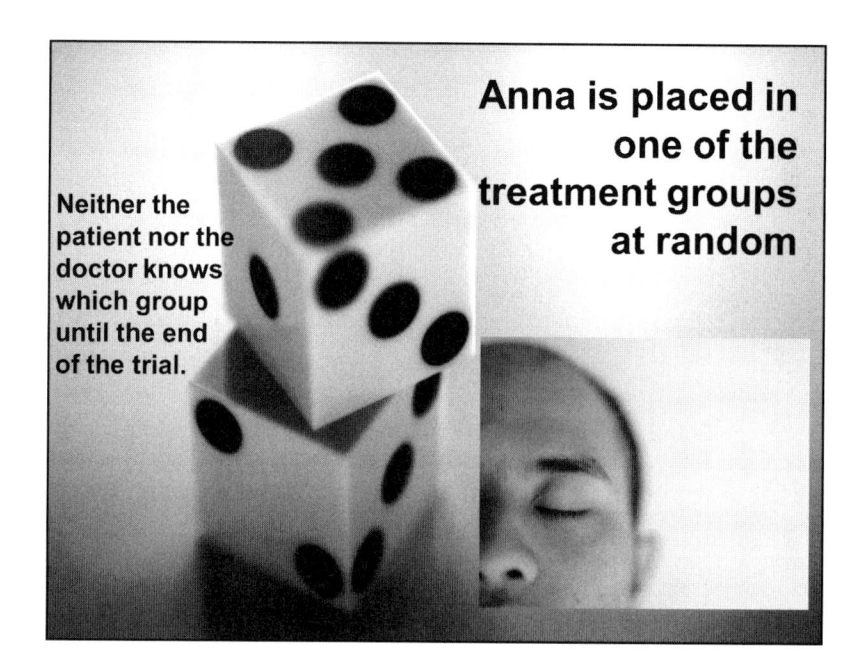

Anna is placed in one of the treatment groups at random

Neither the patient nor the doctor knows which group until the end of the trial.

How is Anna protected in the trial?

- The protocol is approved by an ethics committee

- Good Clinical Practice guidelines

- All side effects are reported

- Insurance provided against medical negligence

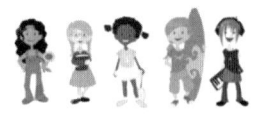

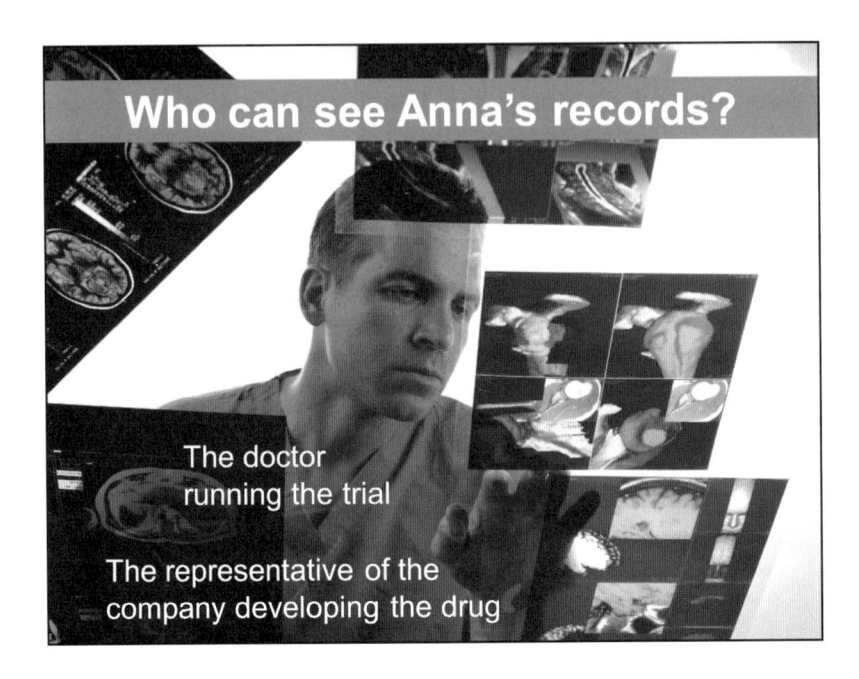

Who can see Anna's records?

The doctor running the trial

The representative of the company developing the drug

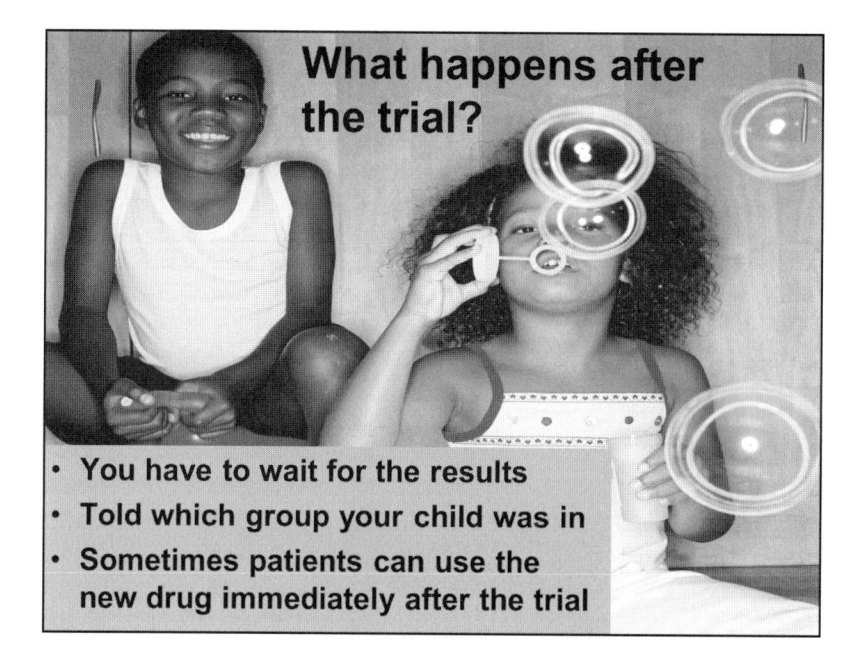

Appendix 3a: Pilot education package for parents

What happens after the trial?

- You have to wait for the results
- Told which group your child was in
- Sometimes patients can use the new drug immediately after the trial

What to consider before giving consent

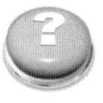

- Do I – and my child – understand what the study is about?
- Have we received enough information?
- Do we accept all parts of the informed consent?
- Is there any reason why my child would not be able to participate for the full length of the study?
- Will we have time for all the clinic appointments?

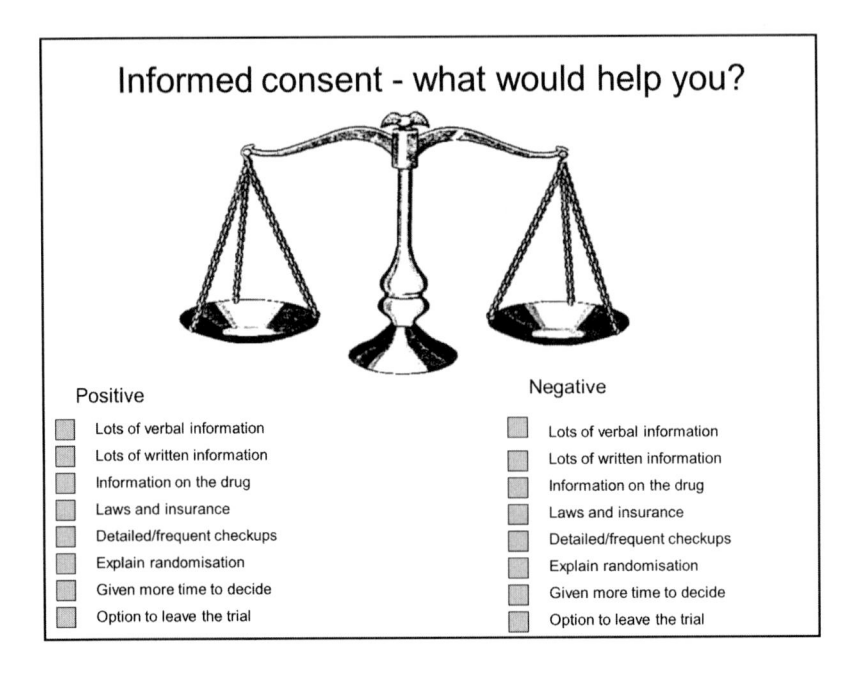

Informed consent - what would help you?

Positive
- Lots of verbal information
- Lots of written information
- Information on the drug
- Laws and insurance
- Detailed/frequent checkups
- Explain randomisation
- Given more time to decide
- Option to leave the trial

Negative
- Lots of verbal information
- Lots of written information
- Information on the drug
- Laws and insurance
- Detailed/frequent checkups
- Explain randomisation
- Given more time to decide
- Option to leave the trial

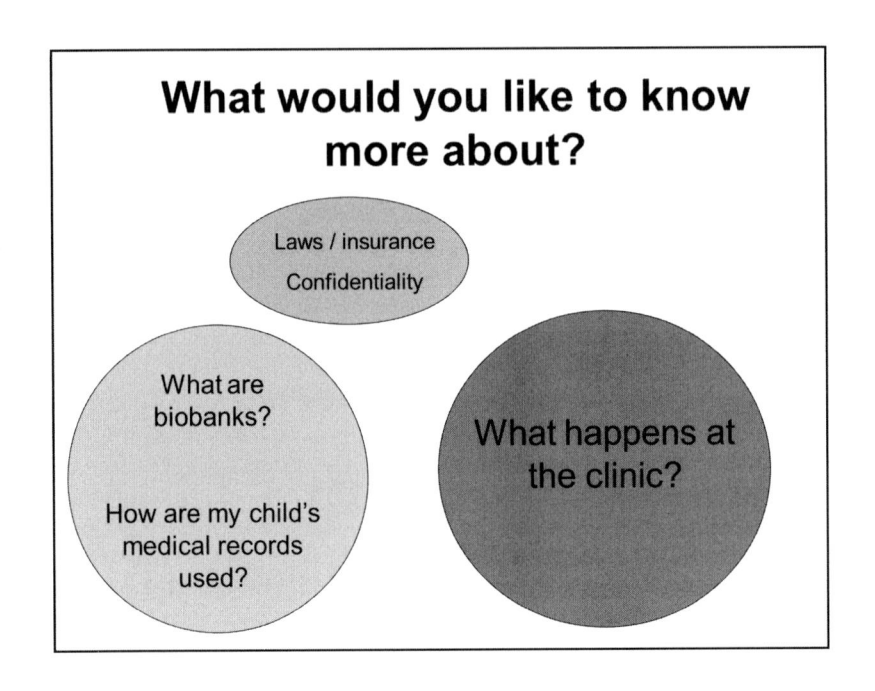

What would you like to know more about?

- Laws / insurance
- Confidentiality
- What are biobanks?
- How are my child's medical records used?
- What happens at the clinic?

Appendix 3b:

Pilot education package for children

(Short example based on the parent version)

CONTRIBUTORS:

Andrea Sandberg
John E. Chaplin

RESPECT

Appendix 3b: Pilot education package for children

NOTE! Outline example only

Andrea Sandberg
Sept. 2010

EDUCATION PACKAGE FOR CHILDREN

We need to make medicines for children so that they can stay healthy

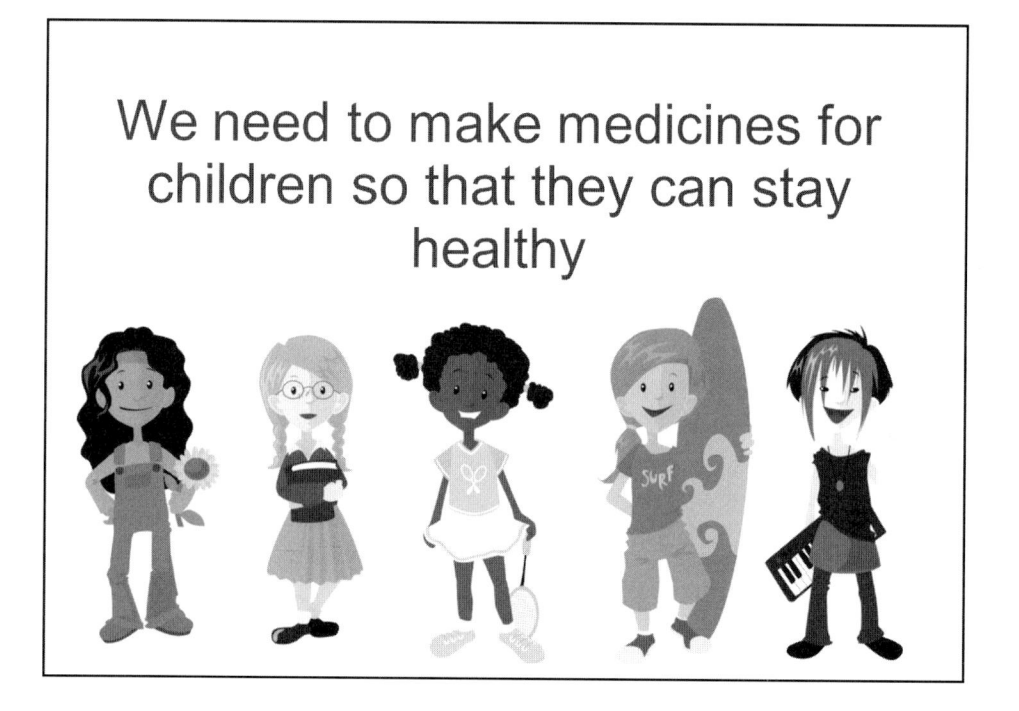

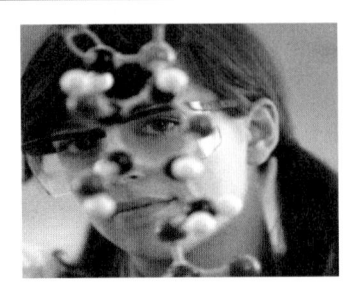

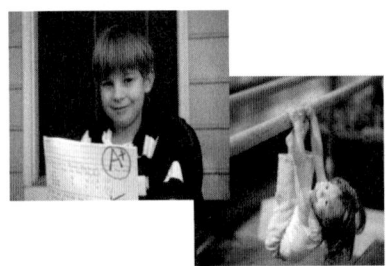

Scientists are working hard to come up with new ideas of how to develop medicines that might cure childhood illnesses or at least improve their health condition

The new medicines that are in development need to be tested in children to assure that they are effective and safe to use. This is done through a clinical trial

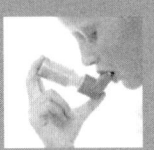

Appendix 3b: Pilot education package for children

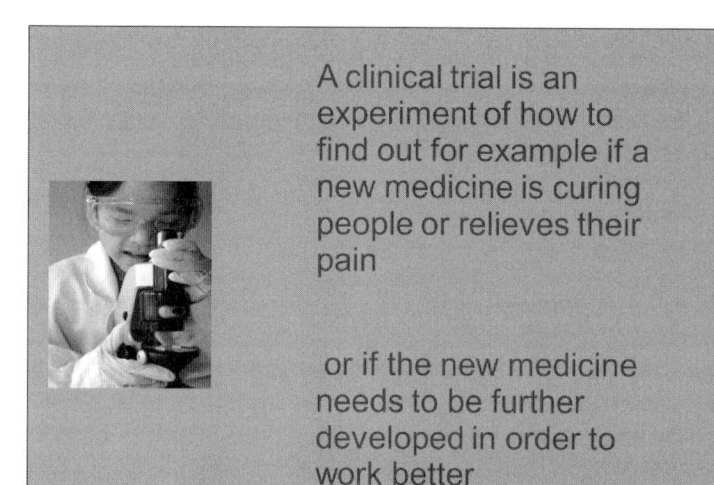

A clinical trial is an experiment of how to find out for example if a new medicine is curing people or relieves their pain

or if the new medicine needs to be further developed in order to work better

In a clinical trial a lot of children try out the new medicine

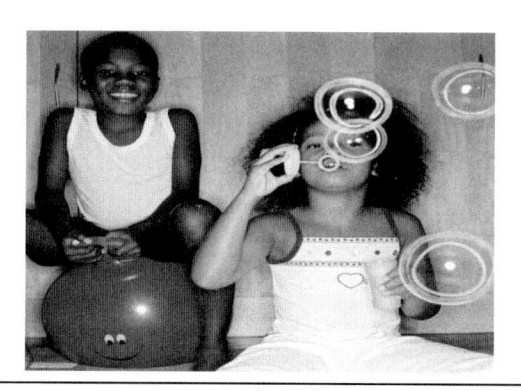

RESPECT

> As a participant you will either be in a group trying the new medicine or in a group who tries anot similar medicine that is already used.
>
> Which medicine you receive is decided by a computer.

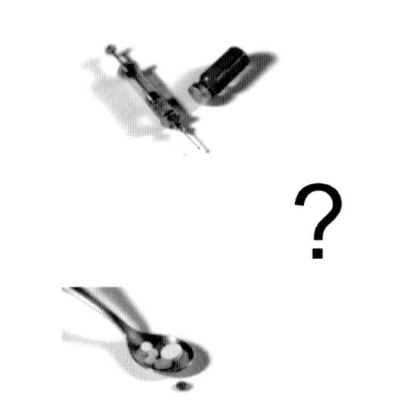

In a clinical trial, no one knows which medicine in the study will turn out to be best in the end

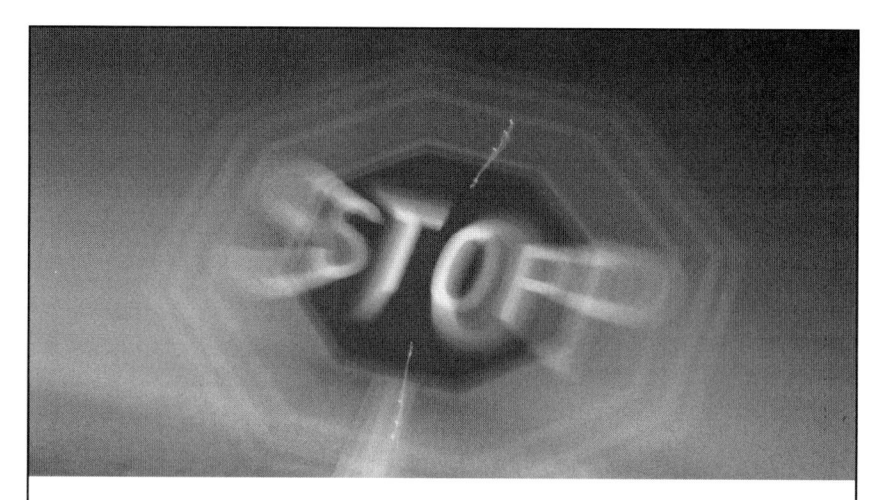

You always have the right to say: "Stop, I do not want to continue in the study". This may be for any reason and you do not need to explain why.

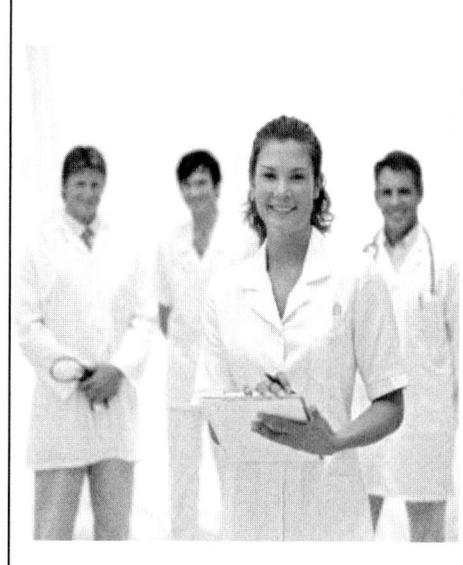

When the children have tried the medicines for a fixed time, the scientists will be able to see which medicine works the best

RESPECT

Each clinical trial is different. Some are short, just a couple of weeks and some are long, and last for several years.

Some trials might require many visits at the clinic and some trials might just require a few visits.

Some trials require you to give blood samples or x-rays or just answer questions.

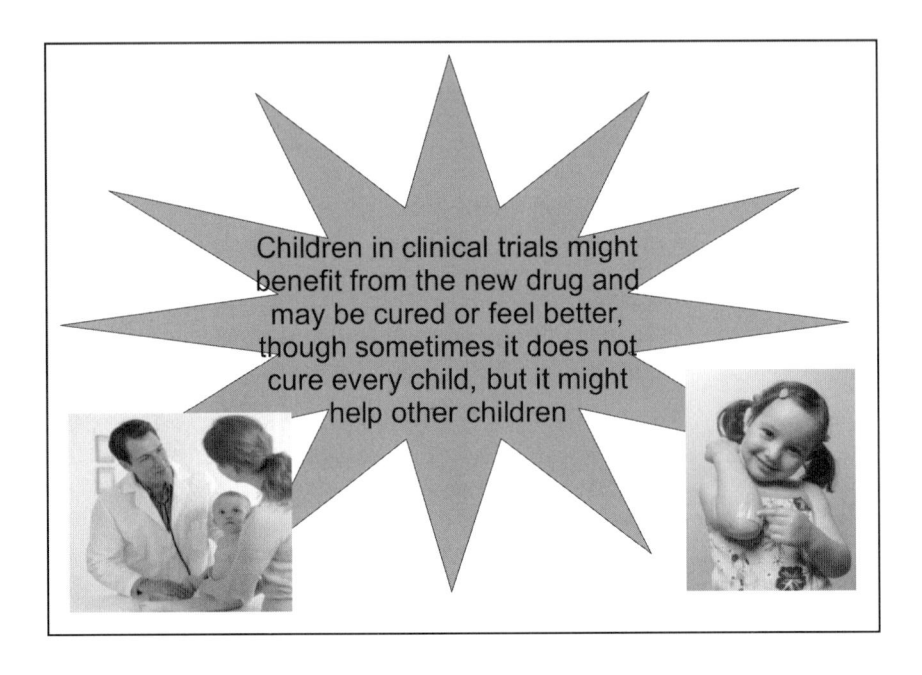

Children in clinical trials might benefit from the new drug and may be cured or feel better, though sometimes it does not cure every child, but it might help other children

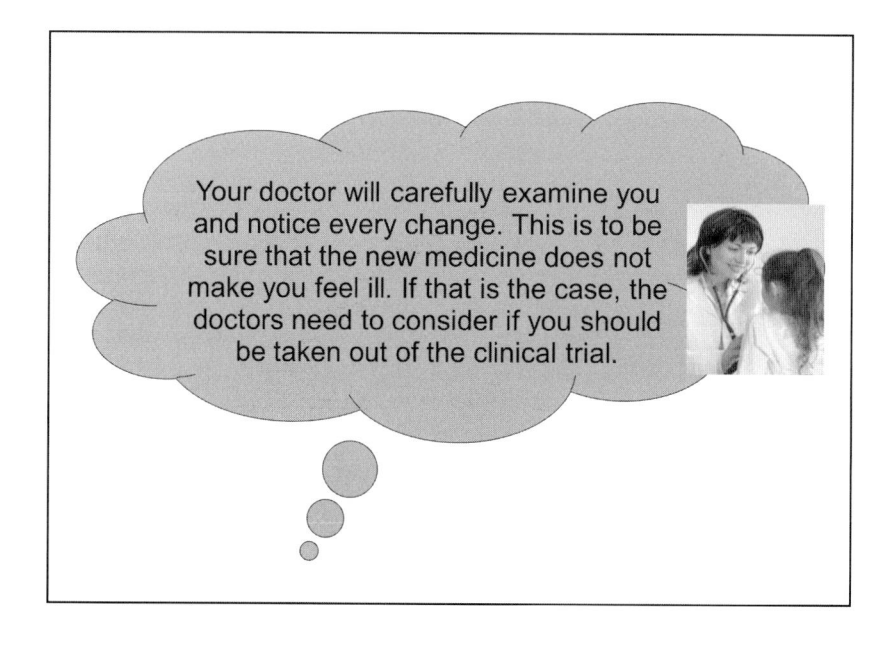

Appendix 3b: Pilot education package for children

> Your doctor will carefully examine you and notice every change. This is to be sure that the new medicine does not make you feel ill. If that is the case, the doctors need to consider if you should be taken out of the clinical trial.

> Children in a clinical trial help the researchers to find out how well the medicine works. In this way, they can develop new drugs to help even more children in the future

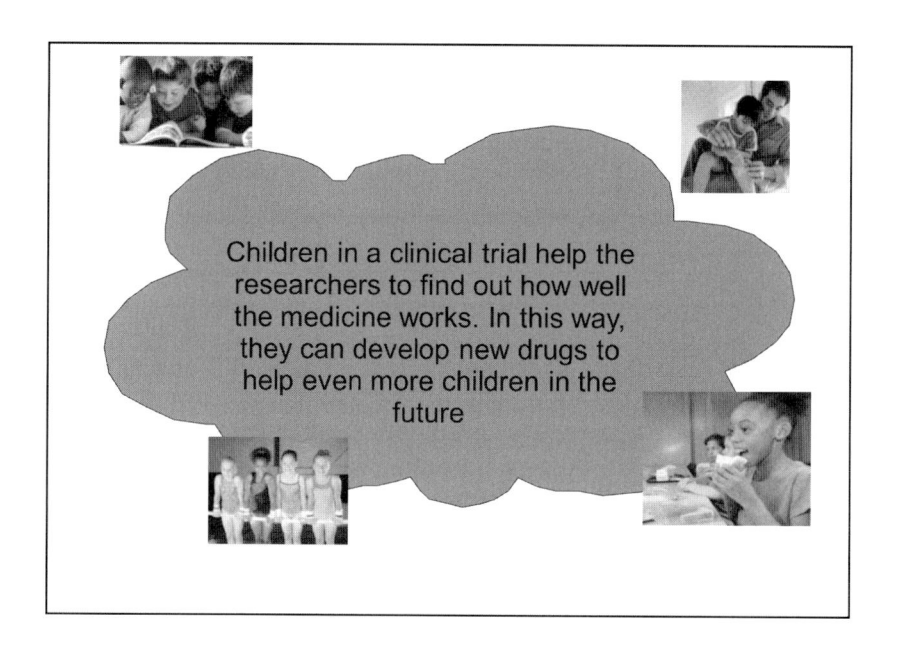

T. G. Baudson, A. Seemüller & M. Dresler (Eds.)

Chronobiology and Chronopsychology

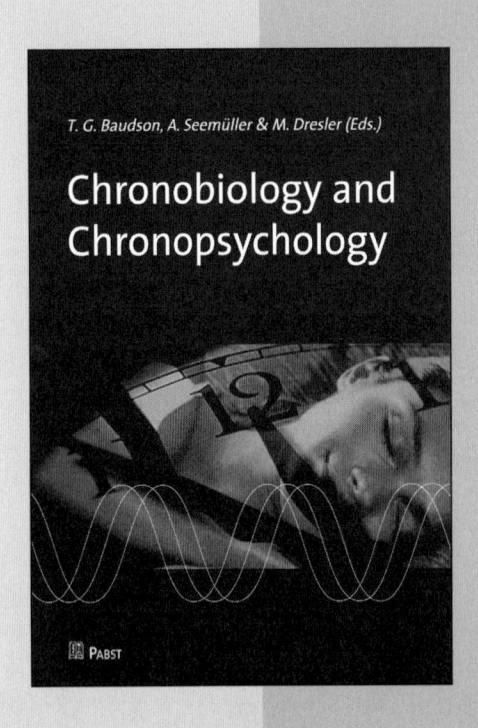

Night and day, sleep and wake, death and birth: All living organisms are subject to external biological cycles and inner clocks that influence our experience and behavior. But how exactly does this influence become manifest, and how can we deal with it? What are the mechanisms underlying such periodic recurrences? Or, more generally: Why is time so important - and what makes it so fascinating?

The contributions to this volume represent a broad and multi-faceted approach not only to the chronosciences in the narrower sense, but also to the way we experience and deal with the passing of time in general. Authors from psychology, neuroscience, biology, medicine and philosophy approach the subject from many different angles, thus providing intriguing insights into a truly interdisciplinary research topic.

PABST SCIENCE PUBLISHERS
Eichengrund 28
D-49525 Lengerich,
Tel. ++ 49 (0) 5484-308,
Fax ++ 49 (0) 5484-550,
pabst.publishers@t-online.de
www.pabst-publishers.de

156 pages, ISBN 978-3-89967-586-3
Price: 20,- Euro

The DISABKIDS Group Europe

The DISABKIDS Questionnaires
Quality of life questionnaires for children with chronic conditions

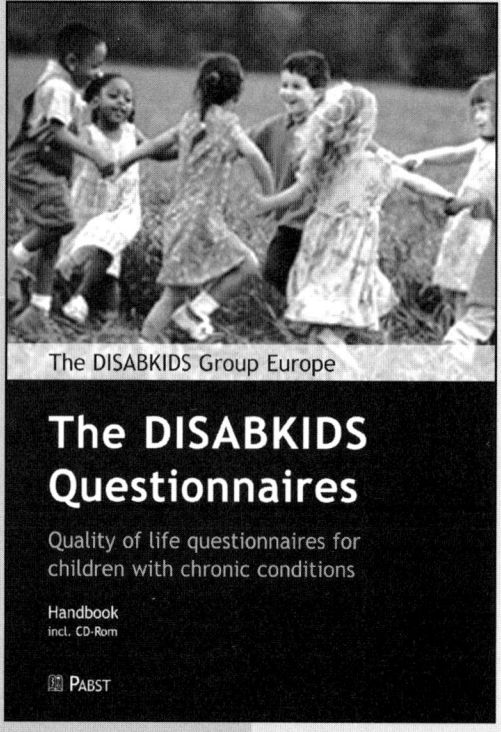

Quality of life (QoL) assessment in children with chronic health conditions and disabilities needs to be age-appropriate and address health-related as well as disease-specific concerns of children in a balanced way. The proposed DISABKIDS modular approach has tackled these challenges of international paediatric OoL research by providing modules that are on the one hand applicable for children of specific age groups and specific health conditions, and on the hand can be applied across different subgroups. The DISABKIDS questionnaires have been developed within a European cross-cultural multi-centre study in order to be able to compare different conditions across health care systems from different countries and in order to be able to conduct multinational clinical studies. The DISABKIDS groups used a simultaneous approach towards cross-cultural instrument development that ensures the cross-cultural applicability of the measures. The current handbook describes all relevant user information (e.g. psychometrics or reference data), necessary for applying the DISABKIDS questionnaires.

The authors:
Silke Schmidt, Corinna Petersen, Holger Mühlan, Marie Claude Simeoni, David Debensason, Ute Thyen, Esther Müller-Godeffroy, Athanasios Vidalis, John Tsanakas, Elpis Hatziagorou, Paraskevi Karagianni, Hendrik Koopmann, Rolanda Baars, John Chaplin, Mick Power, Clare Atherton, Peter Hoare, Michael Quittan, Othmar Schuhfried and Monika Bullinger
THE DISABKIDS Group Europe

2006, 212 pages + CD-ROM, Price: 35,- Euro
ISBN 978-3-89967-166-7

PABST SCIENCE PUBLISHERS
Eichengrund 28, D-49525 Lengerich
Tel.: ++ 49 (0) 5484-308, Fax: ++ 49 (0) 5484-550
E-mail: pabst.publishers@t-online.de, Internet: http://www.pabst-publishers.de

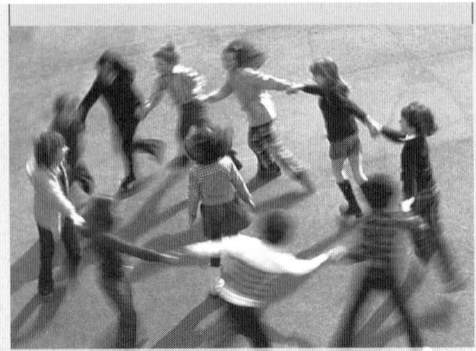

The KIDSCREEN Group Europe

The KIDSCREEN questionnaires

Quality of life questionnaires for children and adolescents

Quality of life (QoL) assessment in children and adolescents needs to be age-appropriate and to address health-related concerns to identify children and adolescents who are at risk from health problems, and to determine the burden imposed by a particular disease or disability. The KIDSCREEN approach has tackled the challenges of international paediatric QoL research by providing measures that are applicable for children and adolescents as well as their parents and that can be used to monitor and evaluate health-related QoL in public-health surveys, in clinical studies, and in research projects.

The generic KIDSCREEN questionnaires were developed in the context of a European cross-cultural representative health survey in order to be able to compare health-related QoL across different countries and in order to be able to monitor the health status of children and adolescents. The KIDSCREEN group used a simultaneous approach to develop its cross-cultural instrument, which ensures the cross-cultural applicability of the KIDSCREEN measures, making them both conceptually and linguistically appropriate for use in many different countries. The current handbook describes all relevant user information necessary for applying the KIDSCREEN questionnaires, e.g. psychometrics, norm data for group and individual comparisons, and instructions on how to score the instrument and how to interpret the results.

232 pages + CD
978-3-89967-334-0, Price: 40,- Euro

PABST SCIENCE PUBLISHERS
Eichengrund 28
D-49525 Lengerich
T. ++ 49 (0) 5484-308
F. ++ 49 (0) 5484-550
E-mail: pabst@pabst-publishers.de
Internet: www.pabst-publishers.de

Let us Sing

more hymns for Unitarians

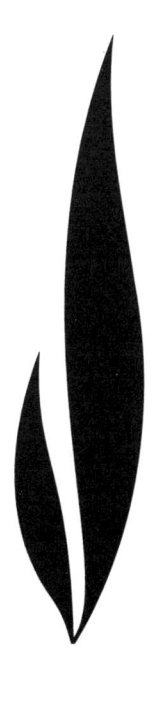

Selection © Unitarian Worship Sub-committee, 1994

Published by the Lindsey Press,
General Assembly of Unitarian and Free Christian Churches,
Essex Hall, 1–6 Essex Street, Strand, London WC2R 3HY

Literary Editor: Peter Sampson

Music Editor: Malcolm Sadler

Music origination and text setting, in New Century Schoolbook, by:
Musonix Typesetting, 2 Avenue Gardens, London SW14 8BP

Printed in England by Caligraving Ltd, Thetford, Norfolk.

ISBN   0 85319 048 8

Contents

PREFACE — *page* iv

ACKNOWLEDGEMENTS — *page* v

INDEXES
    Thematic index — *page* vi
    Index of first lines — viii
    Metrical index — ix
    Index of titles of tunes — x
    Index of authors — xi
    Index of composers of tunes — xii

LET US SING — *numbers* 1–39

Preface

One sign of the health of a religious movement is its eagerness to produce new worship material which matches its developing sense of a distinctive vision and mission. I'm glad to salute all those who are unafraid to meet the challenge of our time by speaking and singing of what lies deep in their hearts.

The hymns included in this slim volume are from a variety of sources but at least half are written by contemporary British Unitarians.

The links between British Unitarians and their sisters and brothers worshipping in the thriving congregations across the Atlantic have inevitably led to wanting to share their devotional material with our own British congregations. The selection included here can only give a taste of the rich fare our friends enjoy.

Many of our own members are always looking out for new songs and hymns to celebrate an occasion or Life itself and have found what they have shared in singing with other religious folk from within and outside the Christian spectrum so memorable that we are glad to be able to offer if only a selection of some 'favourites'.

We started compiling this small collection with the intention of 'filling gaps' perceived in *Hymns for Living* but the Spirit does not always blow to order, although some of the hymns we are confident will supply a long-felt need. We must thank all those authors who have showed such patience in waiting to see their work in print. What we give to fellow Unitarians is an anthology from which to pluck the flowers which are to their taste. May the scent grow ever sweeter over the years!

Sing, let us sing, with a right good will

goes number 60 in *Songs for Living*. We hope that congregations will enjoy learning the new tunes, some of which, again, have been composed by fellow Unitarians, or responding to the challenge to sing new words to well-loved tunes. Participation in worship is an essential aspect of 'the work of the people' and hymn-singing is often the part of our 'liturgy' for which many people feel the greatest warmth and affection and to which they feel they can make their heartiest contribution. Thoughts along these lines have sustained the members of the Unitarian Worship Subcommittee during the sometimes laborious but often more enjoyable process of selecting, trying-out, editing and preparing for publication this latest collection of material for worship in Unitarian congregations.

Peter Sampson
Unitarian Worship Subcommittee

Acknowledgements

Every effort has been made to trace copyright holders but we have not always been successful. If any copyright has been inadvertently infringed we apologise and ask to be informed so that amends may be made in any future edition.

We record thanks to the following who have generously granted copyright permission without fee:
Lena Baxter, June Bell, Don Besig, Richard Boeke, Kate Compston, David Doel, Peter Galbraith, Margaret Hart, Andrew M. Hill, Iona Community / Wild Goose Publications, David Parke, Martha M. Pickrell, Clifford M. Reed, Peter Sampson, John Andrew Storey.

To the following holders of copyright texts:

Stainer and Bell Ltd. for
    One More Step (Carter)
    We Ask That We Live (Swann)
Oxford University Press for
    God, The All-Holy (Wren)
World Library Publications Inc. for
    Sent Forth By God's Blessing (Westendorf)

To the following for their musical compositions or arrangements:
Frank Clabburn, David Dawson, Malcolm Sadler, Margaret Hart, John Taylor, Robert Waller.

To the following holders or administrators of music copyrights:

William Elkin Music Services for
    Little Cornard (Martin Shaw)
Oxford University Press for
    Bunessan (Martin Shaw)
    Wolvercote (William Harold Ferguson)
Stainer and Bell Ltd. for
    One More Step (Carter)
    We Ask That We Live (Swann)
Iona Community / Wild Goose Publications for
    God Who Is Everywhere

Thematic Index

Acceptance	2
Advent (or Christmas)	21
All Faiths	34
Altar, The	26
Animal Life	12
Aspiration	1, 24
Baptism / Child Welcoming / Christening	19, 35
Beauty	2, 8
Benediction	39
Better World	24, 26, 27, 28, 32, 33, 34, 36
Celebration	1
Children	19, 21, 35
Church	27, 36
Circle of Love	17, 30
Commitment	1, 4, 22
Communion	26, 36
Communion with God	9, 36, 37
Compassion	11, 14
Consecration	6, 26
Conservation	see Ecology
Courage	37
Creation	28, 29
Death	2, 32
Dedication	26
Deliverance	21, 33, 37
Design	5
Difficulty	9
Divine Glimpses	14, 20, 21, 24, 35
Ecology	3, 5, 6, 8
Eternity	see Time and Eternity
Exploration	7
Faith	21, 36, 37
Feminine Spirituality	14, 23
Freedom	31, 37
Friendship	22, 30
Fulfilment	7, 23, 28
Future Time	8
Gardening	18
God	5, 9, 14, 15, 20, 23, 24, 28, 29, 33, 37, 38
Goddess	23
Grace	15
Green Peace	3
Growth and Maturity	7, 18, 38
Guidance	38
Harvest	18
Healing and Wholeness	3, 29, 33
Here and Now	2, 16, 31
Home	9, 33
Hope	19, 21
Ideals	4, 26
Incarnation	21, 35
Individual, The	9, 16, 38
Ineffable, The	9
Integrity and Truth	10
Inspiration	11, 13, 36
Jesus	1, 15, 21, 33, 35, 36
Journey of Life	7, 19, 23, 31, 38, 39
Joy in Life	2, 25, 27, 31

Justice	3, 4, 5	Remembrance	32, 36
		Restoration	6, 29
		Revelation	14, 20, 21, 24, 37
Knowledge	9	Rhythms of Life	12, 23

Life and Living	7, 8, 12, 38	Search for Truth	7, 9
Light	13, 20	Seasons of Human Life	2, 7, 12
Love	13, 17, 22, 27, 30		19, 22, 23, 38
Lord's Supper, The	36	Senses and Feelings	2
		Sharing	3, 4, 8, 22, 30
		Sing our Lives	10, 31
Marriage	22	Social Conscience	4
Mercy	23	Space (Outer and Inner)	7, 20, 37
Mystery and Awe	20	Spirit of Life	11, 13, 24

Nature	2, 3, 6, 8, 12, 18, 19, 25	Time and Eternity	7, 12, 16
Night	20		20, 23, 37
		Togetherness	13, 22, 27, 30
Order	5	Transformation	28, 34, 36, 37, 38
Old Age	2	Trinity	15
Opening of Worship	1, 15, 27		
Oneness of Life	12	Union	22
One World / One People		Unitarianism	4
	3, 8, 29, 33, 34, 36	Unrest	9

Partnership	22		
Peace in the World	3, 25, 32, 33, 34	Values	4
Peace Within	9		
Planet Earth	3, 6, 8, 25, 29		
Planting and Sowing	18	War	32, 33
Pollution	6, 8, 29	Wilderness and Wild Places	3, 8, 25
Possibility	16, 19. 38	Women's Spirituality	23
Praise and Thanksgiving	25	Wonderful World	2, 29
Prayer	10, 15	Work and Workers	24, 36
Principles	4	Wrong and Repetance	6, 29, 32, 33

Index of First Lines

Bring flowers to our altar 26
Equity and justice 4
For the earth forever turning 25
God of creation 28
God the All-Holy 15
God who is everywhere present on earth 14
Here in this moment's song 16
Inch by inch, row by row 18
Lady of the seasons' laughter 23
Love is a circle, round and round 17
Loving friends together 30
May the road rise with you 39
Now rejoice! we greet his coming! 21
O beautiful baby, you come here before us 19
O God, O Spirit free 24
O let us now our voices raise 10
O sacred Earth, now wounded 6
One more step along the world I go 38
Our song of joy, for now we join together 27
Red the poppy-fields of Flanders 32
See the mother's desolation 33
Sent forth by God's blessing our true faith confessing 36
So look your last on all things lovely every hour 2
Spirit of Life, come unto me 11
Sweet dreams form a shade 35
The green grass brings the air to life 3
The Spirit lives to set us free 13
There is a place I call my own 31
This day confirms a union 22
Thy darkness descends like a robe on the evening 20
Together now we join as one 1
View the starry realm of heaven 37
We are travellers on a journey 7
We ask that we live and we labour in peace, in peace 34
We set a frame on nature 12
We walk the holy ground of earth 29
Weaver-God, Creator, sets life on the loom 5
Where shall I find that Power 9
Wide, green world, we know and love you 8

Metrical Index

C. M.
  St. Fulbert 1
  Horsley 29

L. M.
  Ombersley 10

5 5. 5 4. D.
  Bunessan 15

5 7. 6 8.
  Sweet Dreams 35

6 5. 6 5. D.
  Ruth 5

6 6. 6 6.
  St. Cecilia 24
  Ravenshaw 4

6 6. 6 6. 8 8. (Dactylic)
  Little Cornard 16

6 6. 6 6. 8 8. 6 6.
  Divine Mysteries 9

6 9. 8 9. 7 11.
  May the Road 39

7 6. 7 6. D.
  Clonmel 3
  Missionary 12
  Passion Chorale 6
  Wolvercote 22

8 5. 8 5. (+ refrain)
  Walk in the Light 13

8 7. 8 7. Trochaic
  All for Jesus 32

8 7. 8 7. 8 7.
  Julion 23

8 7. 8 7 7.
  Dachau Song 1 37

8 7. 8 7. 7 7. 8 8.
  There is a Place 31

8 7. 8 8.
  Blue-green Hills 25

8 7. 8 9. (+ refrain)
  Love is a Circle 17

8 8 7.
  Fellowship 33

8 8. 8 8. D. (Trochaic)
  Schmücke Dich 8

8 8. 8 8. 8 8.
  Joel 21

8 12. 8 12. 8 10.
  Spirit of Life 11

9 9. 7 8. (+ refrain)
  One More Step 38

10 8. 10 9. (+ refrain)
  Here's to the maiden 14

10 11. 11 11. (+ refrain)
  Maccabaeus 28

11 10. 11 10. D.
  Londonderry Air 2
  Our Song of Joy 27

12 10. 11 11. D.
  Mozart 20

12 11. 12 11. D.
  The Ash Grove 36, 26

12 11. 13 12.
  Kremser 19

12 12. (+ refrain)
  Loving Friends 30

Irregular
  Ascension 7
  Peace, Truth and Unity ... 34
  The Garden Song 18

Index of Titles of Tunes

A Blessing	39
All for Jesus	32
Ash Grove (The)	26, 36
Ascension	7
Blue-green Hills of Earth	25
Bunessan	15
Clonmel	3
Dachau Song No. 1	37
Divine Mysteries	9
Fellowship	33
Flying Free	31
Garden Song (The)	18
Here's To The Maiden	14
Horsley	29
Joel	21
Julion	23
Kremser	19
Little Cornard	16
Londonderry Air	2
Loving Friends	30
Love is a Circle	17
Maccabeus	28
Missionary	12
Mozart	20
One More Step	38
Ombersley	10
Our Song of Joy	27
Passion Chorale	6
Peace, Truth and Unity	34
Ravenshaw	4
Ruth	5
Schmücke Dich	8
Spirit of Life	11
St. Cecilia	24
St. Fulbert	1
Sweet Dreams	35
Walk in the Light	13
Wolvercote	22

Index of Authors

Anon	13
Baxter, Lena	26
Bell, June	2, 8, 12
Besig, Don	31
Blake, William (1757–1827)	35
Boeke, Richard – translator of:	
Capek, Norbert (1870–1942)	37
Compston, Kate	5
Carter, Sydney	38
Clabburn, Frank	16
Doel, David	20
Galbraith, Peter	9, 10, 22
Gibbons, Kendyl	23
Hart, Margaret	19, 27
Hill, Andrew M.	3, 4, 7
Hiller, Phyllis	17
Iona Community	14
Mallet, Dave	18
McDade, Carolyn	11
'Missa Gaia'	25
Parke, Mary Boynton	28
Peltz, Diane	30
Pickrell, Martha M.	6
Reed, Clifford M.	1, 21, 24, 29, 32
Sampson, Peter	33
Swann, Donald	34
Traditional	39
Westendorf, Omer	36
Wren, Brian	15

Index of Composers of Tunes

Bancroft, Henry Hugh	7
Besig, Don	31
Carter, Sydney	38
Clabburn, Frank	33
Cruger, Johann	8
Dawson, David	35
English Traditional	14, 26, 36
Ferguson, William Harold	22
Gauntlett, Henry John	1
Gladstone, William Henry	10
Hart, Margaret	27
Handel, George Frederick	28
Haspl, Bodhana	37
Hassler, Hans Leo	6
Hayne, Leighton George	24
Hiller, Phyllis	17
Horsley, William	29
Hurd, David	23
Irish Traditional, arranged D. Dawson	2, 19, 39
Irish Traditional	3
Kremser, Edward (arranger)	19
McDade, Carolyn	11
Mallett, Dave	18
Mason, Lowell	12
Monk, W. H.	4
Mozart, Wolfgang Amadeus	20
Olar, Kim	25
Shaw, Martin Fallas	16
Shaw, Martin Fallas (arranger)	15
Smith, Glenn	30
Smith, Samuel	5
Stainer, John	32
Swann, Donald	34
Stanfield, F.	9
Traditional	13
Waller, Robert	21

Together Now We Join As One — 1

ST. FULBERT C.M. 					Henry John Gauntlett, 1805–76

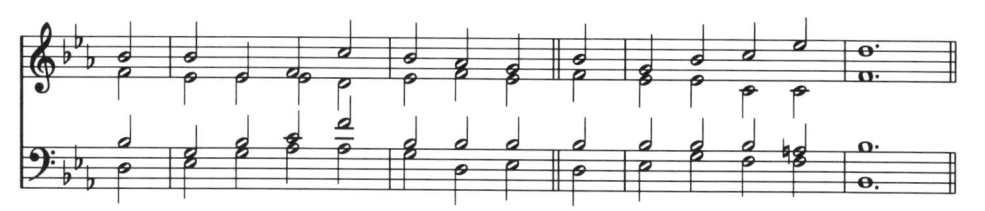

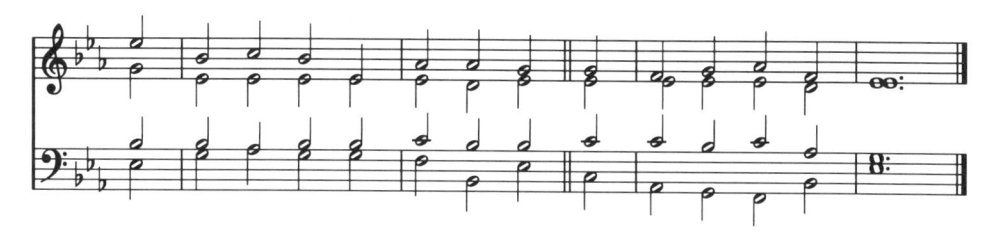

Together now we join as one
  Our common faith to sing;
To render to this pilgrim world
  Our heartfelt offering.

We strive to be a fellowship
  With mind and conscience free,
To search for truth and saving light
  In cosmic mystery.

We worship God – love's source and power;
  We celebrate the life
That all earth's children freely share
  Beyond their sinful strife.

We would, in love, serve humankind
  With caring, justice, peace;
And with the earth seek harmony
  That pride and pillage cease.

We hold in reverence the man
  Who walked in Galilee,
Who healed the sick and loved the poor –
  Revealed divinity.

We welcome truth, we welcome light,
  All prophecy and song,
Whoever they be channelled through
  To all they shall belong.

Clifford M. Reed

2 So Look Your Last

LONDONDERRY AIR   11 10. 11 10. D.

Irish Traditional Melody
Arr. David Dawson
Used by permission

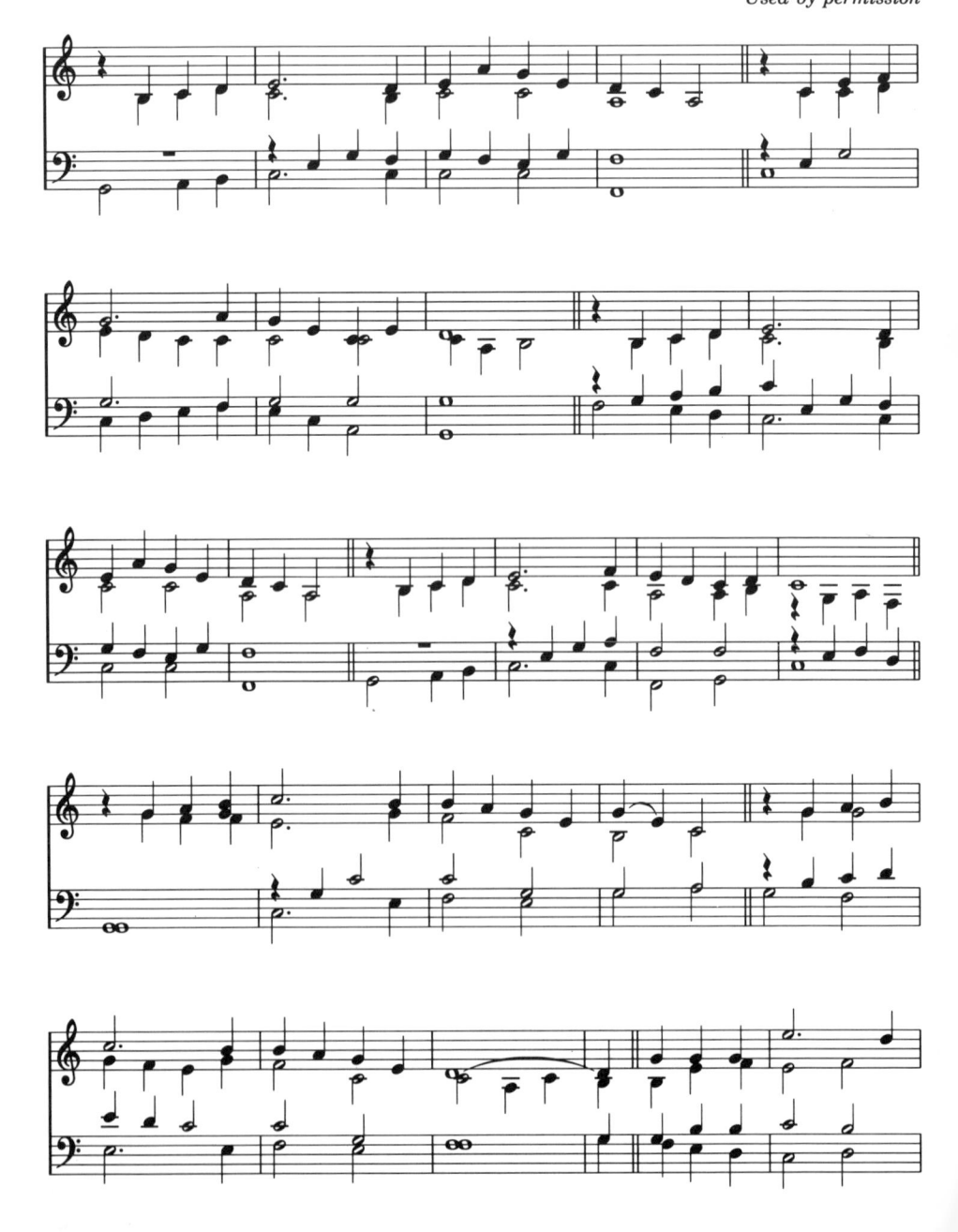

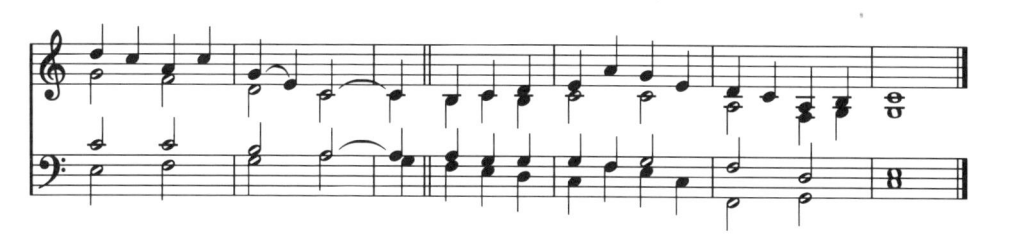

So look your last on all things lovely every hour
   And feel the chill fresh wetness of the burn,
Taste new-baked bread and smell the velvet gilly-flower,
   Hear robins sing, watch autumn colours turn.

Not only human greed and vain endeavour
   May use it up, and wipe it all away:
Your eyes and ears shall one day close for ever –
   Take therefore every earthly beauty of this day.

                                                                                June Bell

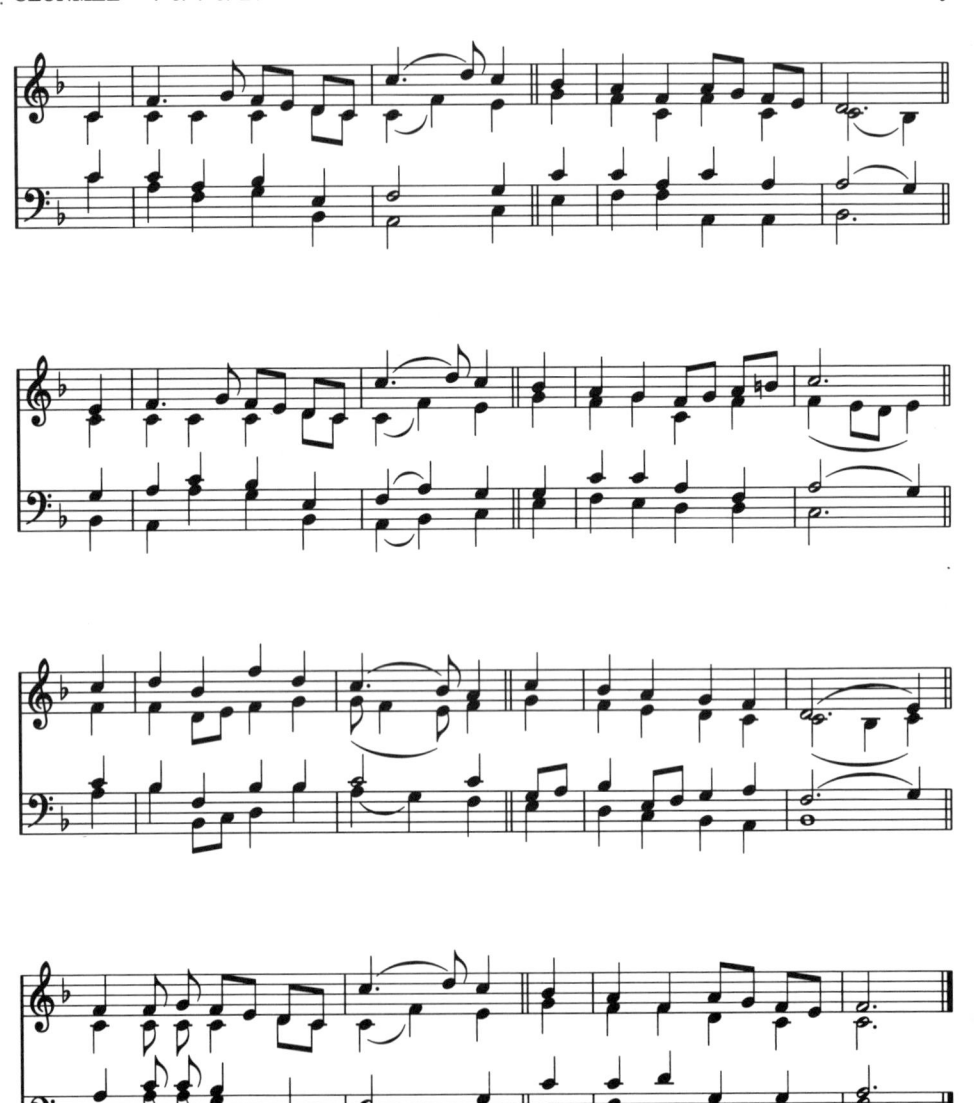

3 The Green Grass Brings the Air to Life

CLONMEL 7 6. 7 6. D. Irish Traditional Melody

The green grass brings the air to life
    Upon this earthly globe,
All living and all growing things
    Are clothed in nature's robe.
Hope for the world, hope for our lives
    Grows in God's wilderness!
So forest, jungle, marsh and moor
    We'll treat with gentleness.

The green earth yields sufficiently
    For every human need;
But not enough when human life
    Is marred by wanton greed;
For each and every one is part
    Of a much greater whole;
The many and the one which make
    The universal soul.

The green peace dwells with planet earth
    When inner spirits rise
To meet the outer world and build
    One home beneath the skies.
Within the garden home of earth
    There grows a gracious tree,
Whose healing leaves the nations calm
    And set their subjects free.

                                        Andrew M. Hill

1. "In God's wilderness lies the hope of the world" *(John Muir, Scottish-born conservationist who founded America's first national park, Yosemite).*

2. "The world has enough for everyone's need, but not enough for everyone's greed" *(Attributed to Gandhi).*

4 Equity and Justice

RAVENSHAW 6 6. 6 6.

Melody abridged by W. H. Monk from *Ave Hierarchia* (M. Weisse, 1480–1534)

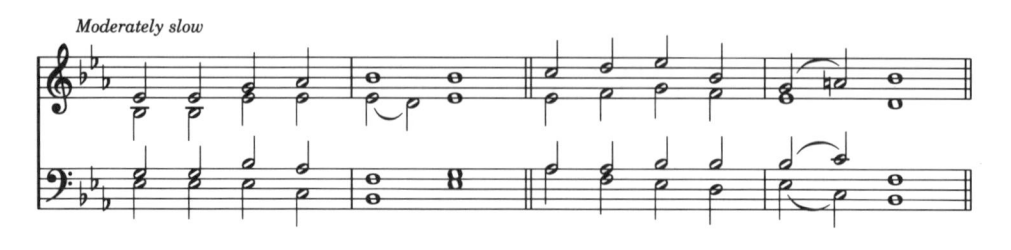

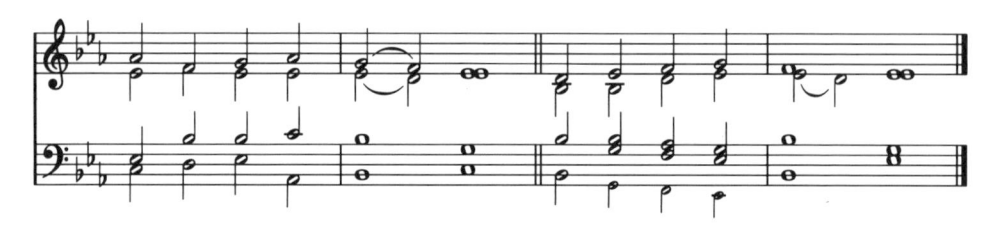

Moderately slow

Equity and justice;
    Service and compassion;
Dignity enhancing;
    Human worth advancing.

Conscience rights considered;
    People's power engendered;
Peaceful earth, expecting;
    Web of life, respecting.

One another, caring
    In a mutual sharing;
Truth, forever growing;
    Life, in spirit, sowing.

Andrew M. Hill

Based on the Unitarian Universalist Association's statement of Principles and Purposes.

Weaver God, Creator   5

RUTH 6 5. 6 5. D.   Samuel Smith, 1821–1917

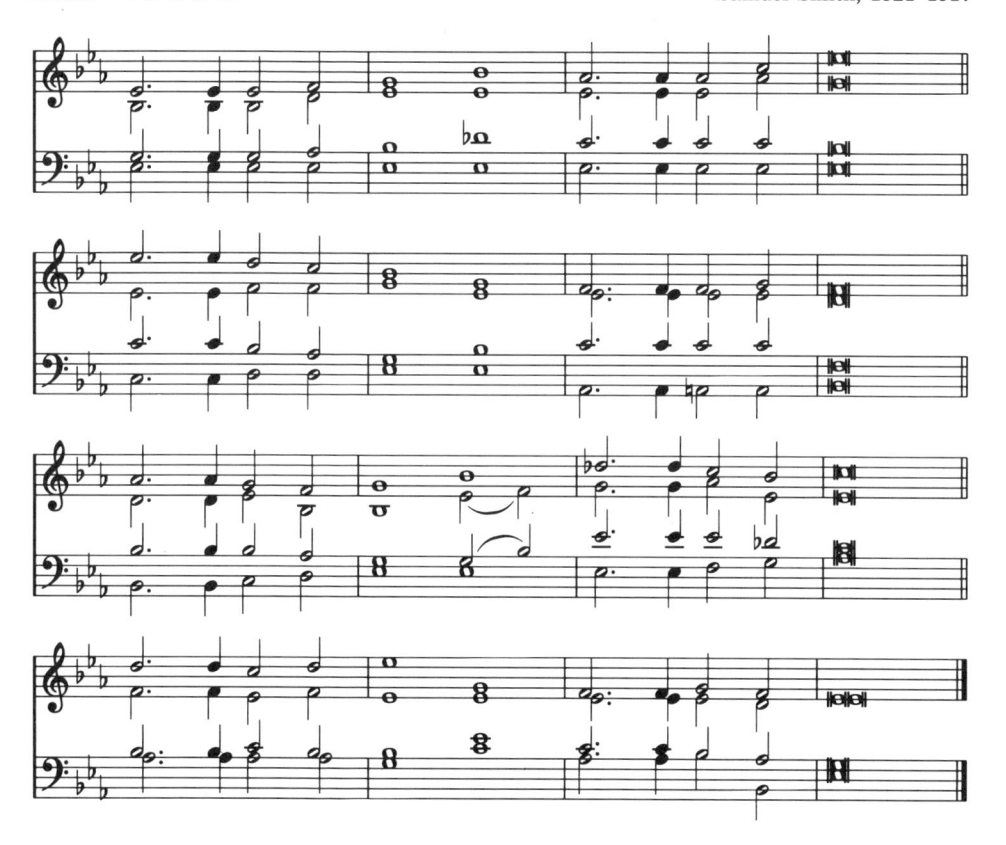

Weaver God, Creator, sets life on the loom,
   Draws out threads of colour from primordial gloom.
Wise in the designing, in the weaving deft;
   Love and justice joined – the fabric's warp and weft.

Called to be co-weavers, yet we break the thread
   And may smash the shuttle and the loom, instead.
Careless and greedy, we deny by theft
   Love and justice joined – the fabric's warp and weft.

Weaver God, great Spirit, may we see your face
   Tapestried in trees, in waves and winds of space;
Tenderness teach us, lest we be bereft;
   Love and justice joined – the fabric's warp and weft.

Weavers we are called, yet woven too we're born,
   For the web is seamless: if we tear, we're torn.
Gently may we live – that fragile Earth be left;
   Love and justice joined – the fabric's warp and weft.

                                          Kate Compston

6   O Sacred Earth, Now Wounded

PASSION CHORALE   7 6. 7 6. D.   Hans Leo Hassler, 1564–1612
harmonised Johann Sebastian Bach, 1685–1750

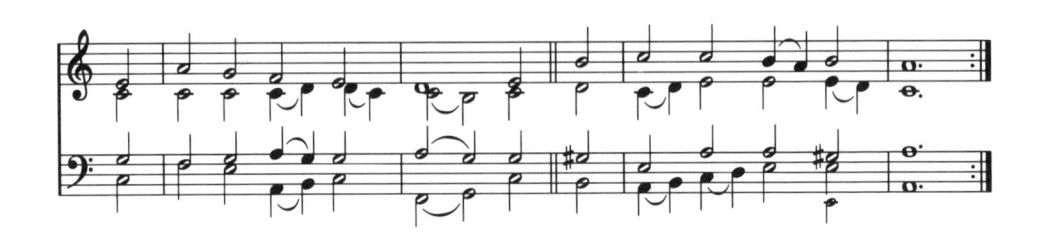

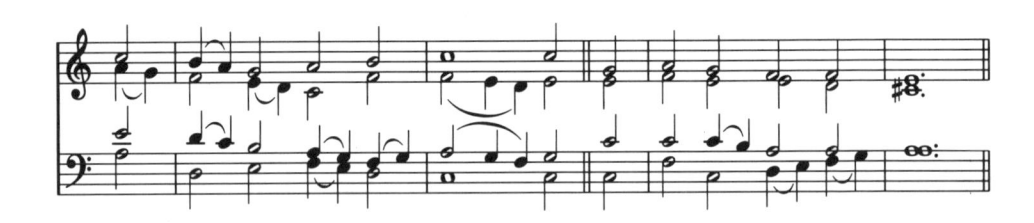

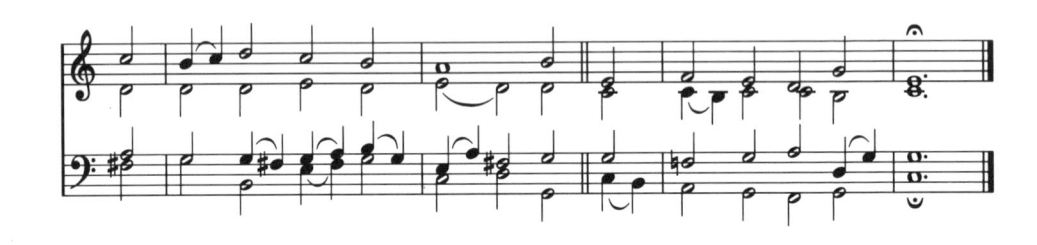

O sacred Earth, now wounded,
    What have we done to thee?
The carnage is unbounded,
    For all our eyes to see.
Thy air and soil and water
    Are poisoned by our greed;
Thy forests we do slaughter
    To serve our every need.

So fierce in our ambitions
    We've entered sunlight's field,
And, armed with strong emissions
    We've torn apart its shield.
And ever there is waiting
    Our bombs' immortal fire,
The flower of all our hating,
    Eternal glowing pyre.

The time has come for grieving,
    To bow our heads, and pause;
And we must cease believing
    That we may break Earth's laws.
The time has come to worship
    This place, where we belong;
To consecrate our Earthship
    With prayer, and poem, and song;

And then to start restoring
    Our Earth, with our own hands,
With work, with love outpouring,
    With laws throughout the lands;
To bring the nations nearer
    With every quest for peace,
Until, as hope grows clearer,
    Our war on Earth may cease.

Martha M. Pickrell

7   We Are Travellers on a Journey

ASCENSION   irregular   Henry Hugh Bancroft, 1904–

We are travellers on a journey
    Which brought us from the sun,
When primal star exploded
    And earth in orbit spun.
But now as human dwellers
    Upon earth-planet's crust,
We strive for living systems
    Whose ways are kind and just.

We are travellers on a journey
    Which grows from human seed,
And through our birth and childhood
    Goes where life's path may lead.
But now we are delving deeper
    In quest of greater worth
And reaching unknown regions
    And planets of new birth.

We are travellers on a journey
    Through realms of inner space
Where joy and peace are planets
    That circle stars of grace.
And when we find the stillness
    Which comes at journey's end,
There'll be complete refreshment,
    A resting place, a friend.

Andrew M. Hill

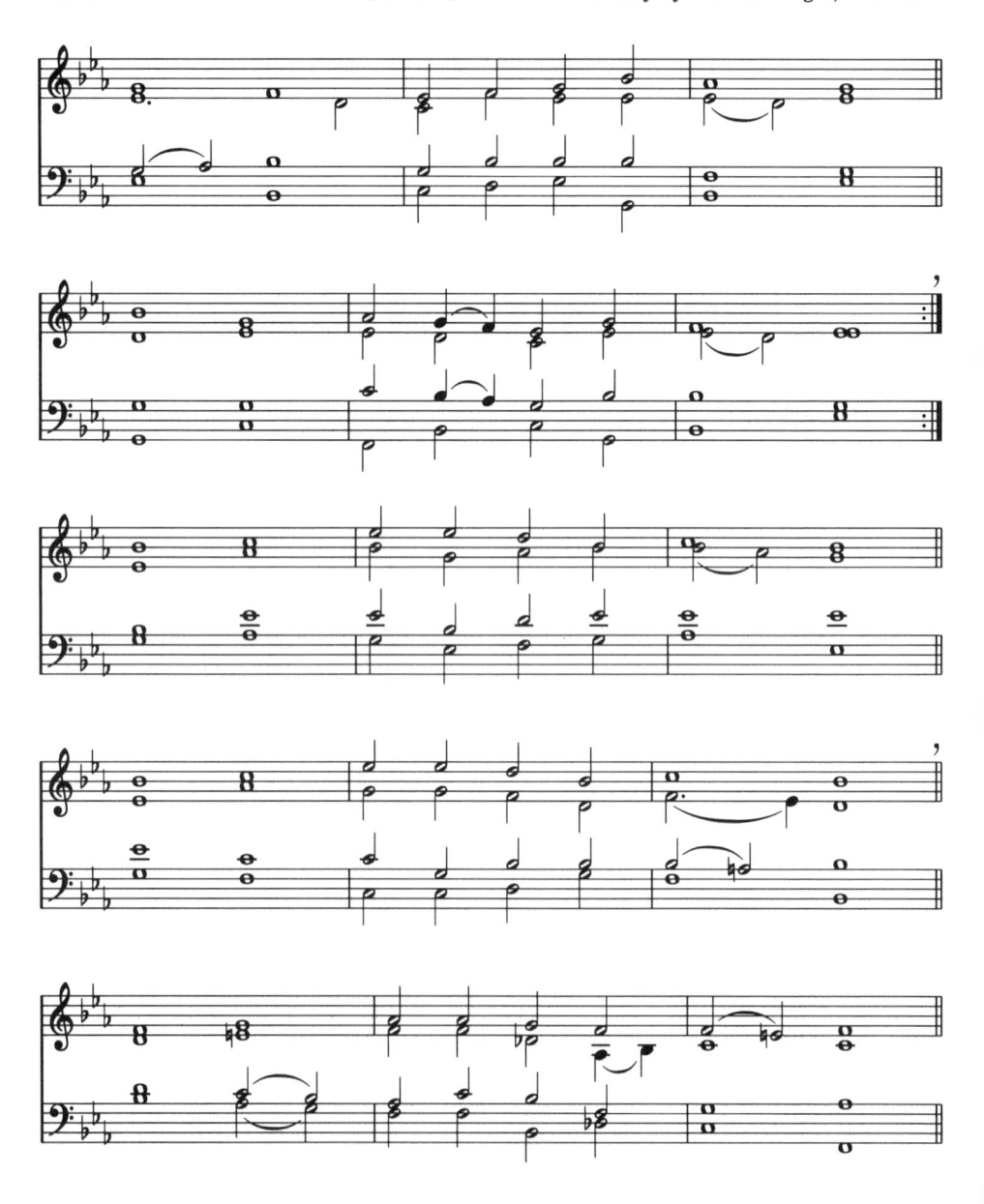

8. Wide Green World, We Know and Love You

SCHMÜCKE DICH   8 8. 8 8. D. (Trochaic)   Melody by Johann Crüger, 1598–1662

8

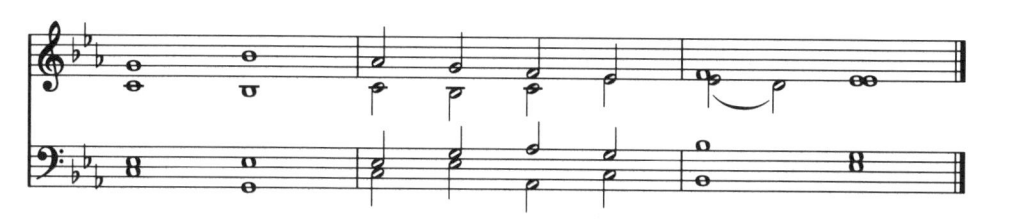

Wide green world, we know and love you:
    Clear blue skies that arch above you,
Moon-tugged oceans rising, falling,
    Summer rain and cuckoo calling.
Some wild ancient ferment bore us,
    Us, and all that went before us:
Life in desert, forest, mountain,
    Life in stream and springing fountain.

We know how to mould and tame you,
    We have power to mar and maim you.
Show us by your silent growing
    That which we should all be knowing:
We are of you, not your master,
    We who plan supreme disaster.
If with careless greed we use you
    Inch by extinct inch we lose you.

May our births and deaths remind us
    Others still will come behind us.
That they also may enjoy you
    We with wisdom will employ you.
That our care may always bless you
    Teach us we do not possess you.
We are part and parcel of you.
    Wide green world, we share and love you.

June Bell

9 Where Shall I Find That Power?

DIVINE MYSTERIES   6 6. 6 6. 8 8. 6 6.   F. Stanfield, 1835–1914

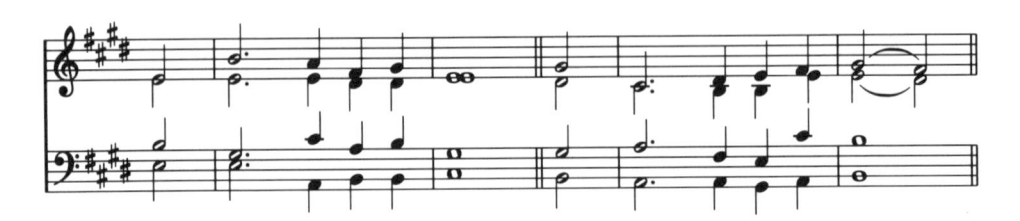

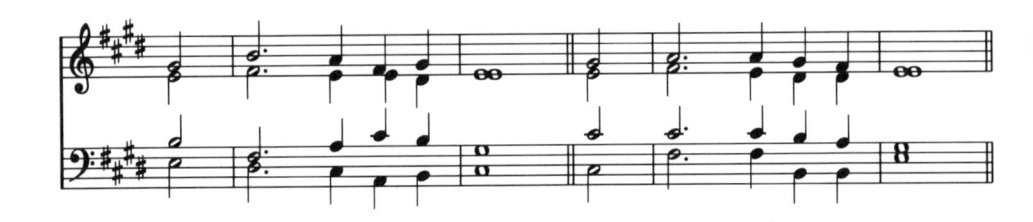

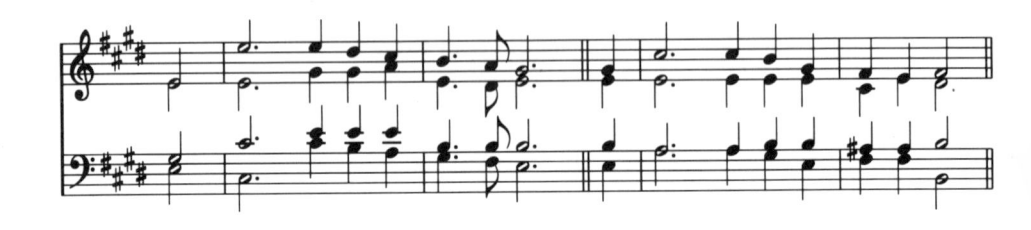

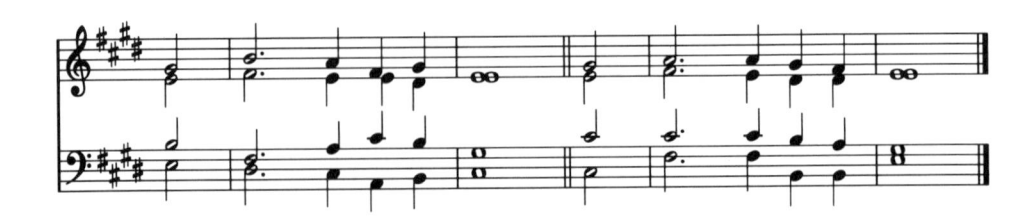

Where shall I find that Power
   Which makes the planets move,
And can I, in this hour,
   Discover Perfect Love?
     Though I am in perplexity,
     May I discern Infinity,
And, though the glass be dark,
   Of Light see just one spark?

Where shall I find that Peace
   Which intellect exceeds,
And can I, in this place,
   Find what my spirit needs?
     Though filled with fears I cannot quell,
     May I escape my private hell,
And, though I cannot move,
   Be rescued by a Dove?

Where shall I find that Home
   Which calls me every day,
And can I, 'twixt the womb
   And death, find out the way?
     And though I, frantic, look around,
     'Midst clamour and despairing sound,
Beneath that awful noise
   I hear a still small voice.

What says this voice, now clear,
   Which I have long ignored?
Can I begin to hear
   The wordless speech of God?
     Vain chatter will I lay aside,
     No longer filled with boundless pride:
The voice of God shall be
   Power, Peace and Home to me.

Peter Galbraith

10 O Let Us Now Our Voices Raise

OMBERSLEY L. M.   William Henry Gladstone, 1840–91

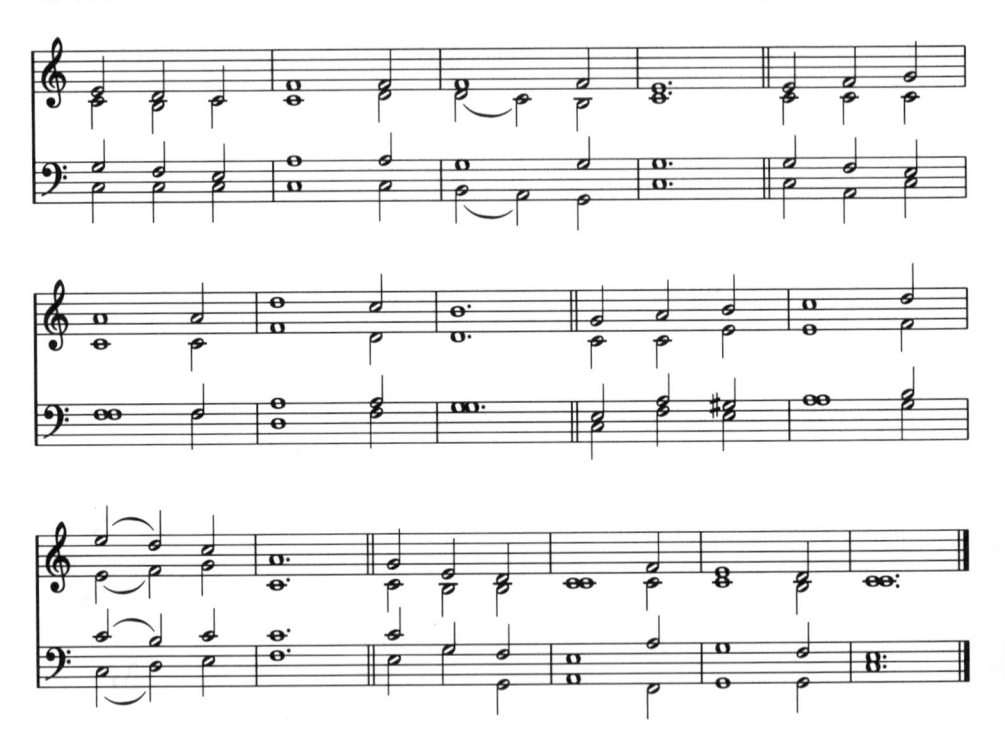

O let us now our voices raise
   In invocation and in praise;
O let us sing with hearts inspired
   By love that's ever mindful fired.

For though we sing a mighty song,
   Louder than any angel throng,
The veil of truth will not be rent
   Unless each word is thought and meant.

For though we sing as angels sweet
   Our melodies will not be meet,
No holy purpose will they find
   Unless our hearts be warm and kind.

So, sing we loud and sing we well,
   Word, thought and heart our loving tell!
Let our compassion fill the air,
   Our hymn a true and worthy prayer!

Peter Galbraith

Spirit of Life   11

SPIRIT OF LIFE   8 12 8. 12 8 10.   Carolyn McDade

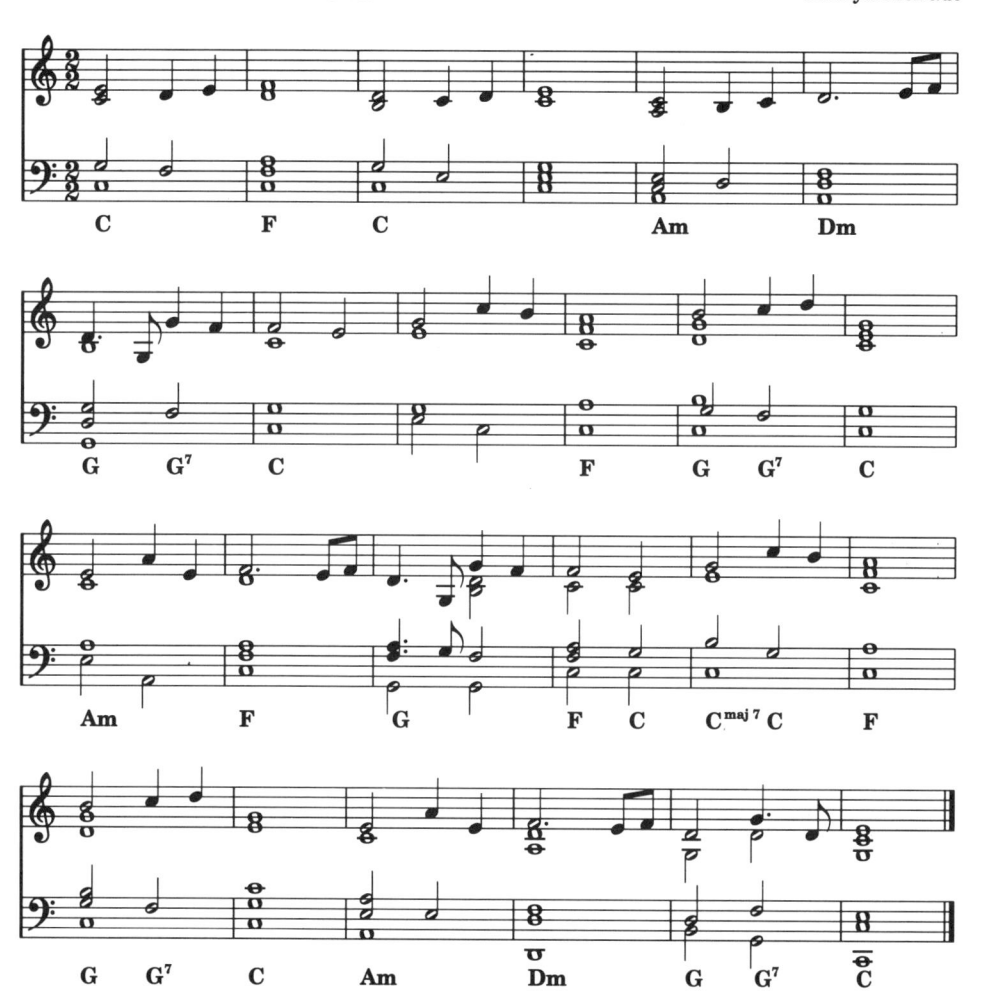

Spirit of Life, come unto me.
   Sing in my heart all the stirrings of compassion.
Blow in the wind, rise in the sea.
   Move in the hand giving life the shape of justice.
Roots hold me close, wings set me free.
Spirit of life, come to me, come to me.

Carolyn McDade

12   We Set a Frame on Nature

MISSIONARY   7 6. 7 6. D.   Lowell Mason, 1792–1872

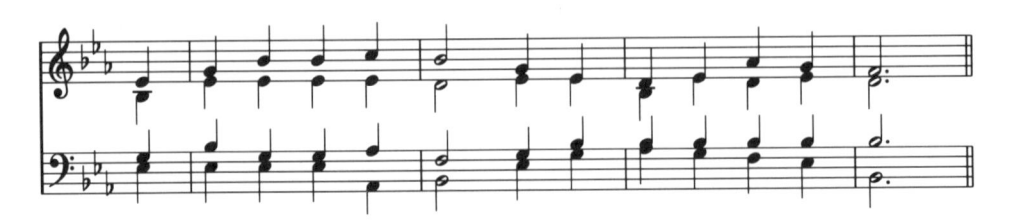

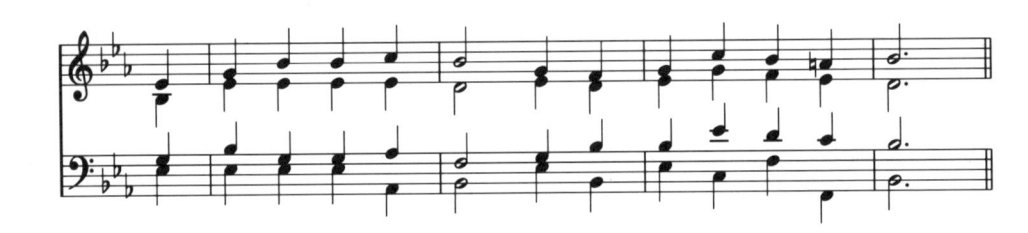

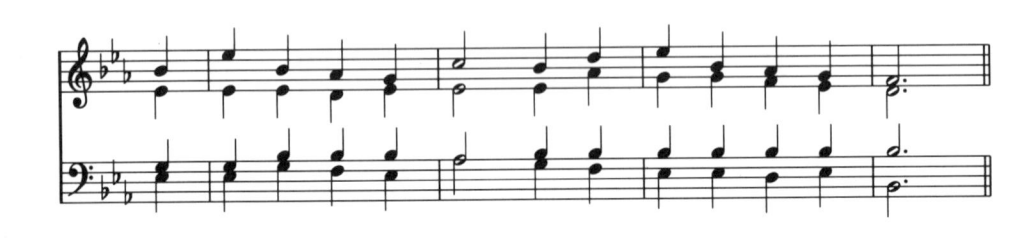

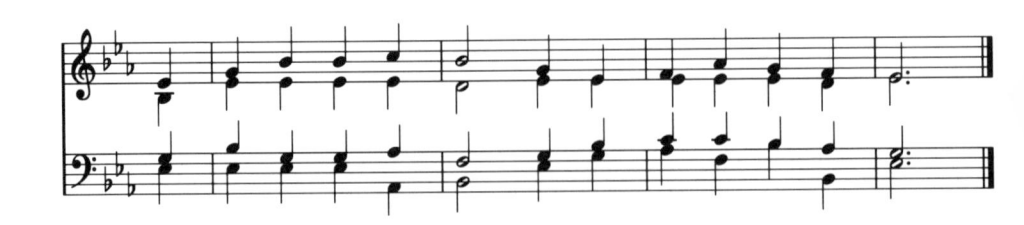

We set a frame on nature
    With hours and months and years,
While each unknowing creature
    Lives on all unwares.
They know the light and darkness,
    They know the moon's four weeks;
The sun in all its starkness
    To them their timing speaks.

We need expedient naming
    And arbitrary dates,
But artificial framing
    Our being alienates
From rhythms that enshrine us
    Like fern or embryo curled,
From forces that align us
    With all the living world.

So let the sun tell seasons
    And grant the moon its phase.
Forget the useful reasons
    For counting hours and days.
We sprang from dark and daylight,
    From ebb and flowing tide.
Our nature is our birthright
    And may not be denied.

                                            June Bell

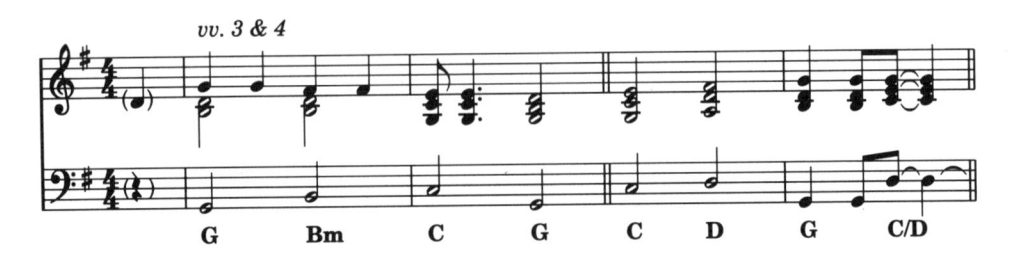

13   Walk in the Light

WALK IN THE LIGHT   8 5. 8 5. + refrain   Traditional

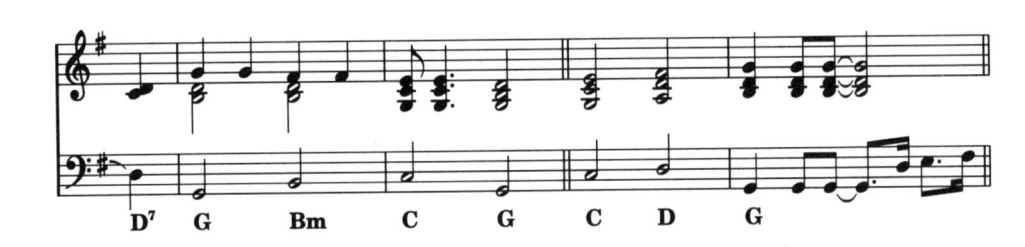

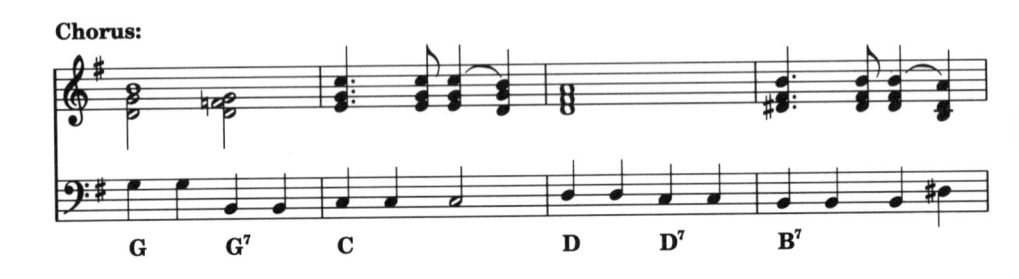

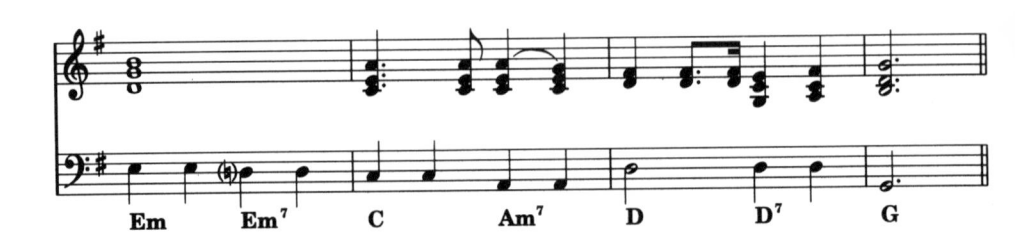

vv. 3 & 4

G   Bm   C   G   C   D   G   C/D

D^7 G   Bm   C   G   C   D   G

Chorus:

G G^7 C   D D^7 B^7

Em Em^7 C Am^7 D D^7 G

The Spirit lives to set us free,
    Walk, walk in the light.
It binds us all in unity,
    Walk, walk in the light.

Chorus:　　Walk in the light,　　*(3 times)*
　　　　　　Walk in the light of love.

The light that shines is in us all,
    Walk, walk in the light.
We each must follow our own call,
    Walk, walk in the light.

Chorus:　　Walk in the light,　　*(3 times)*
　　　　　　Walk in the light of love.

Peace begins inside your heart,
    Walk, walk in the light.
We've got to live it from the start,
    Walk, walk in the light.

Chorus:　　Walk in the light,　　*(3 times)*
　　　　　　Walk in the light of love.

Seek the truth in what you see,
    Walk, walk in the light.
Then hold it firmly as can be,
    Walk, walk in the light.

Chorus:　　Walk in the light,　　*(3 times)*
　　　　　　Walk in the light of love.

The Spirit lives in you and me,
    Walk, walk in the light.
Its light will shine for all to see,
    Walk, walk in the light.

Chorus:　　Walk in the light,　　*(3 times)*
　　　　　　Walk in the light of love.

Anon.

14 God who is Everywhere

HERE'S TO THE MAIDEN   10 8. 10 9. + refrain

English Traditional
Words and Arrangement:
© 1987 The Iona Community

14

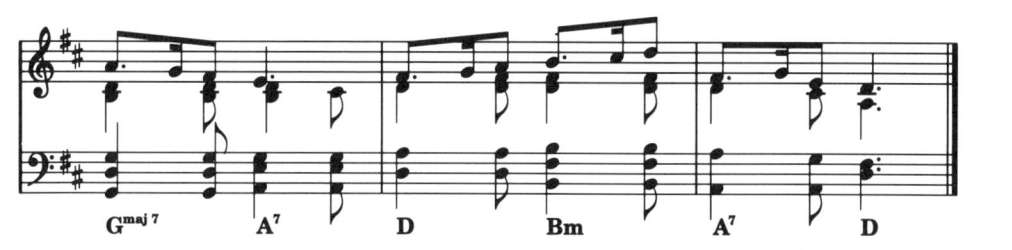

God who is everywhere present on earth,
 No one can picture completely;
Yet to the eye of the faithful she comes
 And shows herself always uniquely.

Chorus: Singing or sad,
 Weeping or glad –
Such are the glimpses of God that we're given.
 Laughter and cheers,
 Anger and tears –
These we inherit from earth and from heaven.

Shrouded in smoke or else high on a hill,
 Quaking with nature's own violence –
Thus was the Lord found, frightening his folk,
 But later he met them in silence.

Chorus: Singing or sad, ...

God is the father who teaches his child
 Wisdom and values to cherish;
God is the mother who watches her young
 And never will let her child perish.

Chorus: Singing or sad, ...

Spear in the hand or with tears on the cheek,
 Monarch and shepherd and lover:
Many the faces that God calls her own
 And many we've yet to discover.

Chorus: Singing or sad, ...

The Iona Community

15 God, the All-Holy

BUNESSAN 5 5. 5 4. D.

Old Gaelic Melody
arranged and harmonized by Martin Fallas Shaw, 1875–1958
From Enlarged Songs of Praise, by permission of Oxford University Press

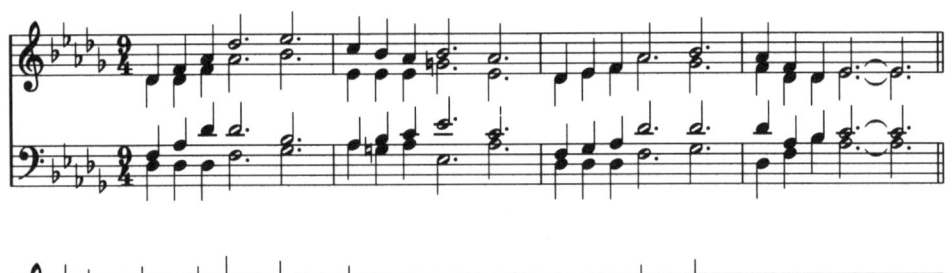

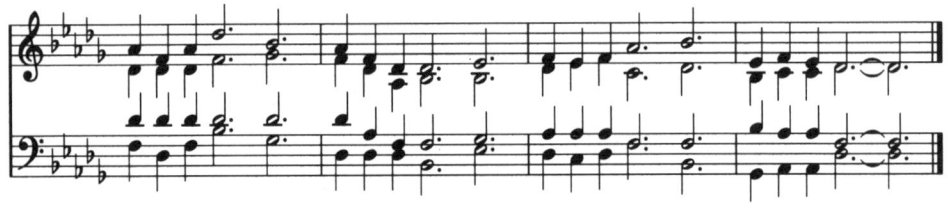

God, the All-Holy,
    Maker and Mother,
Gladly we gather,
    Bringing in prayer
Old hurts for healing
    New hopes for holding,
Giving, receiving
    Loving and care.

Spirit, All-Seeing,
    Knitting and blending
Joy in desiring,
    Friendship and ease,
Make our belonging
    Loyal and lasting,
So that our pledging
    Freshens and frees.

Christ, All-Completing,
    Nature enfolding,
Evil exhausting
    In love's embrace,
Weaving and mending
    Make every ending
God's new beginning
    Glowing with grace.

Brian Wren

Here in This Moment's Song   16

LITTLE CORNARD   6 6. 6 6. 8 8 (Dactylic)   Martin Fallas Shaw, 1875–1958
By permission of William Elkin Music Services

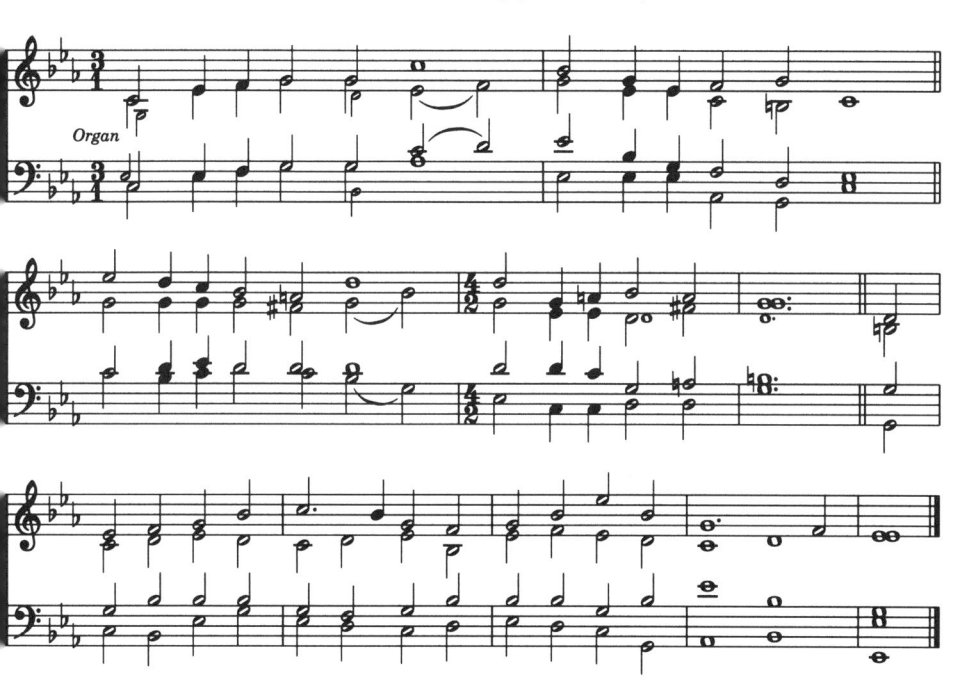

Here in this moment's song
   Great symphonies are sung;
All people we contain,
   Ageless, though old or young:
In passing words and melody
We celebrate eternity.

Thus, in each moment small
   We can contain all hours;
In everyone the All
   Expresses and empowers;
Each person great, a living world
From whom uniqueness is unfurled.

Hope shall admit no bounds,
   As Love no limit knows;
Each new-born dream made real
   In our commitment grows;
The possible, the yet-to-be
Is Now, is Here, is You and Me.

Frank Clabburn

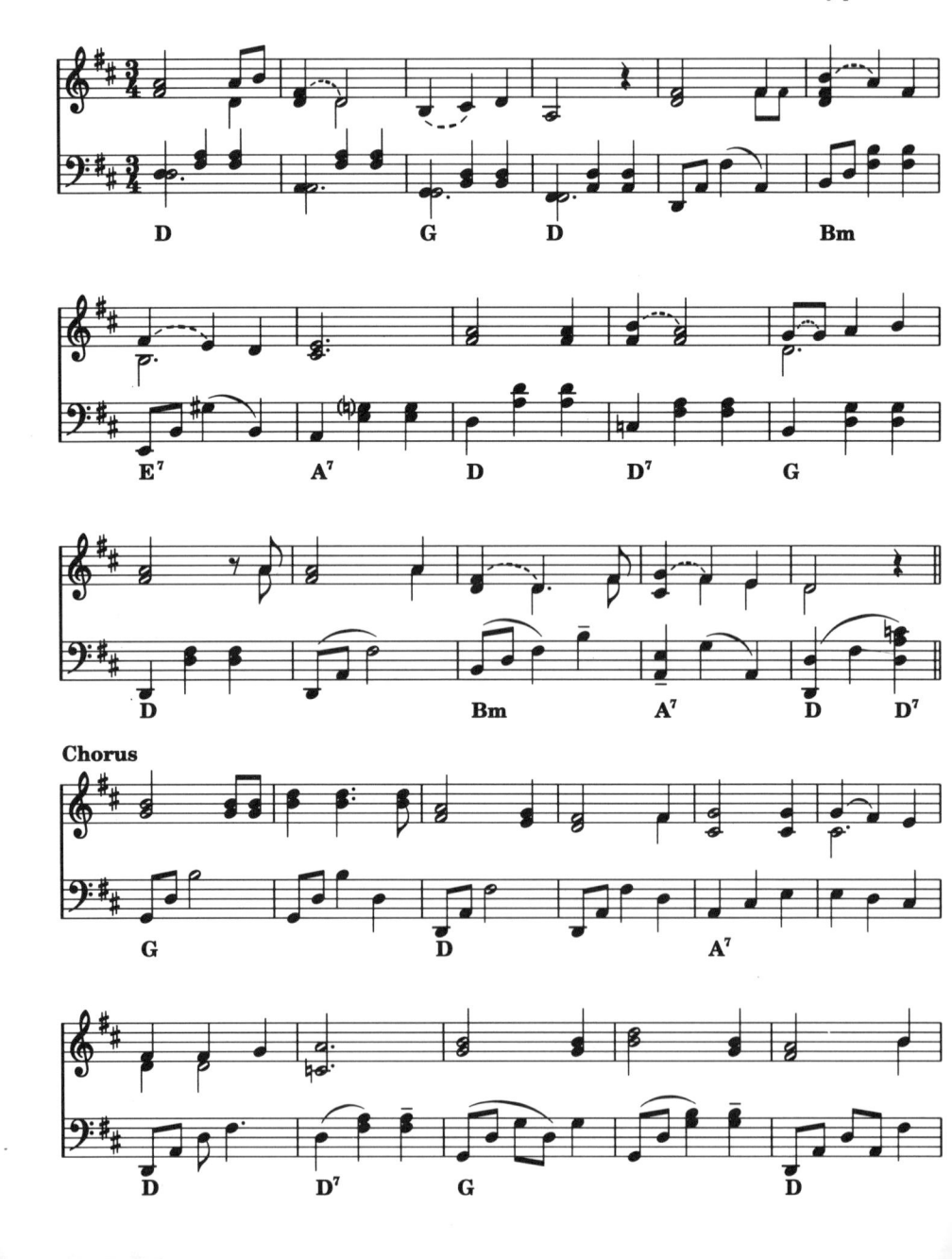

17 Love is a Circle, Round and Round

LOVE IS A CIRCLE 8 7. 8 9 + refrain

Phyllis Hiller
© 1971 Oak Hill Music Pub. Co.
Used by permission

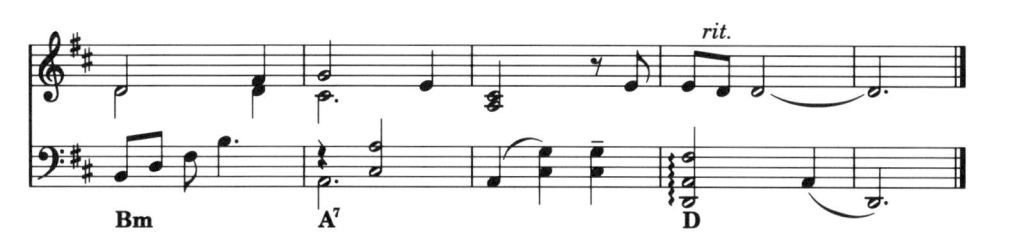

Love is a circle, round and round.
Love is up and love is down.
Love is inside trying to get out.
Love is whirling and twirling about.

Chorus: Love is a circle, it knows no bounds.
The more you give, the more comes around.
Love is ours alone to give.
It lives in us, it's beautiful.

Love is a circle trying to bend.
Love is pieces trying to mend.
Love is darkness waiting for the light.
Love is power and love is might.

Chorus: Love is a circle, it knows no bounds.
The more you give, the more comes around.
Love is ours alone to give.
It lives in us, it's beautiful.

Love is a laugh, love is a look.
Love is the chance that somebody took.
Love will hide, love will show.
The more you give, the more it'll grow.

Chorus: Love is a circle, it knows no bounds.
The more you give, the more comes around.
Love is ours alone to give.
It lives in us, it's beautiful.

Phyllis Hiller

18   Inch By Inch, Row By Row

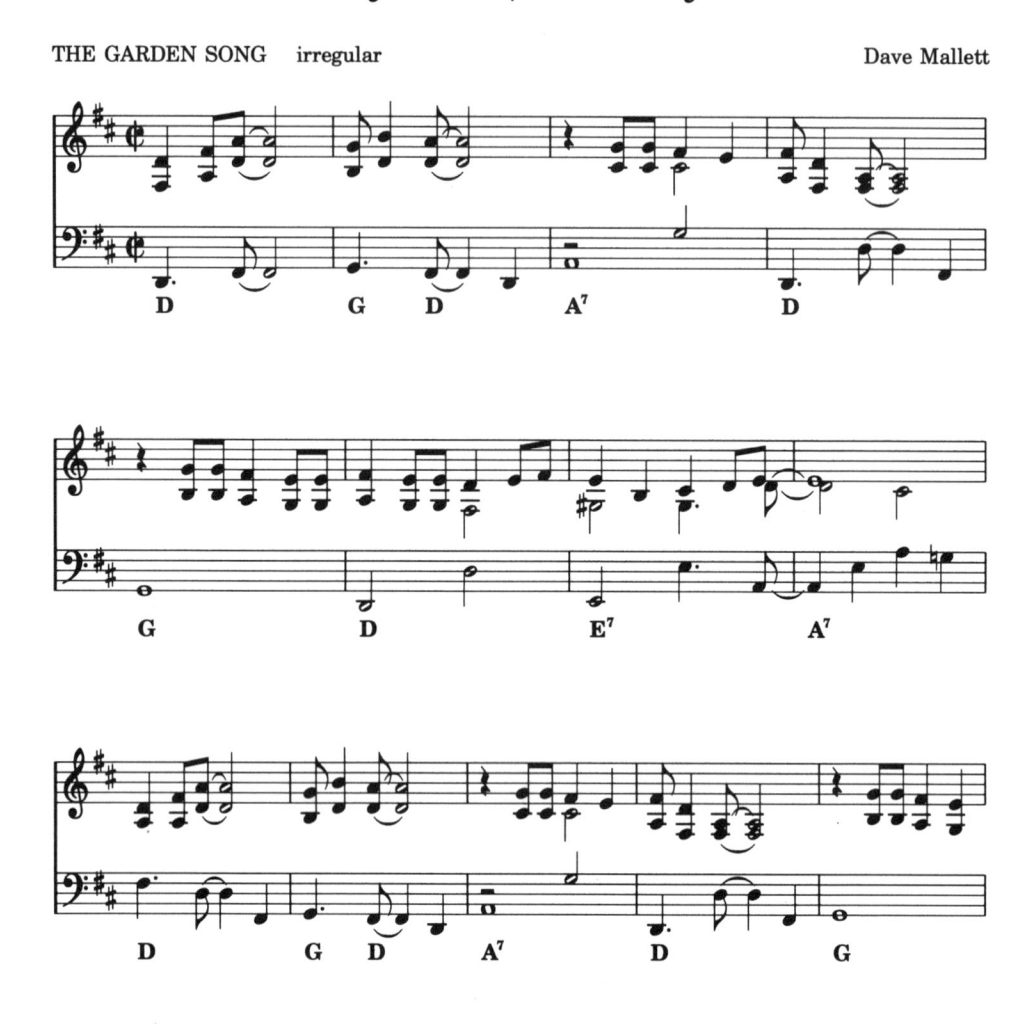

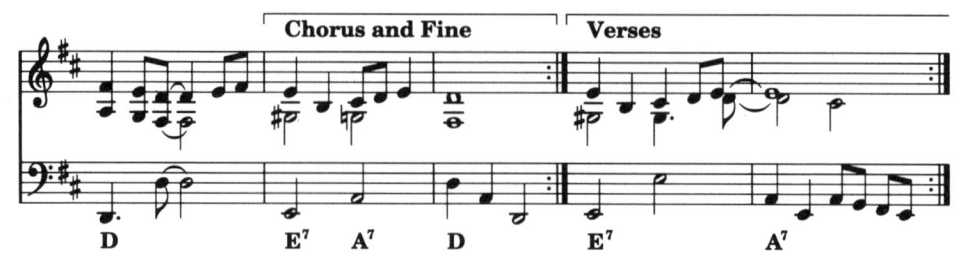

THE GARDEN SONG   irregular   Dave Mallett

Chorus: Inch by inch, row by row,
Gonna make this garden grow,
All it takes is a rake and a hoe
    And a piece of fertile ground.
Inch by inch, row by row,
Someone bless these seeds I sow,
Someone warm them from below,
    Till the rains come tumbling down.

Pulling weeds and picking stones,
We are made of dreams and bones.
Feel the need to grow my own,
    'Cause the time is close at hand...
Grain by grain, sun and rain,
Find my way in Nature's chain:
Tune my body and my brain
    To the music from the land.

Chorus: Inch by inch, row by row,
Gonna make this garden grow,
All it takes is a rake and a hoe
    And a piece of fertile ground.
Inch by inch, row by row,
Someone bless these seeds I sow,
Someone warm them from below,
    Till the rains come tumbling down.

Plant your rows straight and long;
Temper them with prayer and song.
Mother Earth will make you strong
    If you give her love and care.
An old crow watching hungrily
From his perch in yonder tree...
In my garden I'm as free
    As that feathered thief up there.

Chorus: Inch by inch, row by row,
Gonna make this garden grow,
All it takes is a rake and a hoe
    And a piece of fertile ground.
Inch by inch, row by row,
Someone bless these seeds I sow,
Someone warm them from below,
    Till the rains come tumbling down.

Dave Mallett

19   O Beautiful Baby

KREMSER   12 11. 13 12.   Adrian Valerius' *Nederlandtsch Gedenckclanck*, 1626
                                                   arranged Edward Kremser, 1838–1914

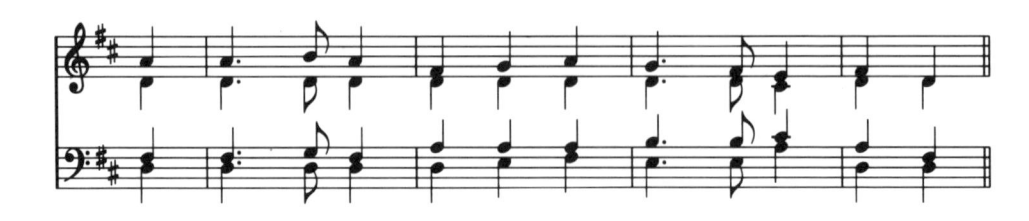

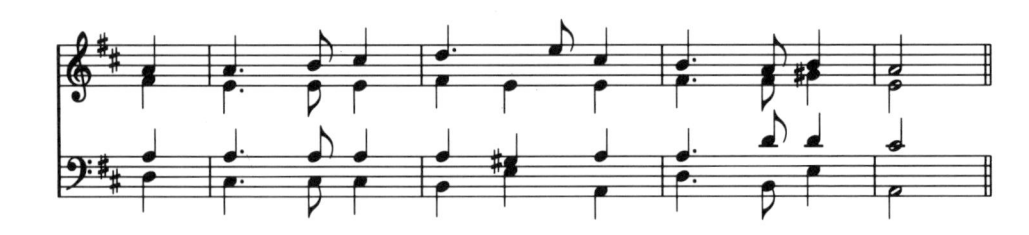

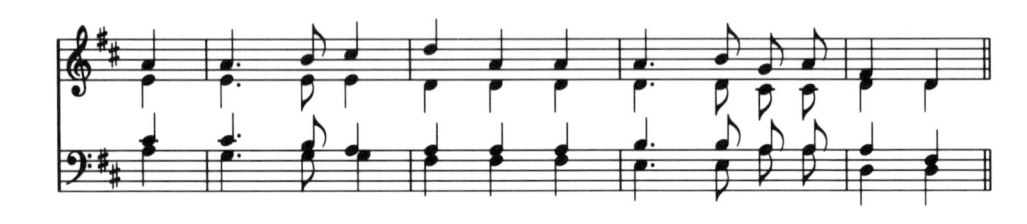

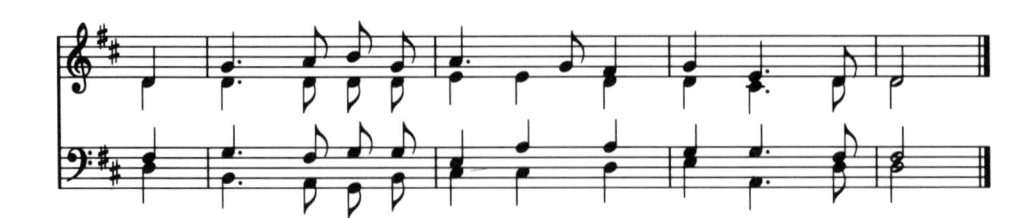

O beautiful baby, you come here before us.
 We wonder at God in his glory in you.
Perfection and beauty we see now before us,
 Simplicity captured, so perfectly new.

Like flowers that show us their beauty in springtime,
 The leaves on the trees which are shed for us all;
The magic of wintertime, frost in its splendour,
 The change in the season, spring, summer and fall.

     him   *his*
O give *her* the strength to o'ercome all *her* labour
 When trials of life seem to gather around.
Grant peace and contentment, strength, purpose and ardour.
 May health and prosperity for *him* abound.
                                    her

                                              Margaret Hart

20 Thy Darkness Descends

MOZART 12 10. 11 11. D.   Wolfgang Amadeus Mozart, 1756–91, arranged by John Taylor

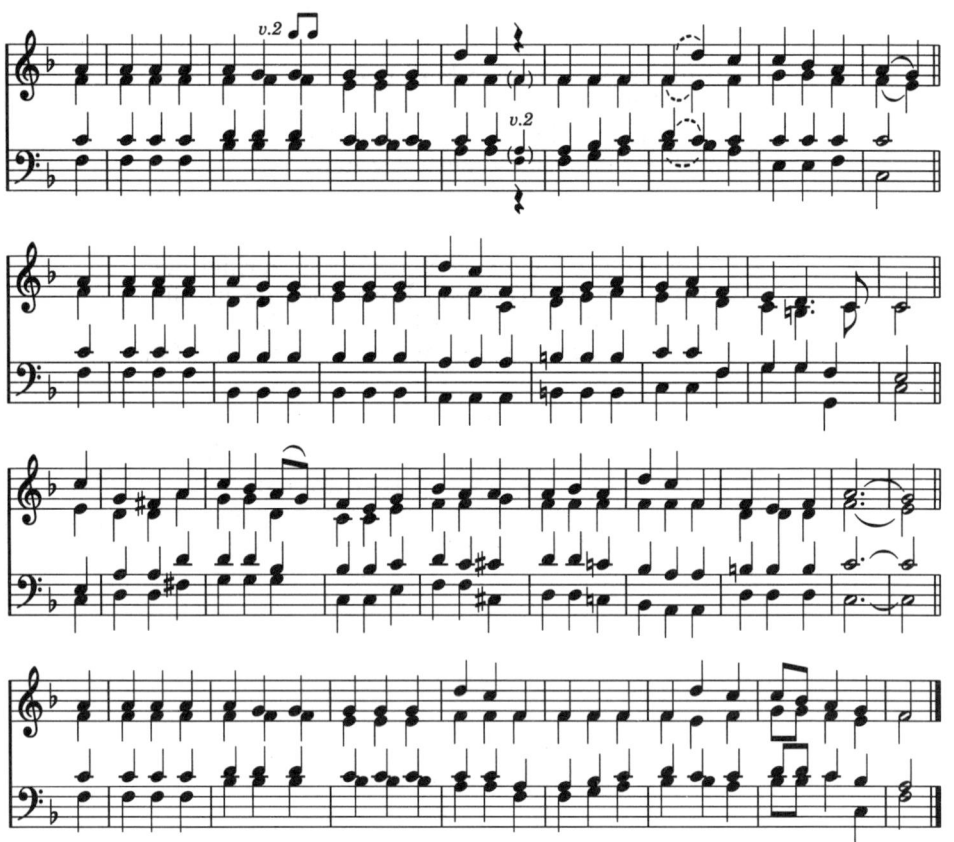

Thy darkness descends like a robe on the evening,
  Clothing our prayers with the silence of night.
Thy stars from the heavens, assurance are sending
  That darkness will ever be blessed by Thy light.
The moon like a goddess her radiance bestowing
  Shines forth without favour, on land and on sea.
Her face bears the light of her consort retiring,
  As souls in their depths bear sweet images of Thee.

Night's mysteries hold us in an awed contemplating
  Of fathomless deeps and infinite space.
Our souls would be lost, whatso'er their intending,
  Saw we not in that void a glimpse of Thy face.
O thou art the flame in our hearts brightly burning.
  Set fire to the chalice which lies in the soul.
Ourselves and our loved ones we give to Thy keeping:
  To Love be the glory, whose Power holds us all.

David Doel

Now Rejoice!   21

JOEL 8 8. 8 8. 8 8.   Robert Waller

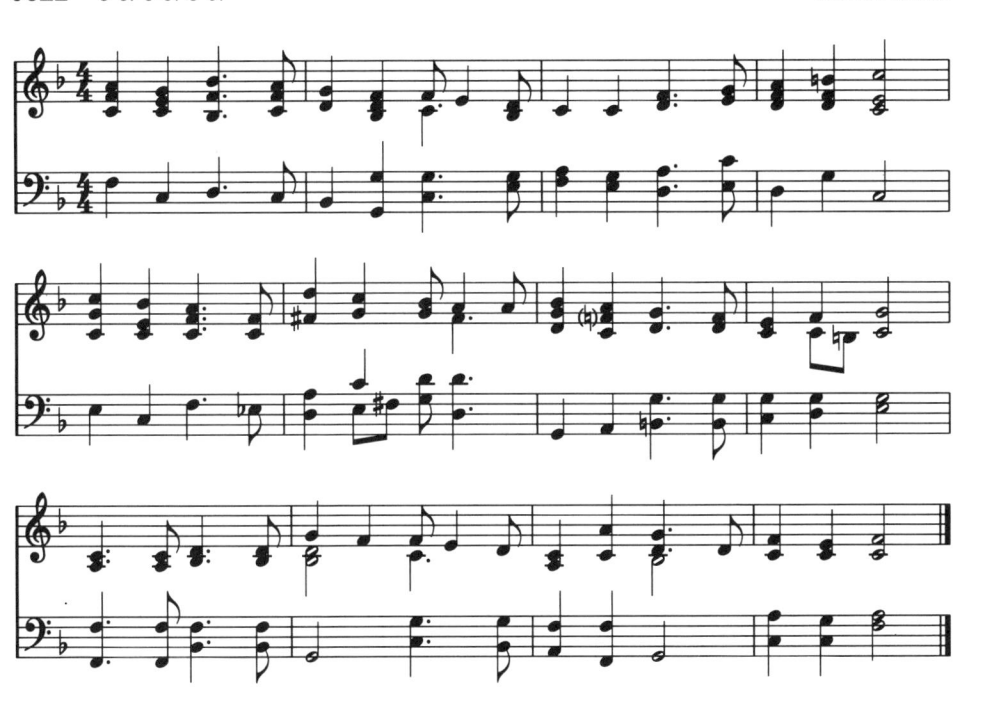

Now rejoice! We greet his coming!
The timeless promise is fulfilled,
Human birth reveals God's glory,
　Hope stirs again where it was stilled.
Once two women praised in Judah –
　We share their joy: our hearts are thrilled.

Humankind is not abandoned
　To hunger's bite, oppression's pride.
In your will for our deliverance
　You take your humble children's side.
Once you sent a babe named Jesus
　To live the love which hate decried.

He – the morning sun from heaven –
　Makes fear of death and darkness cease;
Born again in hearts made ready
　That loving-kindness may increase;
In his birth your Spirit rises
　To guide us in the way of peace.

Clifford M. Reed

22 This Day Confirms a Union

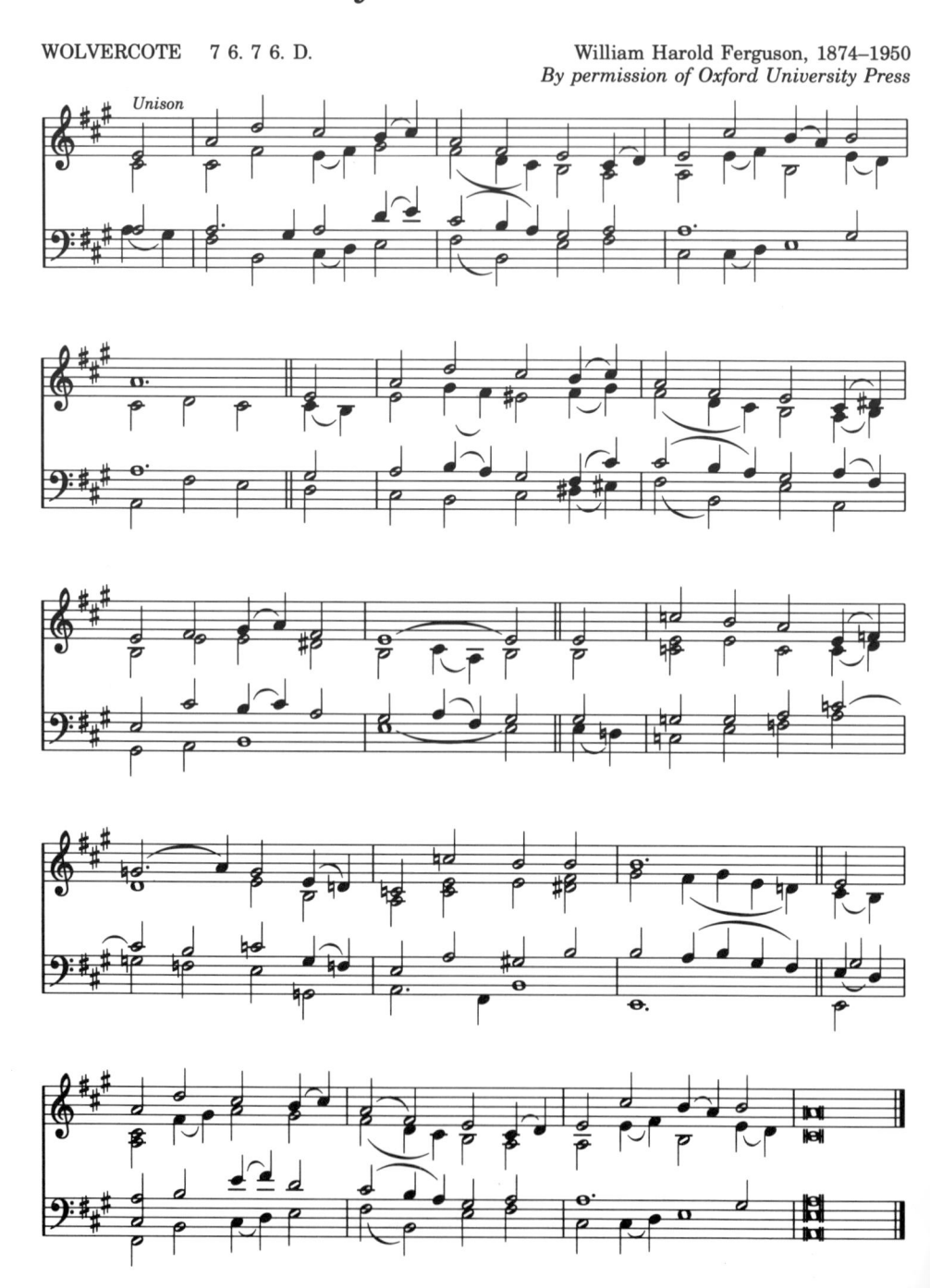

WOLVERCOTE   7 6. 7 6. D.

William Harold Ferguson, 1874–1950
By permission of Oxford University Press

This day confirms a union,
 An act of heart and mind,
And we are met to witness
 The promises that bind.
A binding that brings freedom
 To care and serve and give,
To share in thought and action
 That love may grow and live.

This day confirms a union
 From which each may gain power
To live a life of courage,
 Yet tender as a flower:
Two lives of peace and passion,
 Two lives of work and joy
Which, joined today before us,
 May all that's good employ.

This day confirms a union;
 It is a day of hope,
A day to be remembered
 When it is hard to cope.
So may these two in good times
 And times of trouble prove
That partnerships will triumph,
 Sustained by holy love.

Peter Galbraith

23 Lady of the Seasons' Laughter

JULION   8 7. 8 7. 8 7.

David Hurd
© 1983 G. I. A. Publications, Inc.
Used by permission.

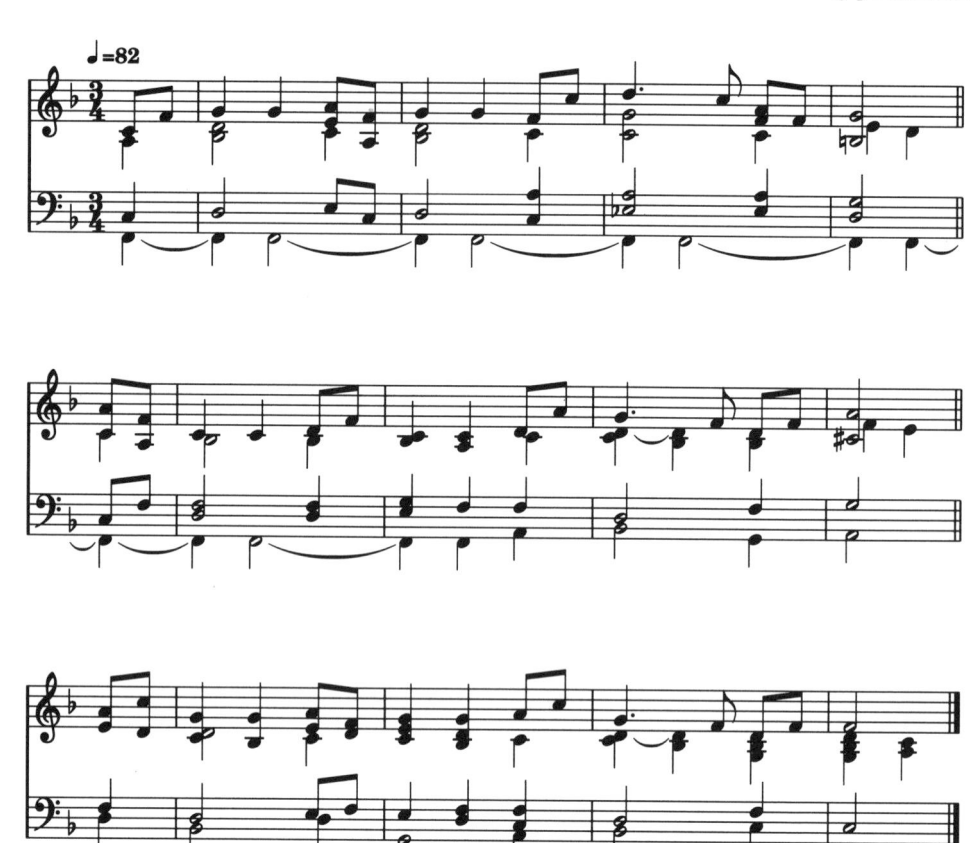

Lady of the seasons' laughter,
   In the summer's warmth be near;
When the winter follows after,
   Teach our spirits not to fear.
Hold us in your steady mercy,
   Lady of the turning year.

Sister of the evening starlight,
   In the falling shadows stay
Here among us till the far light
   Of tomorrow's dawning ray.
Hold us in your steady mercy
   Lady of the turning day.

Mother of the generations,
   In whose love all life is worth
Everlasting celebrations,
   Bring our labours safe to birth.
Hold us in your steady mercy
   Lady of the turning earth.

Goddess of all time's progression,
   Stand with us when we engage
Hands and hearts to end oppression,
   Writing history's fairer page.
Hold us in your steady mercy,
   Lady of the turning age.

Kendyl Gibbons

© 1990 Unitarian Universalist Association

24 O God, O Spirit Free

ST. CECILIA 6 6. 6 6. Leighton George Hayne, 1836–83

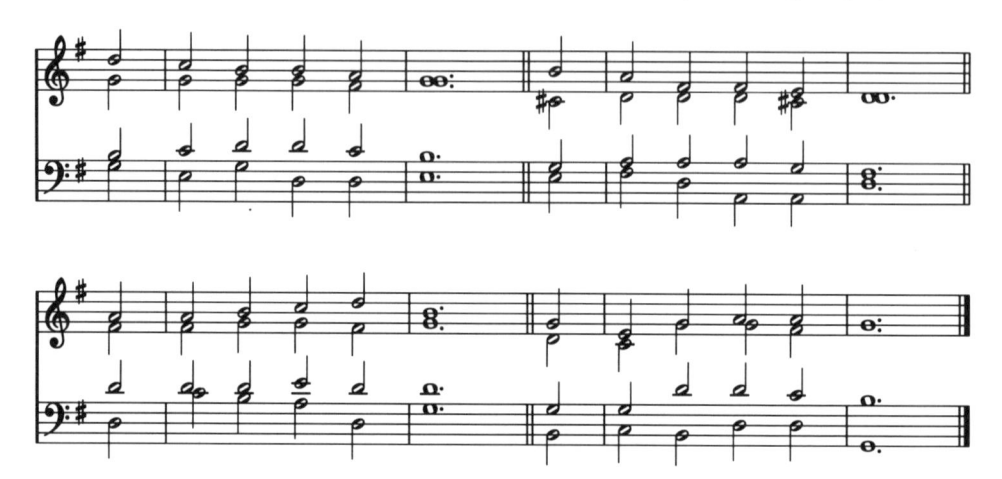

O God, O Spirit free,
> Source of unfolding life,
Through you all comes to be,
> Creative mystery.

You have revealed your will
> Where we create and care,
Where folk are striving still
> With love their lives to fill.

Your gift – a vision bright
> Of people loving, new,
And we, in darksome night,
> Find courage at the sight.

Your kingdom, like a star,
> Illuminates the soul,
And building it we are,
> Though glimpsing it afar.

This earth – my labour's field,
> Its loving care my task,
Help me my heart to yield
> Now that my way's revealed.

O Thou, O God within,
> Who gave your prophets strength,
Come pour your Spirit in,
> Make me their worthy kin.

Clifford M. Reed

The Blue-Green Hills of Earth 25

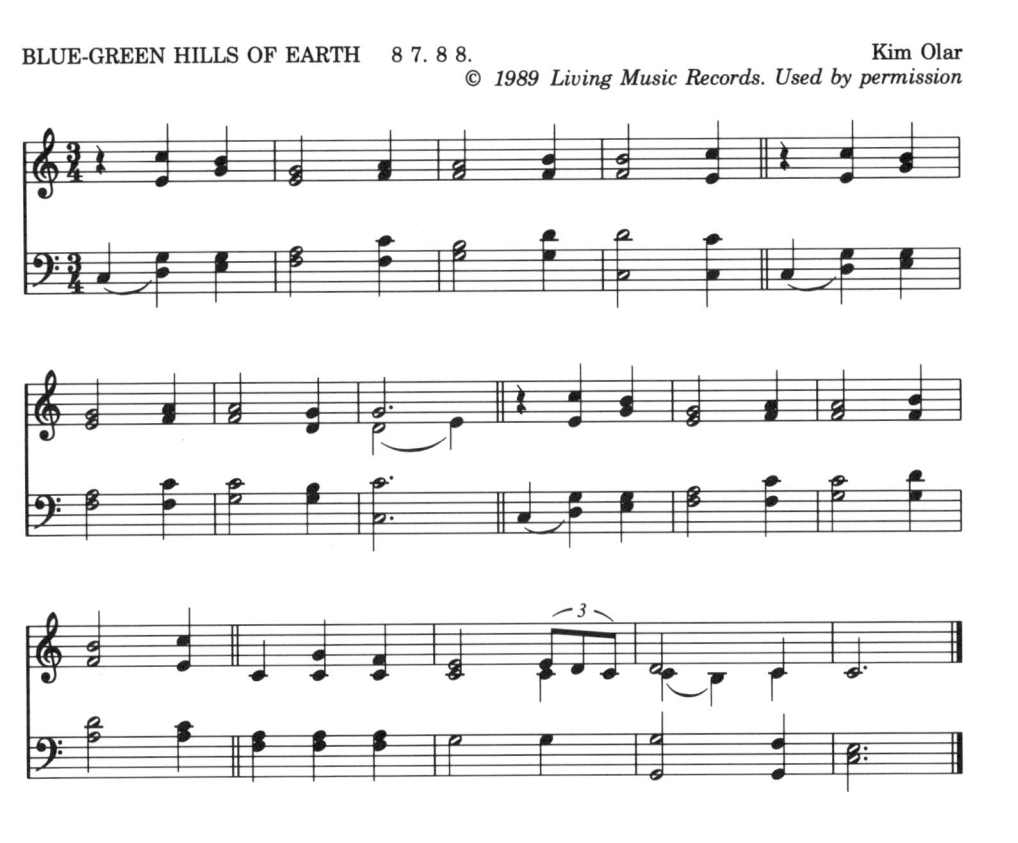

BLUE-GREEN HILLS OF EARTH   8 7. 8 8.   Kim Olar
© 1989 Living Music Records. Used by permission

For the earth forever turning,
   For the skies, for ev'ry sea,
For our lives, for all we cherish,
   Sing we a joyful song of peace.

For the mountains, hills and pastures,
   In their silent majesty,
For all life, for all of nature,
   Sing we a joyful song of peace.

For the world we raise our voices,
   For the home that gives us birth;
In our joy we sing, returning
   Home to our blue-green hills of earth.

from *Missa Gaia*

26 Bring Flowers to our Altar

THE ASH GROVE   12 11. 12 11. D.

Traditional

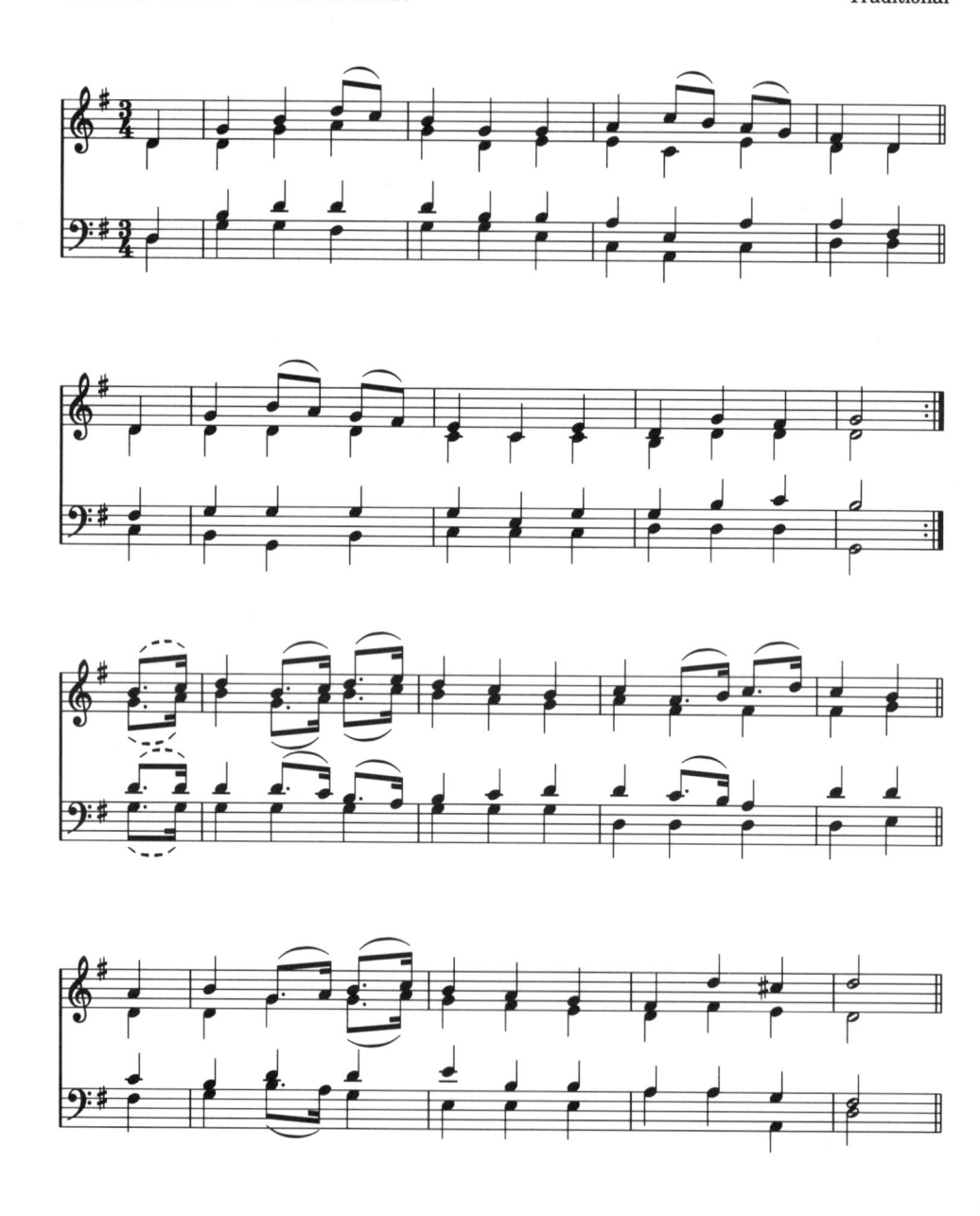

26

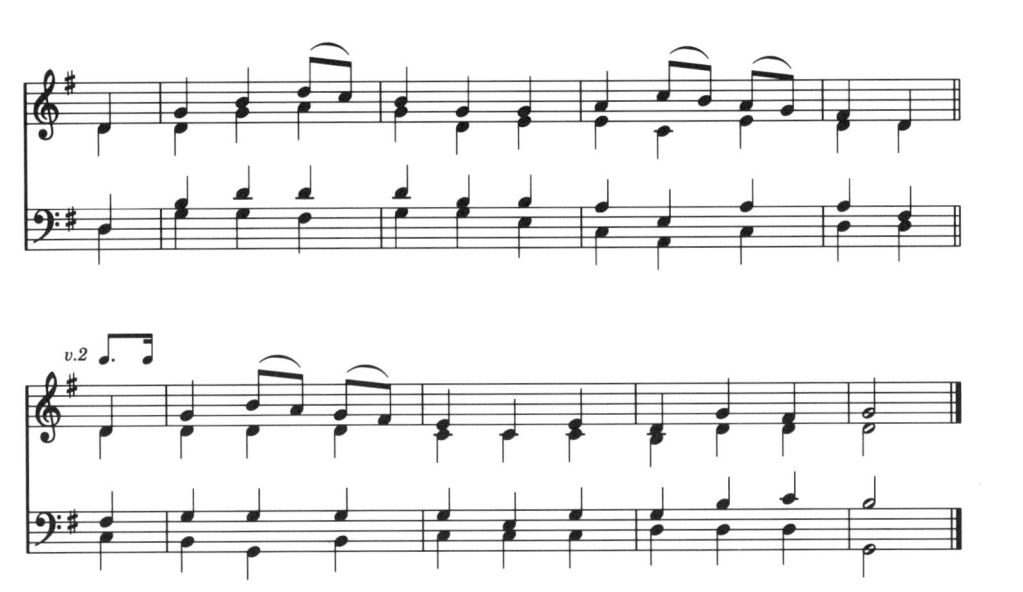

Bring flowers to our altar to show nature's beauty
   The harvest of goodness in earth, sky and sea.
Bring light to our altar to guide every nation
   From hatred to love and to humanity.
Bring a dove to our altar its wings ever flying
   In permanent quest for the peace all may share.
Bring bread to our altar the hungry supplying
   And feeding the poor who depend on our care.

Bring hope to our altar in your cheerful dreaming
   Of all the good things that will make your heart glad.
Bring love to our altar, a bright witness beaming
   To all who are burdened, or lonely and sad.
Bring work to our altar to help every nation
   And celebrate all that's already achieved.
Come yourself to our altar in true dedication
   To all the ideals we in common believe.

Lena Baxter

27 Our Song of Joy

OUR SONG OF JOY 11 10. 11 10. D.

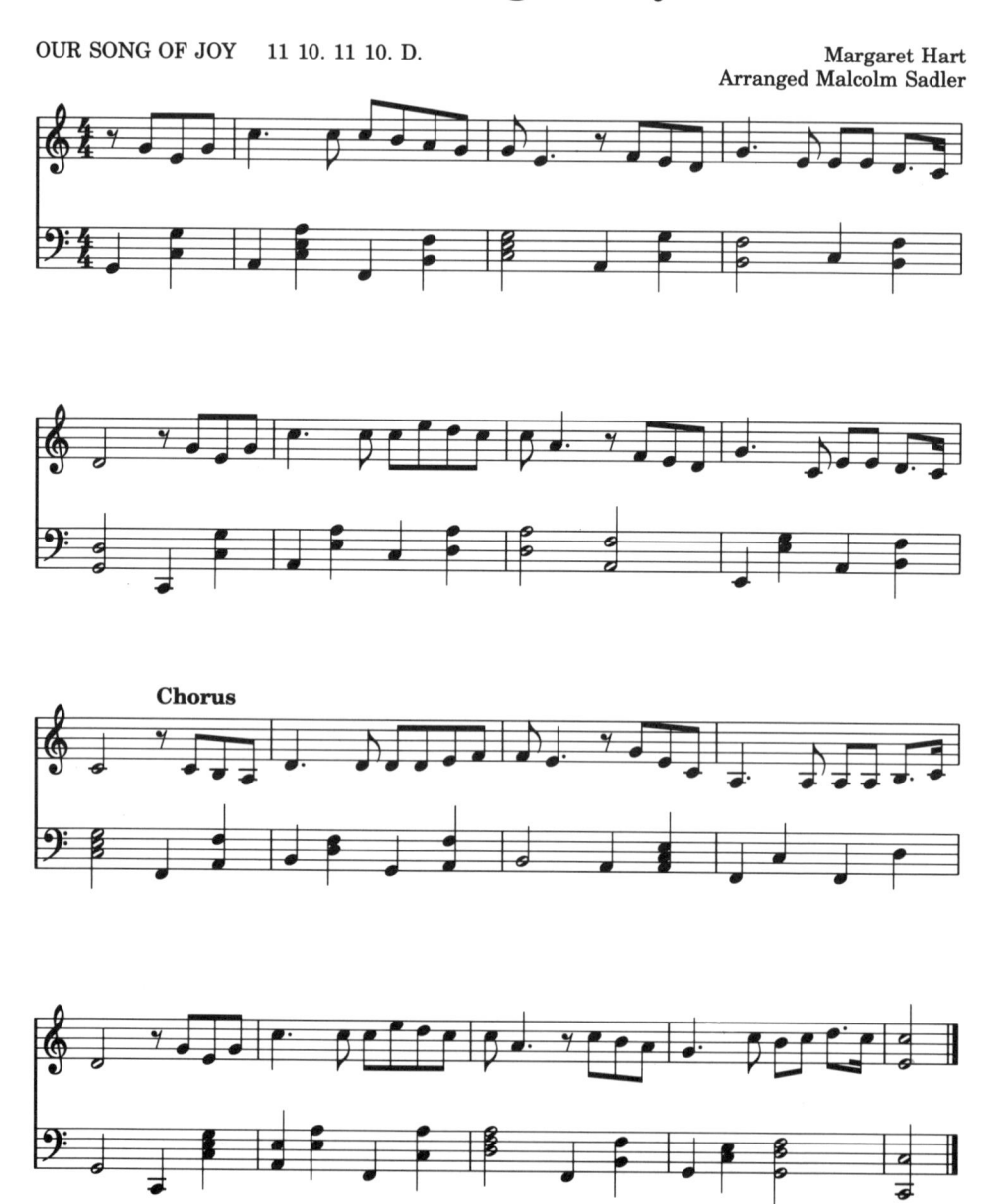

Margaret Hart
Arranged Malcolm Sadler

Our song of joy, for now we join together
   As one, in heart, for love of God we come
To this great House as now we join in singing
   Our joy, our song; our hearts together, one.

Chorus: This House of God, where others went before us.
        They trod the path for us to follow on.
       Our song of joy; we sing as friends together
        May we go forth and join our hearts in song.

Our song of love, which binds us all, one family.
   We come as one, to worship and to pray.
May we find care among our friends here gathered
   As we go on through each and every day.

Chorus: Our House of God, where others went before us.
        They trod the path for us to follow on.
       Our song of joy; we sing as friends together
        May we go forth and join our hearts in song.

Our song of peace, we pray in times of trouble
   That love and God will o'er all peoples reign,
And that our world will be a place of heaven
   On earth, for those who suffer hurt and pain.

Chorus: This House of God, where others went before us.
        They trod the path for us to follow on.
       Our song of joy; we sing as friends together
        May we go forth and join our hearts in song.

We sing for freedom, love and peace for ever
   That our wide world may be like heaven above
For those who follow, may they find contentment
   To do the right, through goodness, truth and love.

Chorus: Our House of God, where others went before us.
        They trod the path for us to follow on.
       Our song of joy; we sing as friends together
        May we go forth and join our hearts in song.

Margaret Hart

28   God of Creation

MACCABÆUS   10 11. 11 11. + refrain

G. F. Handel, 1685–1759
from *Judas Maccabæus*

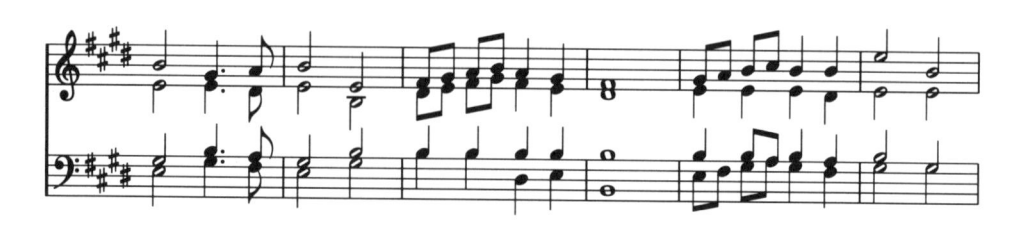

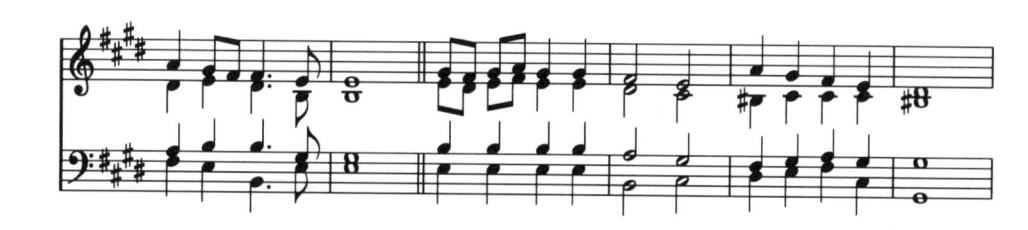

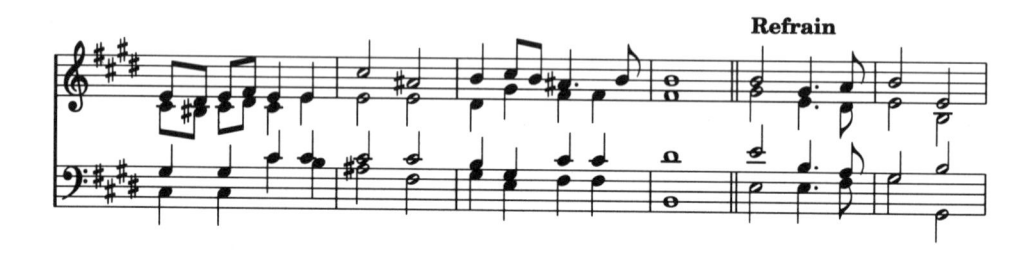

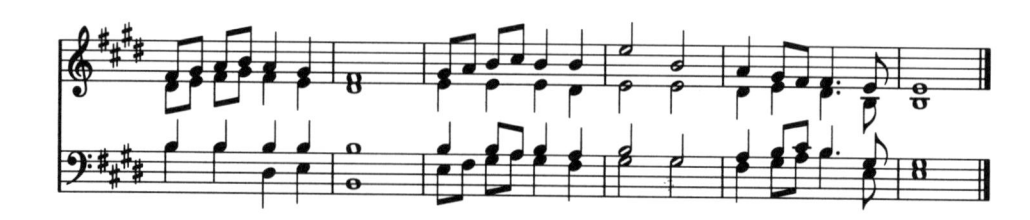

God of creation,
　　Primal, final one;
Through our transformation
　　Let thy will be done.
Firm against temptation,
　　Modest in the sun,
May each soul and nation
　　See thy task begun.

Chorus:　　　　God of creation,
　　　　　　　　　　Primal, final one;
　　　　　　　Through our transformation
　　　　　　　　　　Let thy will be done.

Far do we seek thee,
　　Rarely understand
How through pain and folly
　　Speaks the great command.
When we cry against thee,
　　Fear thy forming hand,
Light us through the valley
　　To the promised land.

Chorus:　　　　God of creation,
　　　　　　　　　　Primal, final one;
　　　　　　　Through our transformation
　　　　　　　　　　Let thy will be done.

God of our growing,
　　Pure and perfect seed,
Fructify our knowing,
　　Glorify our deed;
Set our purpose flowing
　　Free from hate and greed,
Still with thy bestowing
　　All our human need.

Chorus:　　　　God of creation,
　　　　　　　　　　Primal, final one;
　　　　　　　Through our transformation
　　　　　　　　　　Let thy will be done.

　　　　　　　　　　　　　　　　Mary Boynton Parke

29 We Walk the Holy Ground of Earth

HORSLEY C. M.
William Horsley, 1774–1858

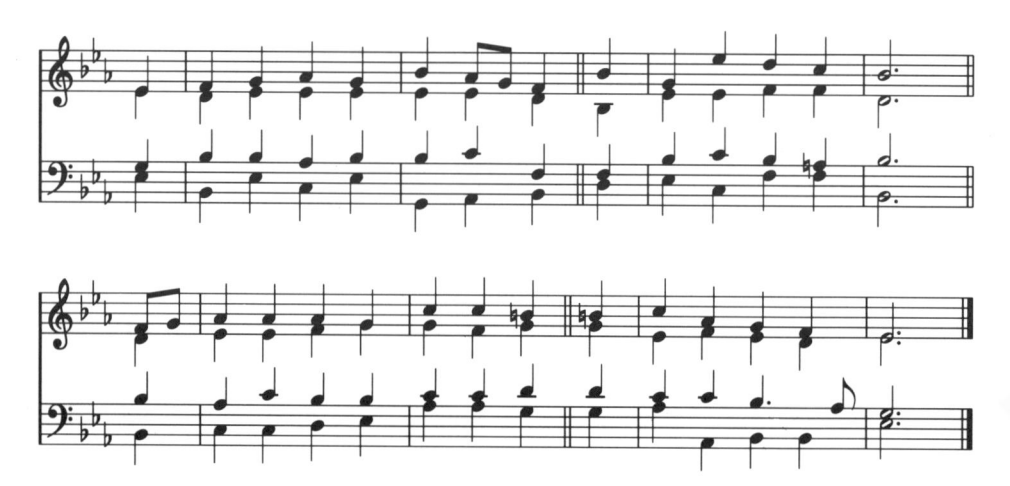

We walk the holy ground of earth,
 Which you, O God, have made;
A jewel in space to be our home,
 In velvet darkness laid.

In endless miracle of life
 A wondrous web you weave,
And, for creation's tapestry,
 Your people's thanks receive.

But we have torn its subtle threads,
 Befouled its colours bright,
Our pride has led us to destroy
 Where wisdom should delight.

We now repent the foolishness
 Which led us to despoil,
Which made us aliens in the world,
 Though moulded from its soil.

Creator Spirit, God of Love,
 Complete what you've begun,
Restore our fractured consciousness
 That this world may be one.

Clifford M. Reed

Loving Friends Together

30

LOVING FRIENDS 12 12. + refrain

Glenn Smith

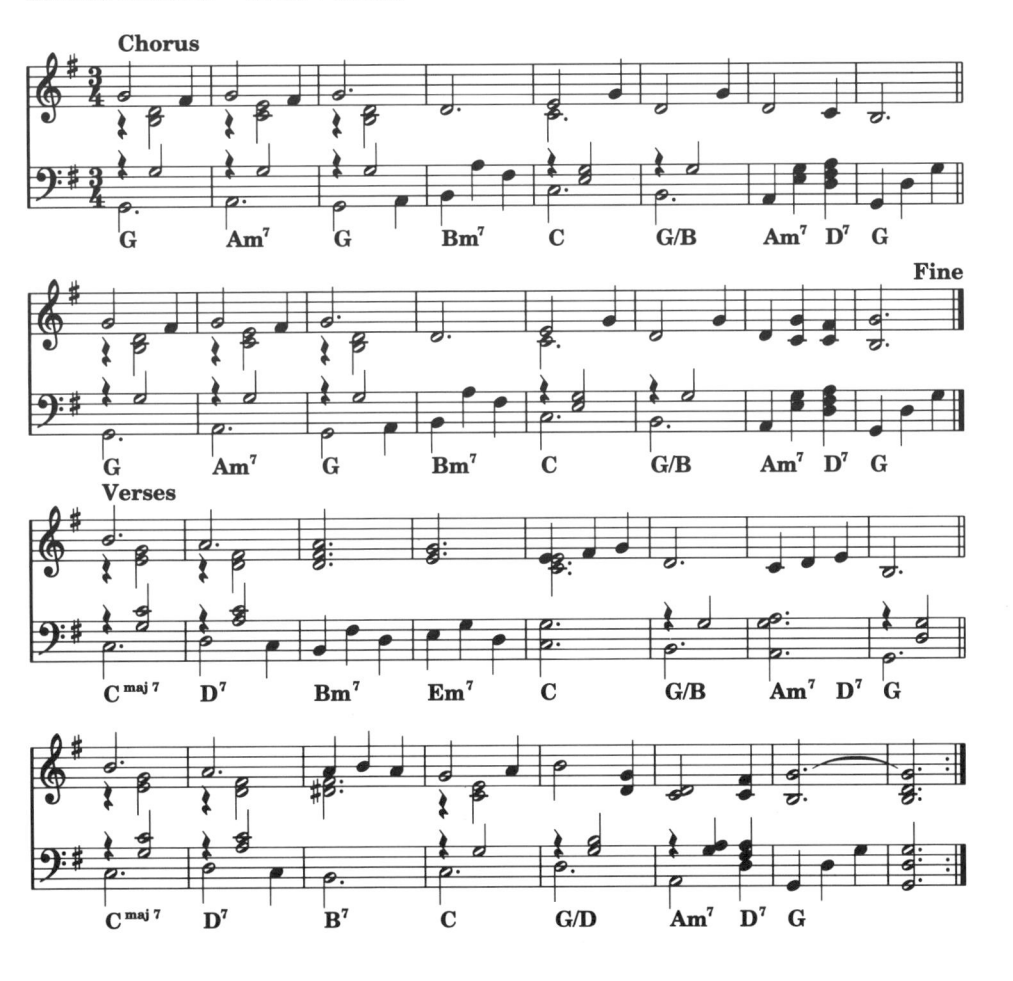

Chorus: Loving friends together, reaching out and touching souls,
        Holding hands for ever one on one yet part of the whole.

   We can stand tall sharing ourselves, sharing ourselves.
   No one soul is an island standing by itself.

Chorus: Loving friends together, reaching out and touching souls...

   Join our singing. Souls intertwine speaking one mind.
   Come and join in the circle, loving humankind.

Chorus: Loving friends together, reaching out and touching souls...

Diane Peltz

31 There is a Place I Call My Own

FLYING FREE   8 7. 8 7. 7 7. 8 8

Don Besig
Arranged David Dawson

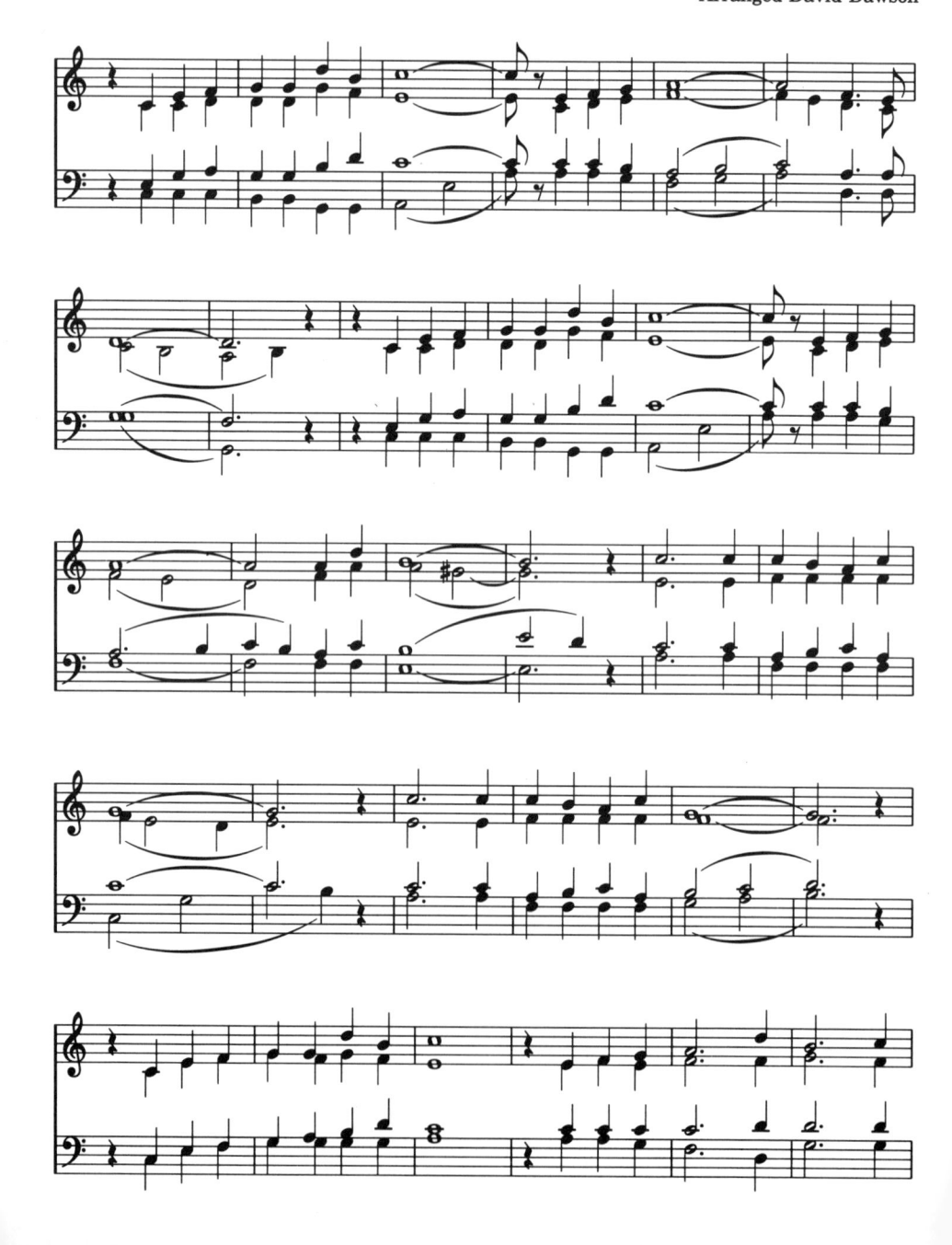

31

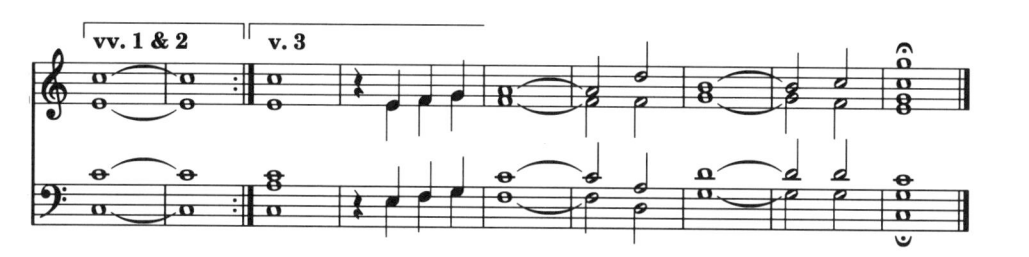

There is a place I call my own
   Where I can stand by the sea,
And look beyond the things I've known
   And dream that I might be free.
Like the bird above the trees
   Gliding gently on the breeze,
I wish that all my life I'd be
   Without a care and flying free.

But life is not a distant sky
   Without a cloud, without rain,
And I can never hope that I
   Can travel on without pain.
Time goes swiftly on its way;
   All too soon we've lost today,
I cannot wait for skies of blue
   Or dream so long that life is through.

So life's a song that I must sing,
   A gift of love I must share;
And when I see the joy it brings
   My spirits soar through the air,
Like the bird up in the sky,
   Life has taught me how to fly.
For now I know what I can be
   And now my heart is flying free –
   And now my heart is flying free.

Don Besig

32 Red the Poppy-Fields of Flanders

ALL FOR JESUS   8 7. 8 7. Trochaic   John Stainer, 1840–1901

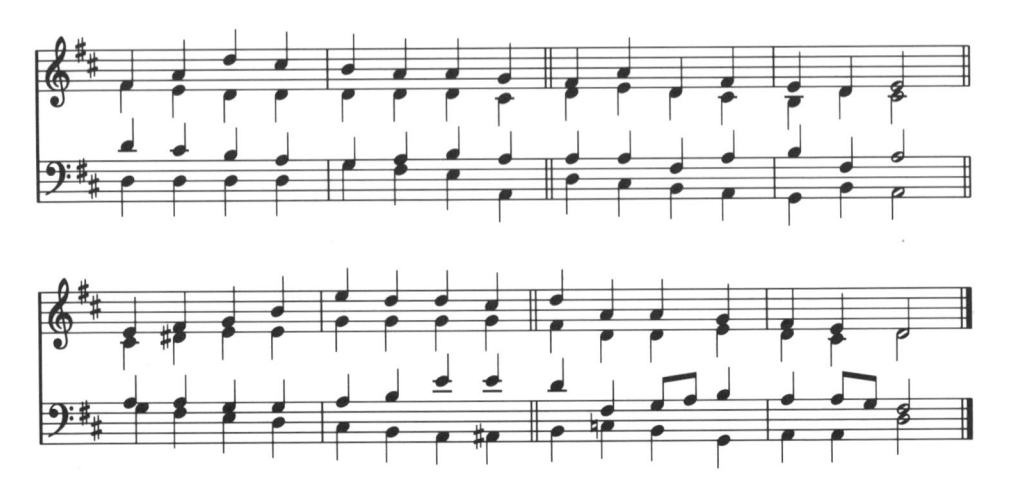

Red the poppy-fields of Flanders,
   Red the Western Desert sands,
Red the snows of Mother Russia:
   Red with blood spilled by cruel hands.

We remember those who died there.
   We must not forget their pain.
We remember all earth's children
   Whom the gods of war have slain.

Some have died for truth and justice,
   Died so others might be free.
Some have died for cause ignoble,
   Died the tools of tyranny.

Red the mud-drowned filth of trenches,
   Red the ruins once so fair,
Red the jungles, red the oceans,
   Red the one blood that we share.

We would heed the pleading voices
   Of the folk who died for peace;
Grant us now your loving Spirit,
   That in us all strife may cease.

                                               Clifford M. Reed

See the Mother's Desolation 33

FELLOWSHIP 8 8 7. Frank Clabburn

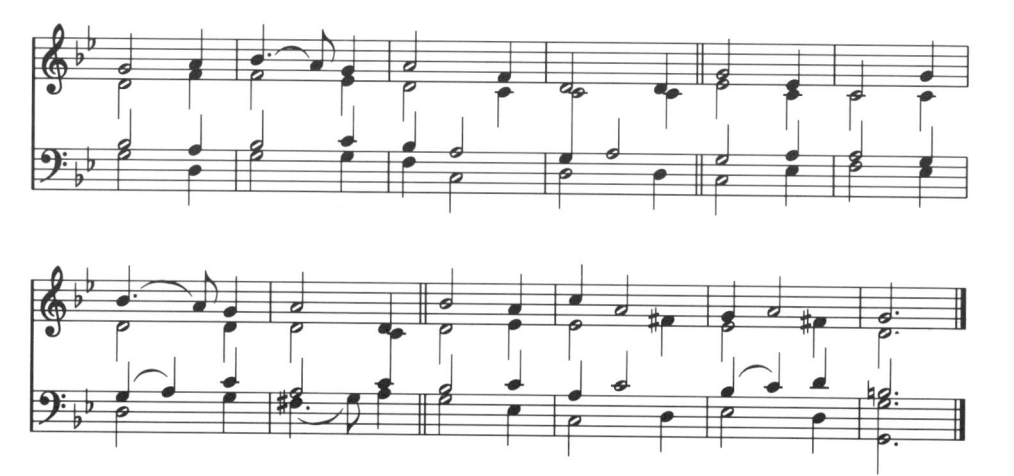

See the mother's desolation
Underneath the cross dejected
Where the child of her womb hangs.

Centuries of sacrificing
On the altar of our own cause
Have not slaked the thirst for blood;

So this hatred still destroys us
Numbs our minds and kills compassion
Sure of only what we fear.

Help, O help us, God of healing,
Help us in our self-willed blindness;
Come to aid us trapped in pride.

Hold us, keep us, warm us, cure us,
Lead us to embrace our kindred
In one worldwide loving home.

Peter Sampson

34

We Ask That We Live and We Labour

PEACE, TRUTH AND UNITY irregular

Donald Swann
© 1965 Donald Swann

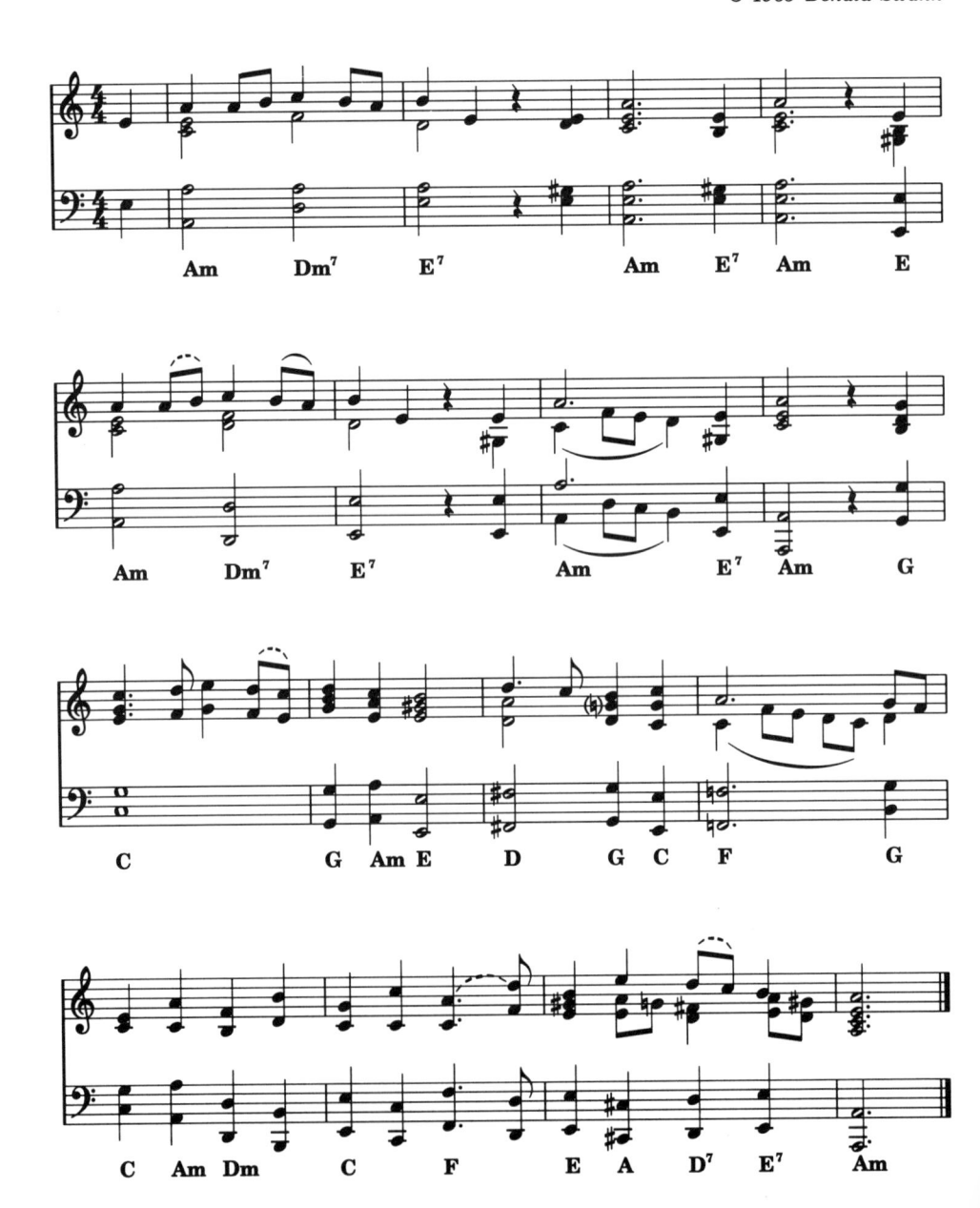

We ask that we live and we labour in peace, in peace;
   That all shall be our neighbours in peace, in peace;
Distrust and hatred will turn to love,
   All prisoners freed,
And our only war will be the one
   Against all human need.

We work for the end of disunion in truth, in truth;
   That all may be one in communion in truth, in truth;
We choose the road of peace and prayer
   Countless pilgrims trod,
So that Hindu, Muslim, Christian, Jew
   Are together in God.

We call to our sisters and brothers, unite, unite!
   That all may live for others, unite, unite!
And so the nations will be as one,
   One the flag unfurled,
One law, one life, one hope, one goal,
   One people and one world.

                                        Donald Swann

35 Sweet Dreams Form a Shade

SWEET DREAMS   5 7. 6 8.

David Dawson

Sweet dreams, form a shade
  O'er my lovely infant's head;
Sweet dreams of pleasant streams
  By happy, silent, moony beams.

Sweet sleep, with soft down
  Weave thy brows an infant crown.
Sweet sleep, Angel mild,
  Hover o'er my happy child.

Sleep, sleep, happy child,
  All creation slept and smil'd;
Sleep, sleep, happy sleep,
  While o'er thee thy mother weep.

Sweet babe, in thy face
  Holy image I can trace.
Sweet babe, once like thee,
  Thy Maker lay and wept for me,

Wept for me, for thee, for all,
  When He was an infant small.
Thou His image ever see,
  Heav'nly face that smiles on thee,

Smiles on thee, on me, on all;
  Who became an infant small.
Infant smiles are His own smiles;
  Heaven and earth to peace beguiles.

William Blake

36 Sent Forth By God's Blessing

THE ASH GROVE 12 11. 12 11. D.   Traditional

36

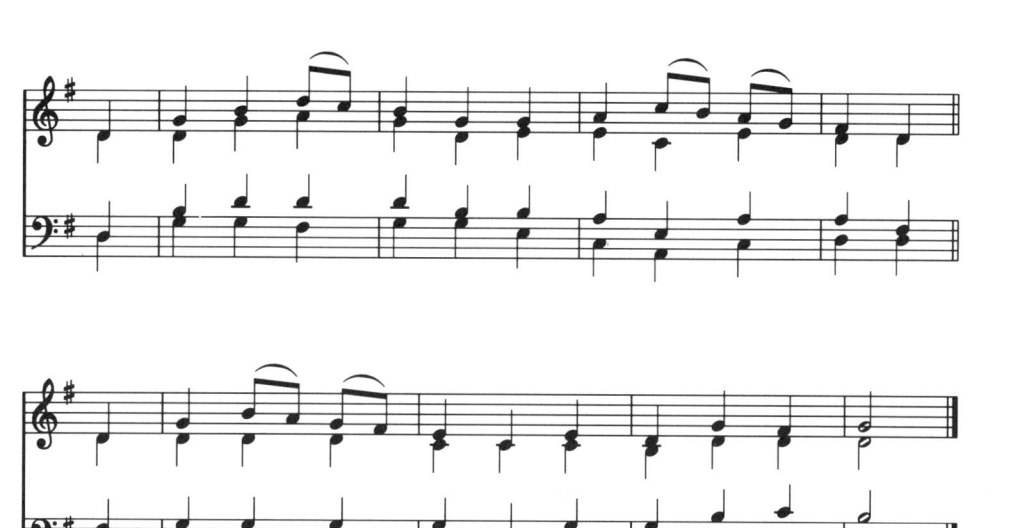

Sent forth by God's blessing, our true faith confessing
    The people of God from his dwelling take leave.
The supper is ended; O now be extended
    The fruits of his service in all who believe.
The seed of his teaching our hungry souls reaching
    Shall blossom in action for God and for Man.
His grace shall incite us, his love shall unite us
    To work for his Kingdom and further his plan.

With praise and thanksgiving to God ever living
    The task of our everyday life we will face;
Our faith ever sharing, in love ever caring
    Embracing as kindred all folk of each race.
One feast that has fed us, one light that has led us
    Unite us as one in the life that we share.
Then may all things living with praise and thanksgiving
    Give honour to Christ and true saints everywhere.

Omer Westendorf

37 View the Starry Realm of Heaven

DACHAU SONG No. 1

Bodhana Haspl
Adapted by Richard Boeke, harmonised by Malcolm Sadler

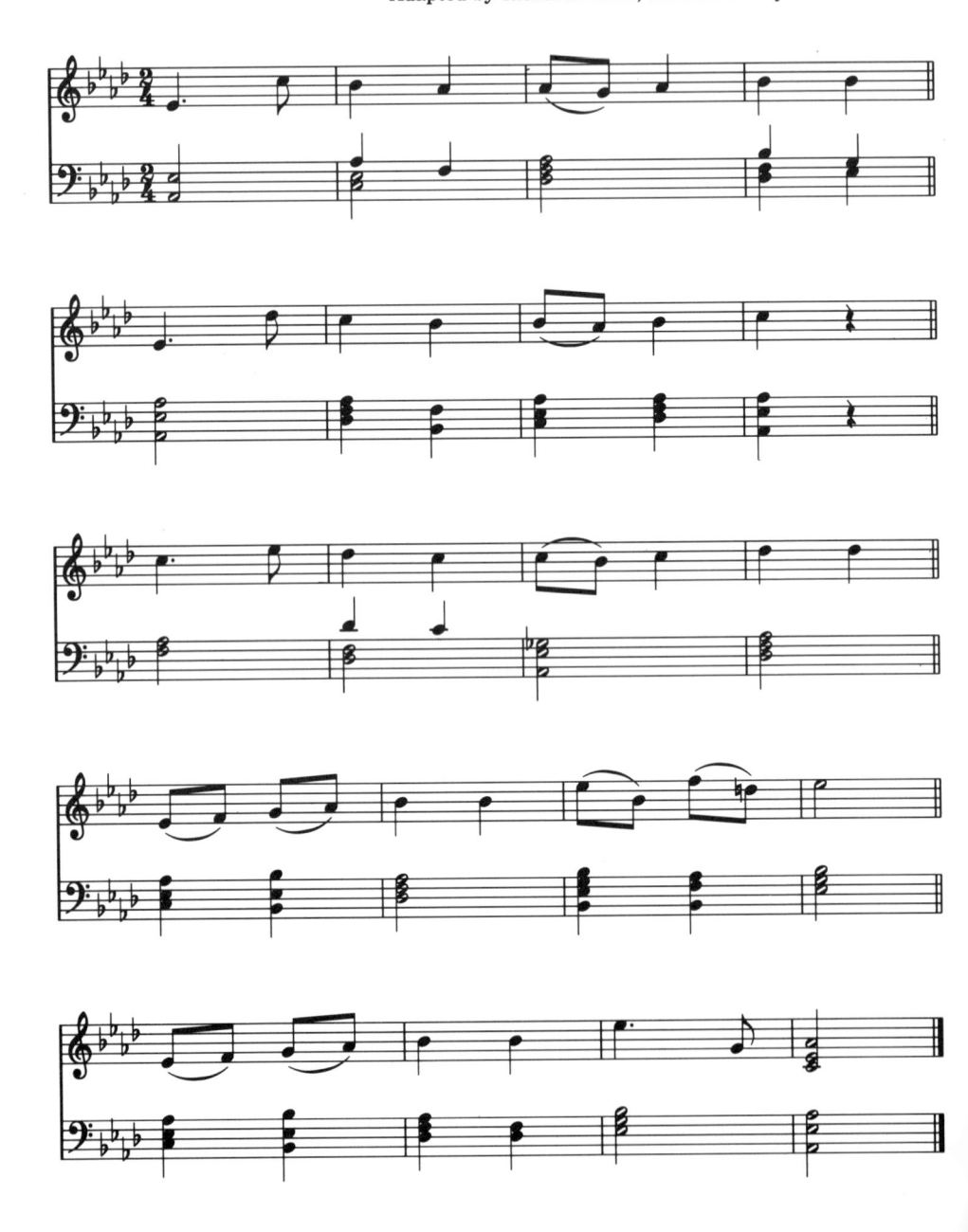

View the starry realm of heaven,
    Shining distant empires sing.
Skysong of celestial children
    Turns each winter into spring.
    Turns each winter into spring.

Great you are, beyond conception,
    God of gods and God of stars.
My soul soars with your perception,
    I escape from prison bars.
    I escape from prison bars.

You, the One within all forming
    In my heart and mind and breath.
You, my guide through hate's fierce storming,
    Courage in both life and death.
    Courage in both life and death.

Life is yours, in you I prosper,
    Seed will come to fruit I know.
Trust that after winter's snowfall,
    Walls will melt and Truth will flow.
    Walls will melt and Truth will flow.

Written in Dachau Concentration Camp
by Czech Unitarian Minister, Norbert Capek,
translated by Richard Boeke.
Music by his daughter, Bodhana Haspl.

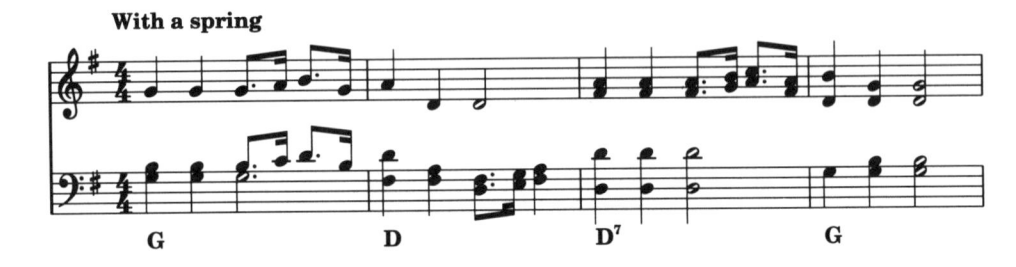

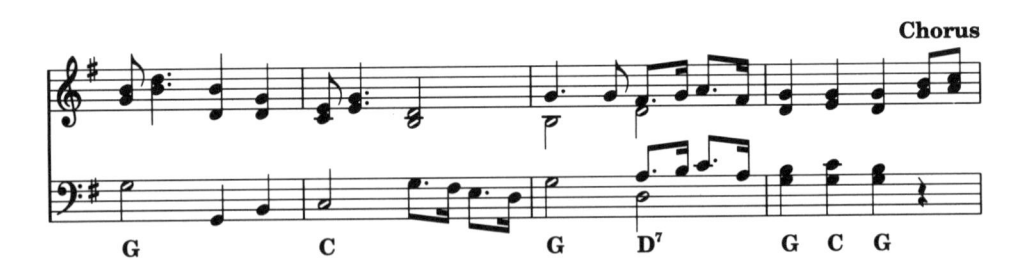

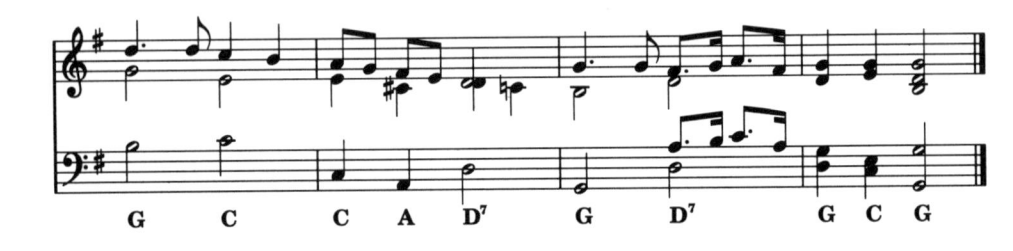

38 One More Step Along the World I Go

ONE MORE STEP 9 9. 7 8. + refrain

Sydney Carter
arranged by Douglas Coombes

One more step along the world I go,
  One more step along the world I go,
From the old things to the new
  Keep me travelling along with You.
Chorus: And it's from the old I travel to the new,
  Keep me travelling along with You.

Round the corners of the world I turn,
  More and more about the world I learn.
And the new things that I see
  You'll be looking at along with me.
Chorus: And it's from the old I travel to the new,
  Keep me travelling along with You.

As I travel through the bad and good,
  Keep me travelling the way I should.
Where I see no way to go
  You'll be telling me the way, I know.
Chorus: And it's from the old I travel to the new,
  Keep me travelling along with You.

Give me courage when the world is rough,
  Keep me loving though the world is tough.
Leap and sing in all I do,
  Keep me travelling along with You.
Chorus: And it's from the old I travel to the new,
  Keep me travelling along with You.

You are older than the world can be,
  You are younger than the life in me.
Ever old and ever new,
  Keep me travelling along with You.
Chorus: And it's from the old I travel to the new,
  Keep me travelling along with You.

Sydney Carter

39 May the Road Rise With You

A BLESSING   6 9. 8 9. 7 11.   Traditional, arranged by David Dawson

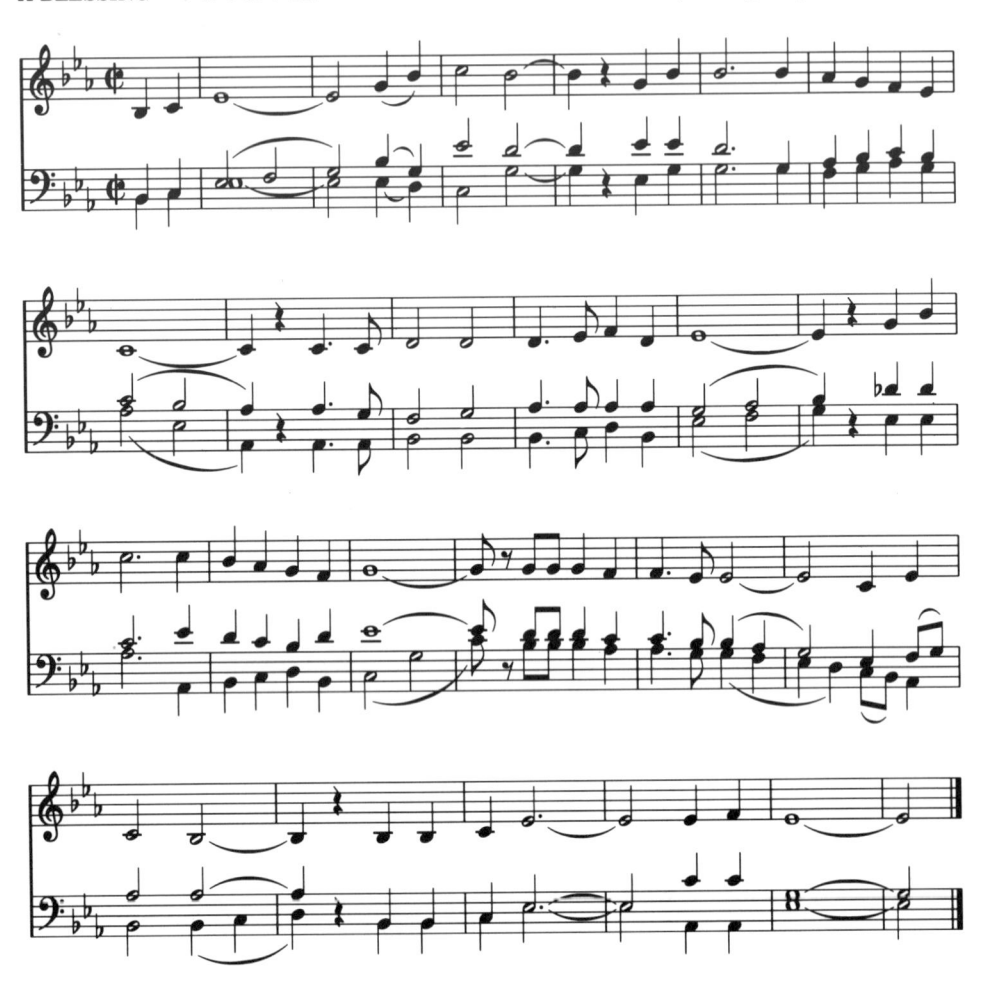

May the road rise with you,
    May the wind be always at your back.
May the sun shine warm upon your face,
    May the rain fall soft upon your fields,
And until we meet again –
    May God hold you in the hollow of $\frac{his}{her}$ hands.

Traditional